BETA$_2$-AGONISTS IN ASTHMA TREATMENT

LUNG BIOLOGY IN HEALTH AND DISEASE

Executive Editor

Claude Lenfant
Director, National Heart, Lung and Blood Institute
National Institutes of Health
Bethesda, Maryland

ADDITIONAL VOLUMES IN PREPARATION

The opinions expressed in these volumes do not necessarily represent the views of the National Institutes of Health.

BETA$_2$-AGONISTS IN ASTHMA TREATMENT

Edited by

Romain Pauwels
University Hospital
Ghent, Belgium

Paul M. O'Byrne
McMaster University
Hamilton, Ontario, Canada

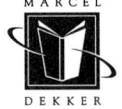

MARCEL DEKKER, INC.   NEW YORK · BASEL · HONG KONG

Library of Congress Cataloging-in-Publication Data

Beta$_2$-agonists in asthma treatment / edited by Romain Pauwels, Paul M. O'Byrne.
   p. cm. — (Lung biology in health and disease ; 106)
   Includes bibliographical references and index.
   ISBN 0-8247-9496-6 (hardcover: alk. paper)
   1. Asthma—Chemotherapy. 2. Adrenergic beta-agonists—Therapeutic use. I. Pauwels, Romain. II. O'Byrne, Paul M. III. Series.
   [DNLM: 1. Adrenergic beta-Agonists—pharmacology. 2. Adrenergic beta-Agonists—therapeutic use. 3. Bronchodilator Agents—pharmacology. 4. Bronchodilator Agents—therapeutic use. 5. Asthma—drug therapy. W1 LU62 v.106 1997 / QV 129 B563 1997]
   RC591.B47 1997
   616.2'38061—dc21
   DNLM/DLC
   for Library of Congress

                                                         97-11742
                                                            CIP

The publisher offers discounts on this book when ordered in bulk quantities. For more information, write to Special Sales/Professional Marketing at the address below.

This book is printed on acid-free paper.

MARCEL DEKKER, INC.
270 Madison Avenue, New York, New York 10016
http://www.dekker.com

Current printing (last digit):
10 9 8 7 6 5 4 3 2 1

PRINTED IN THE UNITED STATES OF AMERICA

INTRODUCTION

Who breathes must suffer . . .

Matthew Prior (1664–1721)

This gloomy bit of wisdom, penned about three centuries ago, must have special significance for the many people who, then as now, were afflicted with asthma. Healers and physicians from all ages have looked for ways to restore free breathing in asthma sufferers—from the Chinese and the Egyptians, who in 3000 B.C. appeared to have been the first to talk about, and to treat, asthma, to contemporary researchers and clinicians. For nearly 5000 years, progress was slow and difficult, and patients were dispirited. This feeling was well expressed by a famous 13th century French surgeon, Henri de Mondeville, who said, "I am not destined to live long unless, by special grace, God will prolong my existence. I am asthmatic, a cougher, phthisic and in consumption and in consequence, it is preferable for me and also more useful for me to hasten my work."

Fortunately, today's patient need not have such a pessimistic approach to his life and future. Reports from all sectors are telling us that asthmatics can live many years and that their lives can be full of wonderful and stimulating experiences.

Although the primary trigger of asthmatic events is inflammation, the basic constriction of the bronchi is what hampers the well-being of the patient. It is therefore no surprise that so much has been invested in time, resources, and scientific talent in the search of effective bronchodilators. This search has sometimes been disappointing, and at other times frustrating, because bronchodilators also exhibit vasoconstriction effects and adverse actions on the heart. Products of the search are the beta receptor agonists, which over the years have become medications of choice in the treatment of asthma.

Beta$_2$-Agonists in Asthma Treatment, edited by Dr. Romain Pauwels and Dr. Paul M. O'Byrne, is the history of a class of medications that take the suffering out of breathing for many patients. The roster of contributors is truly international, and the Table of Contents is as complete and comprehensive as one can be. Physicians will find in this volume the guidance that they need to enable them to do the most, and the best, for their patients.

I believe the Lung Biology in Health and Disease series is fortunate to be home to this volume. Its topic is important and timely, but even better, the editors and the international cast of authors are premier in the field. As the Executive Editor of this series, I want to express to them my deepest gratitude for their contribution.

Claude Lenfant, M.D.
Bethesda, Maryland

PREFACE

Beta$_2$-agonists have been used in the treatment of asthma for many decades and are still the most widely prescribed anti-asthma treatment in the number of patients treated. Their potent bronchodilator activity and rapid onset of action are the main reasons for this. Even though their efficacy is well understood, there are several reasons to examine the available knowledge about these drugs.

First, new insights have been gained in our understanding of the pathogenesis of asthma, and there is a need to reassess the role of beta$_2$-agonists in view of their effect on these pathogenic mechanisms. It is important to relate clinical and therapeutic experience to conceptual knowledge about a disease. The results of therapeutic intervention studies provide hard evidence to buttress our conceptual knowledge.

Second, new beta$_2$-agonists have become available for the treatment of asthma. The development of long-acting beta$_2$-agonists might result in a reassessment of the role of these drugs in the chronic treatment of asthma.

Third, concerns about the possible harmful effects of beta$_2$-agonists have recently caused intense debate about their use. The publication of a book making available all knowledge, including controversial aspects, about beta$_2$-

agonists in the treatment of asthma is therefore very timely and appropriate. Properly synthesized, this knowledge can be used to make practical therapeutic recommendations. The book starts with an overview of the history of the use of beta-agonists in the treatment of asthma, highlighting the development of more potent, more selective and longer-acting drugs. The molecular mode of action of beta$_2$-agonists and the effects of these drugs on airway effector cells and inflammation are thoroughly reviewed. The interaction of the now well-known molecular structure of the beta$_2$-receptor and the various beta$_2$-agonists, the mechanisms involved in the duration of action, and the cellular events following the binding of the beta$_2$-agonist to the receptor are fascinating. The clinical significance of the effects of beta$_2$-agonists on various inflammatory cells is critically analyzed.

The pharmacokinetics of the various beta$_2$-agonists in their different formulations and ways of administration are discussed extensively. An update on the clinical pharmacological characteristics of these drugs includes their well-known bronchodilating and bronchoprotective effects and their less well known effects on cough and mucociliary clearance. Because beta$_2$-agonists are most frequently administered via inhalation, a review of inhalation techniques and devices is presented.

The largest part of this book is dedicated to the clinical aspects of the use of beta$_2$-agonists in the treatment of asthma in both children and in adults. The evidence derived from clinical studies is used for defining the role of beta$_2$-agonists in the treatment of acute and chronic asthma. Beta$_2$-agonists have been used extensively in the treatment of asthma. Reviews of the clinical studies and the therapeutic recommendations should be very helpful for guiding clinicians.

We thank all who contributed to the book and especially the authors who provided us with thorough and up-to-date reviews of their specific topic. Our special thanks also to to Dr. Claude Lenfant for accepting this book into the prestigious Lung Biology in Health and Disease series. We hope that the current volume will enhance that prestige.

Romain Pauwels
Paul M. O'Byrne

CONTRIBUTORS

Gary P. Anderson, Ph.D.   Lecturer, Department of Pharmacology, The University of Melbourne, Parkville, Victoria, Australia

Peter J. Barnes, D.M., D.Sc., F.R.C.P.   Professor, Department of Thoracic Medicine, National Heart and Lung Institute, Imperial College School of Medicine, London, England

Richard Beasley, M.B.Ch.B., D.M., F.R.A.C.P.   Professor, Department of Medicine, Wellington School of Medicine, Wellington, New Zealand

Lars Borgström, Ph.D.   Associate Professor, Astra Draco AB, Lund, Sweden

Carl D. Burgess, M.D., M.R.C.P., F.R.A.C.P.   Associate Professor, Department of Medicine, Wellington School of Medicine, Wellington, New Zealand

Kenneth R. Chapman, M.D., M.Sc., F.R.C.P.C.   Associate Professor, Department of Medicine, The Toronto Hospital and University of Toronto, Toronto, Ontario, Canada

Kian Fan Chung, M.D., F.R.C.P.   Reader in Thoracic Medicine, National Heart and Lung Institute, Imperial College School of Medicine, London, England

Julian Crane, M.B., B.S., F.R.A.C.P. Associate Professor, Department of Medicine, Wellington School of Medicine, Wellington, New Zealand

Ronald Dahl, M.D. Professor, Department of Respiratory Diseases and Allergy, Århus University Hospital, Århus, Denmark

Eric Derom, M.D., Ph.D. Professor, Department of Respiratory Diseases, University Hospital, Ghent, Belgium

Myrna Dolovich, P.Eng(Elec) Associate Clinical Professor, Department of Medicine, Faculty of Health Sciences, McMaster University, Hamilton, Ontario, Canada

Stuart A. Green, M.D. Assistant Professor, Department of Pulmonary and Critical Care Medicine, University of Cincinnati College of Medicine, Cincinnati, Ohio

Peter Howarth, M.D. Southampton General Hospital, Southampton, England

Jan-Anders Karlsson, D.M.Sci. Head of Research, Bayer Yakuhin Ltd., Research Center Kyoto, Kyoto, Japan

James P. Kemp University of California School of Medicine, San Diego, California

Stephen B. Liggett, M.D. Professor of Medicine, Molecular Genetics, and Pharmacology, Department of Pulmonary Medicine, University of Cincinnati College of Medicine, Cincinnati, Ohio

Anders Lindén, M.D., Ph.D. Department of Respiratory Medicine and Allergology, Institute of Heart and Lung Disease, Gothenburg University, Gothenburg, Sweden

Brian Jonathan Lipworth, M.D., F.R.C.P.(Edin) Senior Lecturer/Honorary Consultant, Department of Clinical Pharmacology and Respiratory Medicine, Ninewells Hospital and Medical School, University of Dundee, Dundee, Scotland

Lars Nyberg, M.Pharm., Ph.D. Scientific Advisor, Astra Draco AB and Associate Professor, Uppsala University, Lund, Sweden

Paul M. O'Byrne, M.D., FRCP(C) Professor, Department of Medicine, McMaster University, Hamilton, Ontario, Canada

Romain Pauwels, M.D., Ph.D. Professor, Department of Respiratory Diseases, University Hospital, Ghent, Belgium

Neil Pearce, B.Sc., Dip.Sci., Dip.ORS., Ph.D. Associate Professor, Department of Medicine, Wellington School of Medicine, Wellington, New Zealand

Søren Pedersen, M.D. Professor, Department of Pediatrics, University of Odense, Odense, Denmark

Carl G. A. Persson, Ph.D. Professor, Department of Clinical Pharmacology, University Hospital of Lund and Astra Draco AB, Lund, Sweden

Dirkje S. Postma, M.D., Ph.D. Professor, Department of Pulmonology, University Hospital, Groningen, The Netherlands

Klaus F. Rabe, M.D. Zentrum für Pneumologie und Thoraxchirurgie, Krankenhaus Grosshanssdorf, Landesversicherungsanstalt Hamburg, Grosshanssdorf, Germany

Malcolm R. Sears, M.D., Ch.B., F.R.A.C.P., F.R.C.P.C. Professor, Department of Medicine, McMaster University, Hamilton, Ontario, Canada

Albert L. Sheffer, M.D., F.A.C.P. Clinical Professor, Department of Medicine, Harvard Medical School, and Director, Allergy and Clinical Immunology Section, Harvard Medical School and Brigham and Women's Hospital, Boston, Massachusetts

F. Estelle R. Simons, M.D., F.R.C.P.C. Professor and Deputy-Head, Department of Pediatrics and Child Health, University of Manitoba, Winnipeg, Manitoba, Canada

Peter J. Sterk, M.D., Ph.D. Professor, Department of Pulmonary Diseases, Leiden University Medical Centre, Leiden, The Netherlands

A. E. Tattersfield, M.D., F.R.C.P. Professor, Division of Respiratory Medicine, University of Nottingham, Nottingham, England

Andrea von Berg, M.D. Department of Pediatrics, Marienhospital Wesel, Wesel, Germany

Bertil Waldeck Astra Draco AB, Lund, Sweden

CONTENTS

BETA$_2$-AGONISTS IN ASTHMA TREATMENT

1

On the History of Sympathomimetics in Asthma

CARL G. A. PERSSON

University Hospital of Lund
and Astra Draco AB
Lund, Sweden

I. Introduction

Most of the current anti-asthma drug principles, being originally plant- or hormone-derived, have a long and partly unknown history. Anticholinergic airway treatment by inhalation of smoke from burning datura plants may date back to ancient Indian Ayurverdic medicine (1). Ephedrine, a reputed antiasthma drug, was first formulated as the *Ephedra vulgaris* drug ma huang in China 3000 years BC (2). How early individuals may have noticed their airway effects of xanthine-containing beverages (tea, coffee, or cocoa) is not known. However, more than 100 years ago, Henry Hyde Salter experienced and described well the clinical efficacy of strong coffee in asthma (3). Cuneiform characters printed on clay tablets in old Assyria (ca. 650 BC) tell us about an early inhalant cromone therapy in chest disorders: ". . . thou shalt bray Ammi, spread it over thorn fire, let the smoke enter his anus, his mouth and his nostrils. . . ." (4). Underscoring the deed of Roger Altounyan (5), this early Iraqi remedy may be the only account of inhaled cromones (Ammi Visnaga contains the cromone-like compound khellin) in asthma prior to his discovery of cromoglycate in the late 1960s.

This chapter focuses on sympathomimetic drugs. The history of this pharmacological principle has been partly confused with that of the corticosteroids. Hence, the latter drug principle also is mentioned here. On a more general note, this chapter is meant to assist the reader in understanding the role of original observations in vivo or in other complex biosystems in the discovery and development of drugs for the treatment of asthma.

II. "Curative Influence of Violent Emotion"

The title above is borrowed from Chapter IX in Hyde Salter's brilliant book *On Asthma: Its Pathology and Treatment* first published in 1860 (6). Salter's descriptions of asthma are unsurpassed, and his work remains a valuable reference also in the field of asthma therapy. The following quote from the book typically reflects the sharpness and healthiness of Salter's scientific writings:

> I must be pardoned for not taking up the reader's time in enumerating the different classifications of asthma adopted by different writers. The chief cause of their failure has been, I believe, a want of a simple reading of nature, its place being supplied by an unquestioning inheritance and adoption of received notions. It seems to me to be a subject in which authors have done more in the way of reading each other's books than scrutinizing their own patients.

I think Salter's work should be recommended reading for today's scientists.

It seems to me that Salter discovered the antiasthma efficacy of epinephrine (adrenaline) several decades before this amine was available for experimentation (Fig. 1). Salter knew well about psychogenic factors that worsen or precipitate attacks of asthma in sensitive individuals. However, he distinctly identified the particular situations when violent (pleasant) emotions or sudden alarm (causing intense activity or excitement) had a beneficial influence on his asthmatic patients. The antiasthma effect was instantaneous and very marked as would be expected from a significant "injection" of epinephrine. Salter also advised some of his patients to carry out prolonged exercises, and he prescribed the cold bath to better the breathing in individual cases of asthma.

III. "Stress Therapies" of Asthma

Girolamo Cardano (1501–1575) (7) secured his place in medical history by "curing" a Scottish archbishop of asthma. Cardano radically changed the local environment for the bishop, most noted is the presumed allergen-avoidance brought about by the removal of feather-filled bedding material. However, Cardano also prescribed the cold bath, regular and less voluptuous exercise, and a restricted diet. Hence, an improved way of living, including the possibility

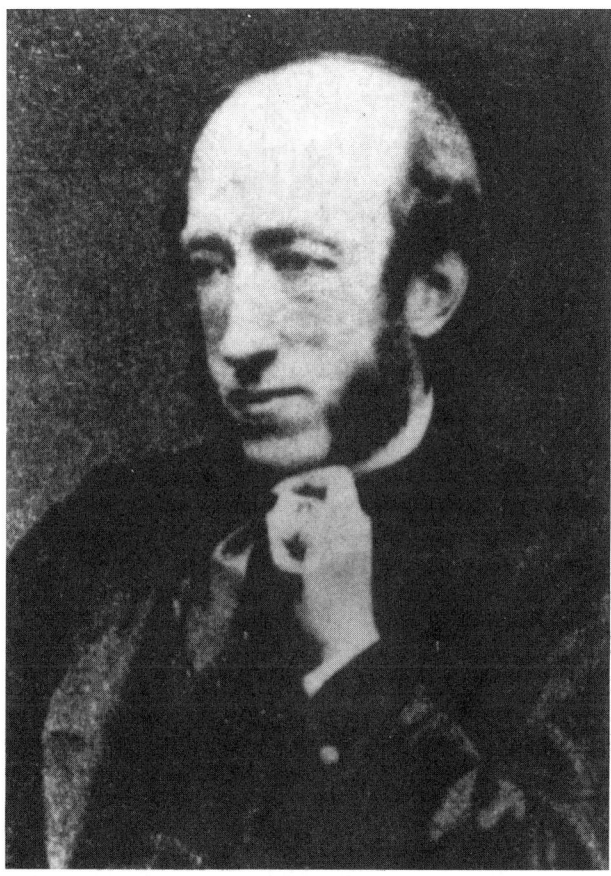

Figure 1 Henry Hyde Salter, MD, FRS (1823–1871) was an astute observer who made many original contributions to our knowledge of asthma. Salter also discovered, evaluated, and predicted important remedies for this disease. For example, he distinguished the antiasthma effect evoked by sudden arousal: "The cure of asthma by violent emotions is more sudden and complete than by any other remedy whatever. . . . I think, too, that mental emotions act, if I may so express it, as a nervous derivative." (Photograph kindly provided by the Royal Society of Medicine, London.)

of endogenous sympathetic and corticosteroid activity, may also have played a role. Already in the first century, Celsus had recommended the bath as a treatment of "cough." Cardano, being a well-read person and a Milanese, may well have been guided by Celsus on this point (medical writings of Celsus had just been retrieved in the Saint Ambrogio Church of Milan). Among asthmatic individuals who used the bodily stress of a cold bath is Sir John Floyer. Beside his famous *Treatise of Asthma*, Floyer (8) wrote a book on the cold bath. Smollett (9) rediscovered this chilling remedy. According to his once famous travel book, Smollett's own asthma became so bad that he desperately, "and against all learned doctors' advice," plunged into the cold, open sea. To his surprise, his asthma got better. William Withering, the founder of clinical pharmacology, recommended "frequent use" (4) and Laënnec (10) "uninterrupted use" of the cold bath. Laënnec also favored prolonged physical exercise in his beautiful landscape of Brittany as a treatment of his own asthma.

Fever may naturally be connected with a bodily effort to overcome a disease and its potentially useful properties have deliberately been employed in the treatment of asthma: During the first century, Ruphos von Ephesos of Rome sent asthmatic patients to areas where they could be sure to attract malaria (11). Fever again received attention in the first decades of this century, following the first suggestions that asthma may be an allergic disease. A great variety of protein-allergen injections was then tried out with the rationale of producing specific desensitization. It was soon discovered, however, that injections of less than innocuous proteins and vaccines could have beneficial effects in asthma whether the asthma was an allergic type of not. Schiff (12) recommended particularly the subcutaneous injection of straight whole milk. Duke (13) included colon bacilli in his nonspecific protein armamentarium, presenting two case reports where the asthmatic patients underwent remarkable improvements along with chill, high fever, and other symptoms following from the subcutaneous and intravenous injections of several millions of these bacilli. One can now only speculate about the antiasthma action of epinephrine release in these bodily stresses. Some of these treatments were used regularly but with intervals that would make a sympathetic contribution less than that of steroids or other perhaps still unknown stress- or injection-induced mechanisms.

IV. Adrenal Extract

George Oliver, a physician from Harrogate in England, was interested in the actions of glycerine extracts of various glands. Curiously, he claimed to have observed that ingestion of adrenal extract reduced the diameter of the radial artery in his son (14). Of greater interest is his report to the Physiological Society (London, March 10, 1894) on the physiological action of this extract (15). Vasoconstriction and increased blood pressure were the most prominent actions of extracts of the adrenals from different species. On April 20, 1896, Bates (16) read a paper before the section of Ophthalmology of the New York Academy of Medicine where he gave a detailed account of 2 years' clinical experience with adrenal extract given topically on the eye. Bates described well how to prepare, sterilize, and maintain stability of the extract. He reported on its powerful vasoconstrictor, blanching effects. He took particular note of the fact that the extract could be applied daily for several months with no tolerance and no ill effect. Bates emphasized that it was without anesthetic action. Thus, Bates clearly distinguished adrenal extract from cocaine, which since 1880 had been widely employed as a decongestant in conjunctivitis, in rhinitis, and occasionally in asthma. Bates also gave a detailed instruction on how to employ the adrenal extract to be used in combination with cocaine to improve distinctly the local mucosal anesthesia that was obtained with the latter agent. The adrenal extract, under labels such as "ischaemin," soon replaced cocaine as a topical decongestant in rhinitis. Oral inhalations of the extract may not have been feasible with the available (nasal) sprays, and I have found no report on topical bronchial treatment of asthma with it. Oral ingestion of the adrenal extract was tried in asthma but the result was equivocal (17–19). Clark (19) also found no good effect of the oral extract in rhinitis; the adverse effect of the ingested extract was even seen as a possible cause of asthma in some of his patients.

V. "Adrenal Substance"

A sufferer from both allergic rhinitis and asthma and a firm believer in the role of "vascular ataxia" in asthma, Solomon Solis-Cohen (Fig. 2) (20) was keen to examine the effects of adrenal preparations. He took first an oral dose of freshly prepared adrenal extract, but the efficacy was poor and side effects appeared. For reasons that remain unexpressed, Solis-Cohen substituted the extract with tabloids containing powder of dried adrenal substance (daily dose ≈2 g). This produced a crucial change in drug. In June 1898, Solis-Cohen himself was helped by his medicine. In 1900, he (21) reported on the success of this treatment in several asthmatic patients. The dose required was up to 6 g of dried adrenal substance daily. The improvement in severe cases could be striking. "The constant dyspnea first disappeared, then the paroxysmal nocturnal attacks became less frequent and less severe. Recovery was not rapid but was continuous." Adrenal substance cannot serve acutely "to cut short a paroxysm. . . . It has, however, been useful in averting the recurrence of paroxysm and in finally bringing about a state of freedom from fear of their recurrence." Solis-Cohen concluded his report with the following statement: "Clinically I have watched closely and critically enough to satisfy myself that neither the susceptibility of patients to suggestion, nor the activity of the observer's imagination are sufficient in themselves to account for the whole of the results." The findings of Solis-Cohen may have been confirmed in the concomitant work of Douglass

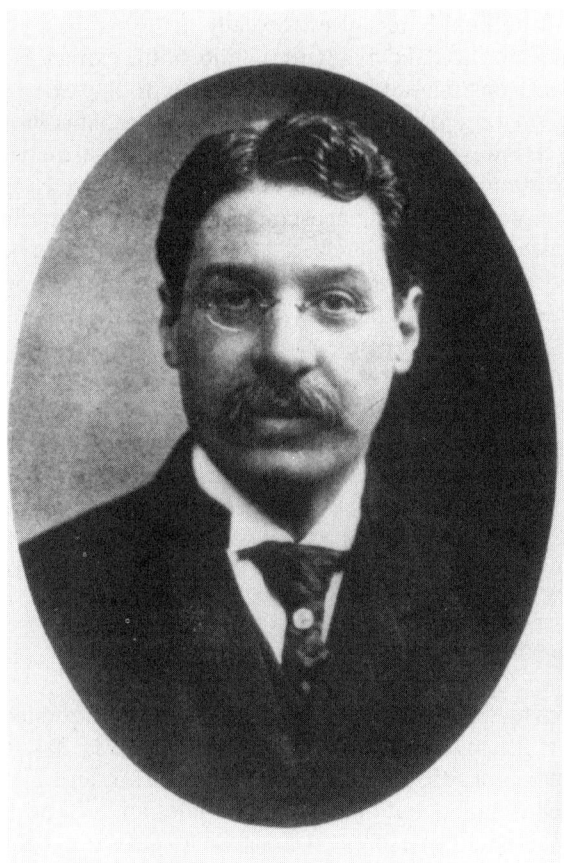

Figure 2 Solomon Solis-Cohen, MD (1857–1948). A Lecturer on Medicine and Therapeutics (Jefferson Medical College, Philadelphia, PA) and Professor of Clinical Medicine, Solis-Cohen designed and delivered a course entitled "Therapeutic Measures Other Than Drugs" (1887–1890), and he edited 11 volumes of *A System of Physiologic Therapeutics* (1901–1905). In between, he published an intriguing report on the anti-asthma effects of the oral intake of desiccated adrenals. Although not previously recognized as such, this report may well have been the original demonstration of the particular efficacy of steroid drugs in asthma (see text). (Photograph kindly provided by Frederick B. Wagner, Jr., MD, University Historian of Thomas Jefferson University.)

(18). In allergic rhinitis and asthma, Douglass "cannot speak overenthusiastically of the benefit and apparent specific effect of this remedy when administered in full doses." However, the report by Douglass confusingly deals with the internal administration of both dried suprarenal gland and adrenal extracts.

The experience with adrenal preparations around the turn of the century may be summarized: The aqueous extract was an effective vasoconstrictor and decongestant in rhinitis, but after oral ingestion, its effect in either rhinitis or asthma was poor or not beneficial. These aspects agree well with the physico-chemical, pharmacological, and pharmacokinetic properties of epinephrine. In contrast, dried adrenal substance appeared to be an effective therapy by the oral route; particularly in the hands of an experienced and astute observer such as Solis-Cohen. Solis-Cohen's observation has been widely considered the original demonstration of the effect of epinephrine in the treatment of asthma. However, I think Solis-Cohen was the first to demonstrate corticosteroid drug actions in asthma and rhinitis (22,23). The steroids contained in the dried adrenals should have been absorbed well, but only a marginal fraction of the oral dose of epinephrine would have survived intestinal and liver catabolism. Solis-Cohen commendably finishes his essay with the following paragraph: "What the active agent is and how much or how little of that active agent is absorbed, I must leave to laboratory students to determine." Owing to the confusion with adrenal extract by researchers, physicians, and eventually also by medical historians, Solis-Cohen's explicit challenge was to be unmet for several decades. It took 50 years before the good effect of purified steroids could be demonstrated in asthma. (By then and for many additional years, Solis-Cohen's original work was forgotten, or it was interpreted to be the first demonstration of the effect of epinephrine in asthma [23].) As we now approach a new millennium, the research on the mode of action of steroids in asthma has been going on for an additional half century and at an increasingly intense level. Proposals abound as to what molecular and cellular mechanisms could be important. However, no one can as yet point out for certain which, if any, of these known mechanisms should be produced by a novel drug principle in order to approach the clinical efficacy of the airway steroids. Also with other established antiasthma principles, such as the cromones and the xanthines, the modus operandi now remains conjectural. This scenario appears perfectly compatible with the possibility that novel anti-inflammatory drug principles to combat asthma also will be discovered before the true molecular and cellular targets have been delineated (24).

VI. Adrenaline

It seems little known that the name *adrenaline* may have been coined by the ophthalmologist and otorhinolaryngologist Norton Wilson, who also described its potent effects on the mucous membranes of the upper airways and the eye (25). Wilson was privileged to call at Takamine's laboratory to obtain and use his crystallised adrenalin chloride. This material was produced from aqueous adrenal extracts by the able research of Takamine (26). (What was produced by Abel and named *epinephrine* apparently was an inactive material.) In 1903, Bullowa and Kaplan (27) demonstrated the effect of subcutaneous injections of adrenalin chloride in asthma. They also found that "much larger doses by mouth do not cause the above effect." Adrenalin injections rapidly became a treatment of choice in asthma. The early attempts made at bronchial inhalation treatment with adrenalin have not been well publicized. When Camps, in 1929 (28), published on the inhalation treatment of asthma, he is referring to the experience of patients who had themselves obtained both adrenalin and the inhalation devices (Spiess-Drager's or Hirth's apparatus) which had been advertized in the lay press.

VII. Sympathomimetics and Mechanisms of Asthma

Why was it that adrenal substance and epinephrine came to be examined in asthma? Probably the answer lies in a favored pathogenetic mechanism in asthma of that time (vasodilatation) and in the well-demonstrated pharmacological action of adrenal extract (vasoconstriction). Solis-Cohen (21) believed in a role of vasodilator mechanisms in asthma and so did Bullowa and Kaplan (27). The latter investigators specifically concluded that epinephrine's efficacy showed that it was vasodilatation and not bronchoconstriction that caused the asthmatic obstruction! Furthermore, the prior demonstration of clinical efficacy in rhinitis of adrenal substance, adrenal extract, and epinephrine contributed significantly to put these important drugs to the trial in asthma.

The medical history of asthma contains many hints as to a role for vascular mechanisms. In 1860, Salter (6) had already realized that it was bronchial and not pulmonary microvessels that contributed to asthmatic reactions. He also distinguished between passive vascular congestion and active vascular responses in inflammatory asthma. The discussion at the end of the 19th century and early in the 20th century specifically referred to Theodor Weber's "Schwellung-Theorie" presented in 1872 (29). Weber talked about asthma as the urticaria of the bronchi, and he found support in nasal mechanisms. Soon thereafter, Stoerk (30) observed an asthmatic attack from the inside of the trachea and the large bronchi through a rigid tube. Reddening and lumenal encroachment occurred almost as in an inflamed nasal mucosa. In 1906, Jesiersky depicted an extremely profuse network of microvessels just beneath the epithelial lining in an asthmatic bronchus. His beautiful, colored drawings also showed a large sinus vein (31). It appeared logical to look for vasoconstrictor drugs to treat both rhinitis and asthma. First on the scene was cocaine, with the adrenal preparations and epinephrine following in the 1890s and early 1900s.

In 1907, Kahn (32), working in a laboratory in Prague, demonstrated the bronchodilator action of epinephrine. For some time, both bronchodilatation and vasoconstriction were considered important actions of epinephrine in asthma. Today, these drugs are widely categorized as bronchodilators, but the possibility is also being considered that even more bronchial actions of sympathomimetics are produced. For example, there has been interest in antiallergic, antiexudative, and other potentially anti-inflammatory actions of beta$_2$-agonists. This interest has naturally increased along with the increasing focus on inflammatory components of asthma (Table 1). However, the term *anti-inflammatory* in this context is probably best reserved for the steroids. Other pharmacological principles obviously cannot replace steroids as treatments for asthma, although they may exert experimental actions which potentially are of an anti-inflammatory nature. A search for additional airway actions of sympathomimetics may, in fact, always be warranted. We may still need to explain why several types of smooth muscle relaxant drugs have failed or been so inferior to the antiobstructive effect of the sympathomimetic drugs. (Xanthines may not be included in this comparison, because they may not primarily be bronchorelaxants in asthma [33] nor may they be given by the inhaled route.)

VIII. Life-Threatening Asthma

Inflammation research and studies of inflammatory changes in asthma were particularly successful in Germany between 1870 and World War I: from Julius Cohnheim's (34) (a pupil of Rudolf Virchow) definition of inflammation as

Table 1 Hypotheses of Asthma and Proposed Modi Operandi of Sympathomimetics

Date	Favored disease feature	Important drug actions
1860	Asthma = CNS disease	"Violent emotions"
1900	Asthma = vasodilation	Vasoconstrictor epinephrine
1907	Asthma = bronchoconstriction	Bronchodilator epinephrine + β-agonists
1970s	Asthma = allergic disease	Antiallergic β-agonists?
1980s	Asthma = inflammation	Anti-inflammatory β-agonists?

Sympathomimetics for the treatment of asthma illustrate our tendency to favor those pharmacological features of drugs that fit with the contemporary notion of what is aberrant and causative in the disease. The bronchodilator effect of sympathomimetics in asthma has remained an important action. However, several other airway effects have been proposed to be of importance in asthma and new aspects of β-agonists continue to be demonstrated in experimental systems.

active vascular exudation of plasma to Felix Marchand's detailed descriptions of the cellular pathology of airways of patients who died of asthma (35,36). Marchand noted the abundance of microvessels in the airway mucosa. He mapped out in great detail the distribution of eosinophils and mast cells in the entire respiratory tract. He discussed local differentiation and turnover of these cells. Marchand remarked that the more superficial the mast cells, the more reduced was their granularity. He saw eosinophils and Charcot crystals where epithelial desquamation occurred. However, Marchand did not agree on denudation with his colleague Fraenkel (37), who was the original champion of the recently revisited idea that epithelial desquamation is a unifying characteristic of asthma (31). Marchand, like many other pathologists between 1900 and 1940, noted that the bronchial epithelium instead could be well preserved even in subjects who had died of asthma. Marchand rather thought that the epithelium could be actively (metabolically) involved in driving the inflammation by releasing inflammatory and chemotactic agents! He also pioneered the view that bronchial, tracheal, and nasal mucosal pathology exhibited many similarities in asthma (38). He called asthma "chronic eosinophilic bronchitis"; he criticized the therapy for not being anti-inflammatory, and he criticized the experimental models of asthma for not being similar to the real disease, because they lacked its inflammatory nature. During their last weeks of life, the patients that Marchand examined had received epinephrine until they no longer responded to this treatment.

It is a fact that epinephrine replaced a very different type of drug in acute asthma: morphine. It is also clear that the use of a respiratory depressant drug such as morphine had been severely criticized by astute asthmologists like Salter. On the other hand, morphine must have helped some patients. Which particular mechanisms were involved in the morphine-induced effects which led to its good reputation? After all morphine was in frequent use for many decades, even centuries, in a condition well supervised by the treatment personnel; that is, the severest attacks of asthma. Very few asthma deaths had been reported in the 19th century and before. Trousseau had stated, "Asthma n'est pas fatale." Salter, who himself probably died of asthma, circumvented a straightforward statement and described all the additional complications "by which asthma kills." Osler coined the aphorism "The asthmatic pants into old age." In a survey published in 1963, Alexander noted that the number of reported deaths appeared to increase after epinephrine had been introduced (39). He received much criticism for this inference. Alexander also remarked about the increased death rate that was recorded between late 1930 and early 1950 (during which time period isoprenaline started to be used). The most dramatic figures emanated from New Zealand where the death rate (per 100,000) from asthma rose from 1.7 in 1939 to 10.4 in 1953. He further thought that the death rate dropped in the 1950s when corticosteroid therapy came to be used extensively in severe asthma. Thus, more than 30 years ago, Alexander brought up subjects that based on novel new data are presently receiving intense attention.

IX. Cocaine and Ephedrine

Bosworth claimed that his report on November 15, 1884, was the first account of cocaine's potent ability to constrict airway blood vessels (40). This action led to the frequent use of cocaine in rhinitis and also to its trial and use in asthma and bronchitis. Cocaine's vascular action is thought to reflect its ability to produce sympathomimetic actions (by blocking the uptake of adrenergic transmitters). However, Bosworth thought that the direct smooth muscle actions of cocaine may contribute to vasoconstriction. Bosworth (41) continued to be very enthusiastic about the cocaine remedy for asthma, and if he were to choose, he unhesitatingly preferred cocaine to the whole of the Pharmacopoeia. He also denied seeing the severe side effects of cocaine that soon were reported by others. As a matter of fact, the cocaine-induced pain and blockage of nasal passages in some patients could be much worse than the condition prevailing when therapy had first been initiated. The "cocaine habit" that eventuated was also much feared. Cocaine as an airway decongestant drug thus had become almost obsolete already before adrenal extracts were made available. Asthma treatment with cocaine had a brief renaissance in the years around 1920. Sluder (42) then published a report entitled "Asthma as a nasal reflex," and the view that neurogenic asthma originated in the nasal mucous membranes received its peak of attention. Local anesthesia of the nasal mucosa by employment of topical cocaine, often together with epinephrine, appeared a rational treatment. However, local anesthetic drugs have not been shown to be effective in allergic airway diseases. Perhaps reflecting in part the possibility that neurogenic mechanisms of exudative inflammation, which are prominent in rodents, may not be relevant to human airways (38).

Ephedrine, similarly to cocaine, may produce vasoconstriction through the action of adrenergic transmitters (by causing their release). A vasoconstrictor drug, ephedrine was rapidly employed as a nasal decongestant in the 1920s (43). It is widely stated in the 1900 literature that ephedrine, similarly to epinephrine, is also a bronchodilator. The standard reference to support this assertion is the work of Chen and Schmidt (2), who were the first Western pharmacologists to examine the effects of ephedrine in many systems. In one dog and at one occasion, they claimed to have seen a bronchodilator effect of ephedrine. The effect was not sustained, nor was it repeatable despite the fact that epinephrine continued to produce bronchodilation in this dog. Chen working together with Middleton also reported the equivocal effects of ephedrine in asthmatic subjects (44). The ephedrine substance was first available to Miller for clinical testing in asthma. In a series of reports, he and his coworkers reported a good efficacy, particularly in those cases of asthma classified as "reflex nasal" (43). However, together with Piness, Miller also reported that ephedrine was without effect in 24 cases with severe asthma (44). The antiasthma effects of the preparation ephedrine-Merck was widely praised by German investigators (see, e.g., refs. 45 and 46), and McDermont (47) from Montreal reported that in most cases of asthma "relief was obtained in from two to five minutes after swallowing a capsule" containing 25 or 50 mg of ephedrine.

In 1928, Halsey (48) examined the effects of ephedrine but was unable to record bronchial smooth muscle relaxation. More recent pharmacological in vitro studies reveal only a poor bronchorelaxant effect requiring unreasonably high concentrations of ephedrine (49). It is further doubtful whether this small relaxant effect is mediated by the specific sympathomimetic mechanism β-receptor stimulation (50). When made available as a drug, ephedrine's oral activity, longer duration of action, and greater chemical stability were appreciated advantages over epinephrine. These properties are evident and useful when ephedrine is employed as a nasal decongestant drug. Ephedrine-like compounds are still widely used for this latter purpose.

X. "β-Agonists" for Asthma: Drugs Precede Theoretical Developments

In the late 1930s, the Austrian pharmacologist Konzett demonstrated that isoprenaline, an epinephrine analogue, produced potent bronchodilating and cardiac stimulant effects (51). Surprisingly, it lacked the smooth muscle contractile effect of epinephrine, including its vasoconstrictor effect. Isoprenaline's clinical efficacy in asthma corresponded to its bronchodilator potency, and the role of vasoconstriction in the bronchial disease largely ceased to be supported by actions of sympathomimetic drugs. Isoprenaline was a sympathomimetic amine that lacked the part of epinephrine's action that could be antagonized by the pharmacological antagonists available in the 1940s. The synthesis and early pharmacological characterization of isoprenaline were probably crucial to the work by Ahlquist (52), who employed isoprenaline and other amines to introduce his α- and β-receptor concept.

In the mid 1960s, researchers working at Swedish and British drug companies, respectively, synthesized and characterized terbutaline and salbutamol as sympathomimetic β-receptor agonists with less actions on the heart than on smooth muscle preparations such as the tracheobronchial strips. Only after this particular property had been well described and after the patent applications of these compounds had been filed in 1966 was the concept of β_1- and

β_2-receptors introduced by Lands et al. (53). In Sweden (Lund), it was Henry Persson, Ph.D., who initiated and pursued the research that led to the production of terbutaline (54,55). In the early 1960s, Persson was already an experienced pharmacologist in the sympathomimetic area with great creativity in the approach to research, including the design of novel methods. His stubborn disposition, his optimism, and his deep-seated devotion to experimental research are coupled with a sound, skeptical look at findings and interpretations reported by other researchers. Indeed, his advice is that "no data are solid until confirmed by yourself." Persson undoubtedly trusts his own observations whether or not his data may agree with current contentions. To this I will add, from personal experience, I can attest to Persson's overwhelming generosity and ability to give other researchers genuine encouragement. These traits, I believe, may explain the success of the structure-activity research that Persson carried out together with two chemists and that produced terbutaline.

The chemists involved in the terbutaline work have continued to contribute significantly to the development of novel sympathomimetic drugs. Kjell Wetterlin thus worked 15 years on an idea of his own to invent the Turbuhaler, which is a unique multidose system for breath-actuated inhalation of pure drug powders (56). It is clear that the development of the modern inhalation devices has come a long way since Bishop's pocket and office powder insufflators were introduced for inhalation of cocaine in the 1880s. The other chemist involved in the synthesis of terbutaline, Leif Svensson, developed his interest in prodrugs and succeeded in mastering enzyme activation mechanisms by synthesizing the bisdimethylcarbamate of terbutaline (bambuterol). After oral administration and absorption, bambuterol, by a series of hydrolytic and oxidative processes, provides well-controlled terbutaline-mediated antiasthma efficacy for more than 24 hr (57,58). The oral sympathomimetic drugs may have started with ephedrine, although the efficacy and the mode of action of this drug are in doubt (see above). A major development in this field was the introduction of orciprenaline in the 1960s followed by the availability of terbutaline and salbutamol in the 1970s; these three β-agonists being suited both for inhalation and oral administration. By their relatively low airway concentrations, the oral drugs are not as effective acutely as the inhaled β-agonists, which is particularly evident in bronchial provocation studies (59). On the other hand, the oral β_2-agonists may not be associated with mucosal actions which, in the current controversy on the regular use of inhaled β-agonists, are being discussed as potentially less desirable. Oral and inhaled β_2-agonists may thus be distinct classes of antiasthma drugs.

The β-receptor molecule has now been fully described and can be assembled in vitro. Drug receptor interactions and numerous ensuing biochemical reactions are known in abundant detail. At the same time, a significant further step has been taken in the development of novel β-receptor agonists for asthma. Formoterol and salmeterol, given by the inhaled route, have been found to have a much longer duration of action in asthma than salbutamol and terbutaline. Such a long duration in asthmatic subjects of any inhaled β_2-agonist was originally discovered in 1986 administration of formoterol (60). Indeed, the previous animal studies had not identified any impressive duration of action of formoterol. It is only in later, specific airway studies employing topical mucosal drug application that formoterol's long duration of action has been demonstrated in vivo in animals (61). With salmeterol, there is more general agreement between bronchorelaxation in vitro or animal data and clinical observations in asthma (62,63). It is notable that these recently introduced β-agonist drugs were not a result of progress in theoretical β-receptor research. Retrofit explanations of the long duration of action of formoterol and salmeterol are now being offered at the molecular and receptor level.

Much of the development within β-agonists concerns duration of action. Inhaled epinephrine and isoprenaline produced only short-lasting bronchodilatation. Inhaled orciprenaline produced a somewhat longer lasting effect than isoprenaline. But orciprenaline was soon overshadowed by the appearance of terbutaline and salbutamol. The pharmacological β_2-receptor selectivity together with the duration of action (at least 4 hr) thus favored the use of terbutaline/salbutamol. The 12-hr duration of action produced by formoterol and salmeterol has been welcomed but has also fueled a debate on the desirability of a continuous and high topical β-agonist tone in the airways. This debate may currently put a hold on any further prolongation of the duration of action of antiasthma drugs, although once daily inhaled β_2-agonist molecules are feasible. It appears to be a different matter with the ingested bronchodilator drugs. Once daily dosing may even be preferred with these latter drugs.

XI. Conclusions

The generally acclaimed progress in medical research on sympathomimetic drugs may not always focus on truly significant events. Astute, nondogmatic, sometimes even rebellious researchers seem to have made the important contributions; frequently without receiving proper recognition. By his unique insight into the nature of asthma, Salter could describe the antiasthma efficacy of epinephrine some 50 years before this drug became available. Around 1940, several years before the concept of α- and β-receptors was introduced, Konzett described well the particular properties of isoprenaline. In the early 1960s, by sagacious experimental approaches and unflinching convictions, drug industry researchers pursued original research ideas to devise successfully the bronchoselective drugs terbutaline and salbutamol. This occurred well before there was any mention of β_2-receptors. Nils Svedmyr described many clinical pharmacological facts about asthma. By the mid 1980s, he was thus "logically" involved in the original and unexpected discovery of the long duration of action of inhaled formoterol in asthma.

The unadjusted medical history of novel sympathomimetic drugs may offer some insight into the nature of drug discovery work. The importance of generally acknowledged basic research in this field cannot be neglected, but in the individual cases, the academic theories have not preceded but rather been dependent on the drug discoveries. The actual basis for major discoveries has involved astute observations in complex in vivo systems as key ingredients. Further, the major steps forward have been made possible by utilizing heuristic structure-activity work as a basic research tool. New molecules put into complex biosystems have thus provided exciting and surprising readouts upon which progress has been built. (A similar story can be told about steroids for the treatment of asthma.) The success is dependent on individuals who have the ability to observe and also the integrity and the courage to pursue unorthodox, novel pathways.

Another potential lesson to be learned from the drug development research in this field (and in the steroid field) is the compatibility between a significant progress and an incomplete understanding of the true modes of action. Salter naturally saw violent emotions to be acting as "a nervous derivative" to antagonize the proasthmatic inactivity of the central nervous system (see Table 1). (He was well aware of the nocturnal worsening of asthma and he pioneered its treatment with strong coffee.) Then followed a period when the vasoconstrictor effect was considered highly desirable in asthma. After its discovery in 1907, the bronchodilator aspect has remained a major therapeutic action. However, the roles of additional actions, including vascular antipermeability effects, and antimediator release effects (61,64), continue to intrigue us. Such nonbronchodilator airway actions of β_2-agonists, whether potentially good or bad, will likely attract attention in close relation to what is considered most topical in discussions of asthma (see Table 1). Whether right or wrong (cf. epinephrine's vasoconstrictor property a century ago), the new ideas may prompt important progress. Subcellular biochemical actions of β-receptor stimulation also continue to be a field of challenges and controversies particularly concerning linkage with important functions in vivo. Several types of isolated cell systems, including human "inflammatory cells," are now readily accessible and exhibit interesting responses to β_2-agonist molecules (65). A lesson to be learned here may concern limited translatability of isolated cell and cell culture data to in vivo and particularly to the asthmatic airways in vivo (66).

Acknowledgment

I thank Ingegerd Källén and Mai Broman for expertise secretarial assistance.

References

1. Gandevia B. Historical review of the use of parasympatholytic agents in the treatment of respiratory disorders. Postgrad Med 1975; 51(suppl 7):13–20.
2. Chen KK, Schmidt CF. The action of ephedrine, the active principle of the Chinese drug Ma Huang. J Pharmacol Exp Ther 1925; 24:339–357.
3. Persson CGA. On the medical history of xanthines and other remedies for asthma: a tribute to H.H. Salter. Thorax 1985; 40:881–886.
4. Mann RD. Modern Drug Use. An Inquiry on Historical Principles. Lancaster, UK: MTP, 1984.
5. Altounyan REC. Review of clinical activity and mode of action of sodium cromoglycate. Clin Allergy 1980; 10:481–489.
6. Salter HH. On Asthma; Its Pathology and Treatment. London: Churchill, 1860 (1st ed.); 1868 (2nd ed.).
7. Cardano G. De vita propria liber. Pauda, 1575.
8. Floyer J. The ancient psichpolousia revived; or an essay to prove cold bathing both safe and useful. London, 1702.
9. Smollett T. Travels. Introduced and edited by F. Felsenstein (1979). Oxford University Press, 1766.
10. Keers RY. Laënnec, R.T.M. his medical history. Thorax 1834; 36:91–94.
11. Tischer M. Über die Asthmabehandlung mit pflanzlichen Heilmitteln in der Volksheilkunde und in der Medizin seit dem 16. Jahrhundert. Berlin: Ebering, 1939.
12. Schiff NS. Non-specific versus specific therapy in bronchial asthma. Am J Med Sci 1923; 156:664–677.
13. Duke WW. Details in the treatment of hay-fever, asthma and other manifestations of allergy. Am J Med Sci 1925; 166:645–663.
14. Sneader W. Drug Discovery: The Evolution of Modern Medicines. New York: Wiley, 1985.
15. Oliver G, Schäfer EA. On the physiological action of extract of the suprarenal capsules. J Physiol (Lond) 1895; 17:9–14.
16. Bates WH. The use of extract of suprarenal capsule in the eye. NY Med J 1896; 63:647–650.
17. Swain HL. The local use of the aqueous extract of the suprarenal glands of the sheep in the nose and throat. NY Med J 1989; 68:916–918.
18. Douglass B. The treatment of hay fever by suprarenal gland. NY Med J 1900; 71:725–728.
19. Clark JP. The use of suprarenal extract in hay fever. Boston Med Surg 1902; 146: 664–667.
20. Solis-Cohen S. A preliminary note on the treatment of hay-fever with suprarenal substance: with a report of personal experience. Philadelphia Med J 1989; 2:341–343.
21. Solis-Cohen S. The use of adrenal substance in the treatment of asthma. JAMA 1900; 34:1164–1166.
22. Persson CGA. Airway epithelium, microcirculation, and glucocorticoids. In: Schleimer RP, Busse W, O'Byrne P, eds. Topical Glucocorticoids in Asthma—Mechanisms and Clinical Action." Dekker, New York: Marcel Dekker, 1996:

23. Persson CGA. Glucocorticoids for asthma—early contributions. Pulm Pharmacol 1989; 2:163–166.
24. Persson CGA. A cornucopia of drug discovery? Nature Med 1996; 2:5–6.
25. Wilson NL. Clinical notes on adrenalin. Laryngoscope 1901; July:63–66.
26. Takamine J. Adrenalin the active principle of the suprarenal glands and its mode of preparation. Am J Pharm 1901; 73:523–531.
27. Bullowa JGM, Kaplan DM. On the hypodermatic use of adrenalin chloride in the treatment of asthmatic attacks. Med News 1903; 83:787–790.
28. Camps PWL. A note on the inhalation treatment of asthma. Guy's Hosp Rep 1929; 79:496–498.
29. Weber T. Zur Theorie des Bronchialasthma. Tagbl Vers Dtsch Naturf Artzte 1872; 45:159–171.
30. Stoerk K. Asthma bronchiale. Stuttgart: Enke, 1875:1–102.
31. Persson CGA. Airway epithelium and microcirculation. Eur Respir Rev 1994; 4: 352–362.
32. Kahn R. Zur Physiologie der Trachea. Arch Physiol 1907; 398–426.
33. Persson CGA, Pauwels R. Pharmacology of antiasthma xanthines. In: Page CP, Barnes P, eds. Pharmacology of Asthma. Handbook of Experimental Pharmacology. Berlin: Springer, 1991, 98:207–225.
34. Cohnheim JF. Neue Untersuchungen über die Entzündung. Berlin, 1873.
35. Marchand F. Beitrag zur Pathologie und patologischen Anatomie des Bronchialasthma. Beitr Pathol Anat 1916; 61:251–324.
36. Marchand F. Ein neuer Fall von Asthma bronchiale mit anatomischer Untersuchung. Dtsch Arch Klin Med 1918; 127:184–209.
37. Fraenkel A. Zur Patologie des Bronchialasthmas. Dtsch Med Wochenschr 1900; 26:269–276.
38. Persson CGA, Svensson C, Greiff L, Andersson M, Wollmer P, Alkner U, Erjefält I. The use of the nose to study the inflammatory response of the respiratory tract. Thorax 1992; 47:993–1000.
39. Alexander HL. A historical account of death from asthma. J Allergy 1963; 34:305–313 and Comments 313–322.
40. Bosworth FH. A new therapeutic use of cocaine. Med Rec 1884; 26:533–534.
41. Bosworth FH. An additional note on the therapeutic action of cocaine. NY Med J 1886; 43:322–324.
42. Sluder G. Asthma as a nasal reflex. JAMA 1919; 73:589–591.
43. Leopold SS, Miller TG. The use of ephedrine in bronchial asthma and hay fever. JAMA 1927; 88:1782–1786.
44. Chen KK, Schmidt CF. Ephedrine and related substances. Med Anal Rev Gen Med Neurol Pediatr 1930; 9:1–117.
45. Hess O. Ueber Ephedrin. Munch Med Wochenschr 1926; 73:1691–1693.
46. Kämmerer H, Dorrer R. Kurze Mitteilung über die Wirkung des Ephedrin-Merck auf Asthmakranke. Munch Med Wochenschr 1926; 73:1739–1740.
47. McDermont HE. The use of ephedrine in bronchial asthma. Can Med Assoc J 1926; 16:422–423.
48. Halsey JT. Action of ephedrin on intestine and bronchi. Proc Soc Exp Biol Med 1928; 137:343–351.

49. Waldeck B, Widmark E. The interaction of ephedrine with adrenoceptors in tracheal, cardiac and skeletal muscles. Clin Exp Pharmacol Physiol 1985; 12:439–442.
50. Tye A, Baldesberger R, Lapidus JB, Patil PN. Steric aspects of adrenergic drugs VI. Beta adrenergic effects of ephedrine isomers. J Pharmacol Exp Ther 1967; 157:356–362.
51. Konzett H. Neue broncholytische hochworksame Körper der Adrenalinreihe. Naunyn-Schmiedeberg Arch Exp Pathol Pharmacol 1941; 197:2734.
52. Ahlquist RP. A study of the adrenotropic receptors. Am J Physiol 1948; 153:586–600.
53. Lands AM, Arnold A, McAuliff JP, Luduena FP, Brown TG Jr. Differentiation of receptor systems activated by sympathomimetic amines. Nature 1967; 214:597–598.
54. Persson H, Olsson T. Some pharmacological properties of terbutaline (NN), 1-(3.5-dihydroxyphenyl)-2(t-butylamino)-ethanol. A new sympathomimetic β-receptor-stimulating agent. Acta Med Scand 1970; 512(suppl):11–19.
55. Persson H, Johnson B. A dual preparation technique for studying the differentiation of the effect of sympathomimetic agents on heart and tracheal muscle. Acta Med Scand 1970; 512(suppl):21–24.
56. Wetterlin K. Turbuhaler®: a new powder inhaler for administration of drugs to the airways. Pharmaceut Res 1988; 5:506–508.
57. Svensson L.-Å, Tunek A. The design and bioactivation of presystemically stable prodrugs. Drug Metab Rev 1988; 19:165–194.f
58. Smolensky MH, D'Alonzo GE. Administration-time dependence of the kinetics and effect of once daily 20 mg dosing of bambuterol versus placebo in asthma patients. Eur Respir J 1991; 4:555S.
59. Anderson SD, Seale JP, Rozea P, Bandler L, Theobald G, Lindsay DA. Inhaled and oral salbutamol in exercise-induced asthma. Am Rev Respir Dis 1976; 114: 851–859.
60. Löfdahl C.-G, Svedmyr N. Effect duration of inhaled formoterol, a new β_2-adrenoceptor agonist, compared to salbutamol in asthmatic patients. Acta Pharmacol Toxicol 1986; 5(suppl):229.
61. Erjefält I, Persson CGA. Long duration and high potency of antiexudative effects of formoterol in guinea-pig tracheobronchial airways. Am Rev Respir Dis 1991; 144:788–791.
62. Ball DJ, Coleman RA, Denyer LH, Nials AT, Sheldrik KE. In vitro characterisation of the β_2-adrenoceptor agonist salmeterol. Br J Pharmacol 1987; 88:591.
63. Ullman A, Svedmyr N. Salmeterol, a new longacting inhaled β_2-adrenoceptor agonist. A comparison with salbutamol. Thorax 1988; 43:674–678.
64. Svensson C, Greiff L, Andersson M, Alkner U, Grönneberg R, Persson CGA. Antiallergic actions of high topical doses of terbutaline in human nasal airways. Allergy 1995; 50:884–890.
65. Linden M. The effects of β_2-adrenoceptor agonists and a corticosteroid, budesonide, on the secretion of inflammatory mediators from monocytes. Br J Pharmacol 1992; 107:156–160.
66. Persson CGA. *In vivo* veritas. Thorax 1996; 51:441–443.

2

Molecular Biology of the Beta₂-Adrenergic Receptor

Focus on Interactions of Agonist with Receptor

STEPHEN B. LIGGETT and STUART A. GREEN

University of Cincinnati College of Medicine
Cincinnati, Ohio

I. Introduction

Over the last decade, substantial progress has been made in understanding the molecular basis of beta₂-adrenergic receptor (β_2AR) function (1–3). Primarily using the methods of site-directed mutagenesis and recombinant expression, relationships between structural elements of the receptor and their role in receptor function have been established. In this chapter, we briefly review specific aspects of the molecular biology of the β_2AR, and in detail discuss the interaction between agonists and the receptor relevant to our recent finding of the molecular basis of the binding of salmeterol to the β_2AR which results in prolonged receptor activation.

II. Features of G-Protein–Coupled Receptors

Shown in Figure 1 are the features of a prototypic G-protein–coupled receptor. All receptors in this family are composed of stretches of seven hydrophobic residues which putatively represent transmembrane-spanning domains (TMDs). The amino-terminus is extracellular and the carboxy-terminus is intracellular.

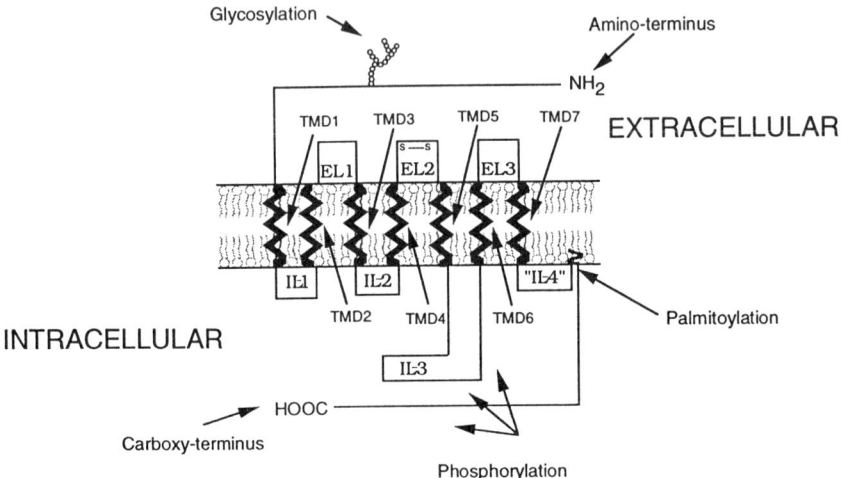

Figure 1 Schematic representation of a prototypic G-protein–coupled receptor. EL-1–EL-3, extracellular loops 1–3; IL-1–IL-3, intracellular loops 1–3; TMD 1–7, transmembrane domains 1–7.

Consequently, there are three extracellular and three intracellular loops. Some receptors have a cysteine in the cytoplasmic tail of the receptor that is palmitoylated. Since this presumably anchors this cysteine to the membrane, a fourth intracellular loop is thereby formed. Other posttranslational modifications common to G-protein–coupled receptors include glycosylation, phosphorylation, and disulfide bonding.

The classic paradigm for signal transduction with these receptors involves agonist binding which alters the receptor conformation leading to the binding and activation of the G-protein. The activated G-protein then alters the activity of an effector such as an enzyme or ion channel. The former is typified by adenylyl cyclase. With receptors such as the β_2AR, which couple to the stimulatory G-protein (G_s), agonist binding results in activation of adenylyl cyclase causing conversion of intracellular adenosine triphosphate (ATP) to cyclic adenosine monophosphate (cAMP). The agonist thus acts as the "first messenger," whereas cAMP acts as the "second messenger." Recent data suggest that in the absence of agonist, coupling of receptor to G-protein can occur spontaneously, thus establishing a "basal" level of cellular activity (4–7). In this model, agonists tend to stabilize this active, G-protein–bound conformation. Antagonists have no effect on this equilibrium, whereas inverse agonists stabilize the inactive conformation. It should be noted that this concept has arisen from studies utilizing marked overexpression of receptors. It is thus unclear at present whether certain aspects of this two-state model are physiologically relevant. For clarity, in the subsequent discussion on agonist-receptor interactions, we refer to receptors being "activated by agonists" (which is the classic model), but this is synonymous with activated receptors being "stabilized by agonists" in the two-state model.

III. Structure/Function Relationships of β_2AR

The general approach for establishing structure/function relationships with the β_2AR has been with site-directed mutagenesis. A hypothesis is made concerning the potential role of a region of the receptor. The cDNA encoding for the receptor is then mutated to result in a deletion of this region of the protein or a substitution with other amino acids. This construct is then transfected into cells, and using the expressed receptor, the consequences of the structural alteration are assessed in parallel studies with wild-type receptor. Most commonly, the host cell for these studies is a mammalian cell which does not endogenously express β_2AR but does have the other components of the signal transduction process. With this approach, the key regions for many features of the β_2AR, including those necessary for proper folding and insertion of the receptor into the membrane, agonist binding, G_s coupling, and desensitization, have been delineated (1,2). A composite depicting these domains is provided in Figure 2.

The binding of typical agonists such as isoproterenol occurs in a binding "pocket" established by the TMDs approximately 11 Å into the membrane (8). Several key contact points between agonist and receptor have been identified. The amine head group of catecholamines interacts with the carboxylate group on Asp113 which is in TMD3 (9,10). Mutant β_2ARs having a serine in this position are not activated by catecholamines but are activated by catechol esters which can form hydrogen bonds to serines. The hydroxyl groups on the catecholamine ring have been shown to form bonds with Ser204 and Ser207 which are localized in TMD5 (11). Mutant receptors where these serines were replaced with alanines have been studied using isoproterenol and isoproterenol derivatives lacking the para- and metahydroxyl groups. The isoproterenol derivative lacking the parahydroxyl group was unable to activate the receptor lacking Ser207, whereas the derivative lacking the metahydroxyl was unable to activate the receptor lacking Ser204. Isoproterenol itself could activate both receptors, and the metaderivative could activate the Ser204 mutant and the paraderivative could activate the Ser207 mutant. This suggests that the catecholamine can be positioned and can activate β_2AR by forming hydrogen bonds with either serines, but with endogenous catecholamines (and most synthetic

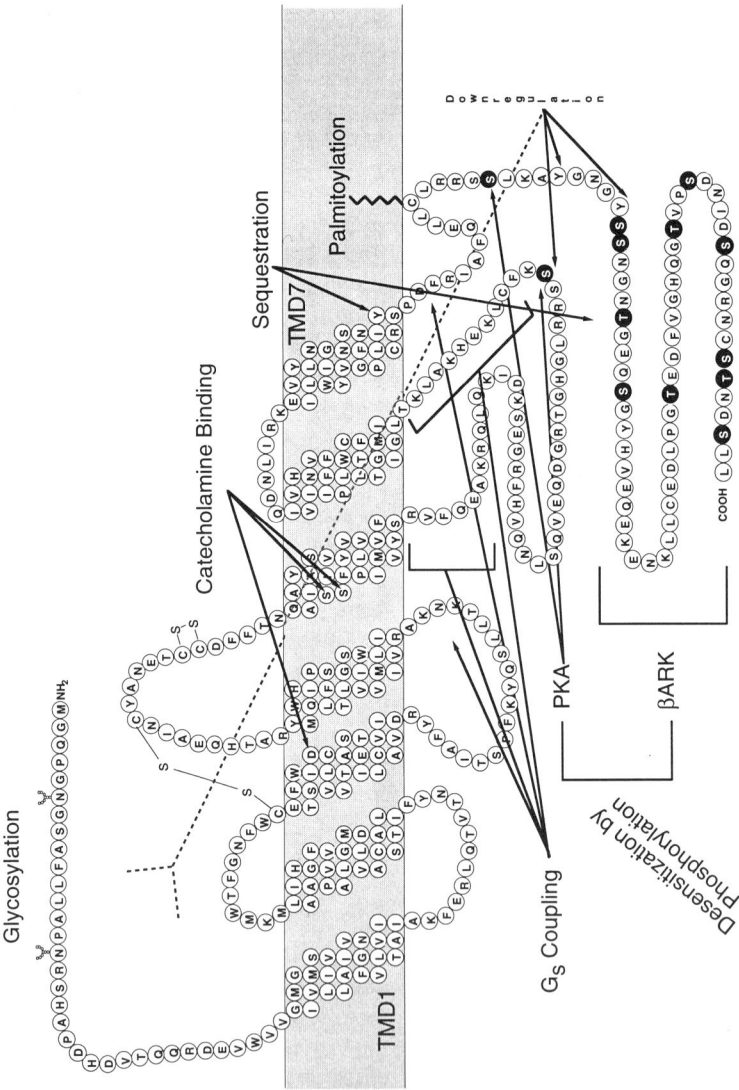

Figure 2   Structural features of the human β₂-adrenergic receptor. Shown is the primary amino acid sequence (using the single amino acid abbreviation) with regions indicated that have been found to be important for agonist binding, G-protein coupling, and agonist regulation. See text for details.

β-agonists), interactions occur at both serines. The determinants of stereospecificity of catecholamines are not known.

There is some evidence that the hydroxyl group on the β-carbon of catecholamines interacts with residues on TMD4 (presumably Ser165), and that this may be an important region for defining stereospecificity (12). However, mutant receptors lacking Ser165 fail to express, suggesting that this may be difficult to approach using mutagenesis. Determinants of agonist specificity for the β₁AR and β₂AR are not known. Thus, it is unclear what specific residues impart the rank order of potency for β₂AR (isoproterenol > epinephrine >> norepinephrine) as compared with the β₁AR (isoproterenol > norepinephrine ≥ epinephrine). This has been addressed with chimeric βAR, in which progressive substitution of β₂AR transmembrane segments into β₁AR was carried out (13). A gradual switch in rank order was noted with such progressive substitutions, with the most dramatic occurring when TMD4 of the β₂AR was substituted into a receptor which had β₂AR sequence from TMDs 1–3 and β₁AR sequence in TMDs 5–7. Nevertheless, the full β₂AR-binding phenotype was not found until a chimera consisting of the TMDs 1–6 of the β₂AR was studied. The data suggest that many residues may be involved in establishing the agonist-binding pocket, and that subtle changes in this milieu may account for different affinities for agonist. Similar observations have also been made for antagonist binding (13). Here, the situation is even more complex, because the critical contact points are not known for antagonist binding, and the diverse structures of synthetic antagonists make it difficult to assess the molecular basis of high-affinity binding.

The regions of the β₂AR which couple to G_s are the second and third intracellular loops (14,15). Given what we know about the agonist-binding sites in TMD 3 and TMD 5, it makes sense that the inner connecting loops contain the G-protein–coupling domains. Agonist binding then promotes (stabilizes) a conformation of these loops which favors interaction with G_s. For the third intracellular loop, it appears that the amino- and carboxy-terminal residues of the loop closest to the membrane insertion sites are critical for G_s coupling. The specific residues within the second intracellular loop that are required for G_s binding and coupling are not known.

During continuous agonist exposure, a number of G-protein–coupled receptors display the property of desensitization, which is the waning of a response despite the presence of a stimulus of constant intensity (1). Such regulation suggests the need for certain receptors to be dynamically regulated in order to maintain homeostasis under normal conditions and during pathophysiological states. It has been proposed that desensitization may limit the therapeutic effectiveness of agonist (termed tachyphylaxis). *In the treatment of asthma, it is not at all clear whether clinically relevant tachyphylaxis to chronic β-agonist treatment occurs.* The reader is referred elsewhere (16) and to other chapters in this volume for further discussion of this topic. Agonist-promoted β_2AR desensitization has been primarily studied using in vitro systems, where three phases have been identified. It is important to note here that the paradigms established thus far have been based almost exclusively on results from studies using full agonists. In studies with partial agonists, desensitization appears to be less pronounced, but the mechanism which accounts for this difference is not known (1). The most rapid phase of desensitization, which occurs within seconds of exposure, is due to phosphorylation of the receptor by the cAMP-dependent protein kinase A and a cAMP-independent kinase termed the βAR kinase (βARK) (17–20). βARK phosphorylation induces binding of another protein, β-arrestin, which serves to uncouple the receptor from G_s. Phosphorylation of the receptor by protein kinase A (PKA) appears to directly induce uncoupling. The sites for phosphorylation by these kinases are shown in Figure 2. A second mechanism of desensitization, termed sequestration or internalization, is brought into play after minutes of agonist exposure and is typically maximal at 30 min. Sequestered receptors have become internalized to a subcellular compartment where they are not available for coupling to G_s. A sequence within the distal portion of TMD 7, which could also lie just within the cytoplasmic portion of the tail, appears to be necessary for agonist-promoted sequestration (21). This motif is similar to the NPXXY sequence in the low-density lipoprotein (LDL) receptor that has been shown to be necessary for ligand-induced internalization. There is also evidence that other portions of the cytoplasmic tail are required, since substitution of the β_2AR cytoplasmic tail into the β_3AR (which does not sequester) results in a chimeric receptor that does sequester (19). In addition, there appears to be an interaction with the third intracellular loop that may be important for modulating the extent of sequestration. This concept is based on the finding that deletion of a proline-rich region of this loop of the β_1AR enhances sequestration, whereas substituting this region into the β_2AR third loop depresses sequestration (22). Internalized receptors appear to have two fates: they can be recycled to the surface or they can undergo degradation. Evidence also suggests that dephosphorylation of β_2AR occurs while the receptor is internalized, so sequestration may also serve as a mechanism of resensitization (23). After more prolonged agonist exposure (hours), the net number of cellular receptors decreases; a process termed receptor downregulation. Downregulation has been proposed to be due to degradation of receptor protein, a loss of mRNA stability, and/or a decrease in the rate of transcription. Which mechanism predominates appears to be dependent on several factors, including agonist concentrations, the cell type, and whether the studies are carried out using natively expressing or recombinantly expressing cells. At the level of the receptor protein, two amino-terminal residues at positions 16 and 27 appear to be critical for downregulation (24,25) (see Fig. 2). It should be noted that at these two residues, the β_2AR

displays heterogeneity within the human population due to polymorphisms in the gene encoding for the receptor (26). These different forms of the β_2AR may play a role in establishing the severity of asthma or the overall responsiveness to β-agonist therapy (3,27–31). In addition, the PKA site in the third intracellular loop, an undefined portion of the cytoplasmic tail, and two tyrosine residues in the cytoplasmic tail are required for full agonist-promoted downregulation (19,32,33).

IV. Delineating a Specific Salmeterol Exosite Binding Motif in the β_2AR

The pharmacological characteristics of the long-acting β_2AR agonist salmeterol have suggested that this agent may bind to the receptor in a unique manner (34–36). A single dose of salmeterol produced profound smooth muscle relaxation in cat trachea preparations, which remains constant for 12 hr or more despite removal of the drug from the bath and extensive washing. This is in marked contrast to what is observed with isoproterenol, albuterol and formoterol, where the physiological effect promptly abates when these agonists are removed. Under the same conditions as above, after washout the effects of salmeterol are reversed by the antagonist sotalol but return once the antagonist is removed. Such studies point toward salmeterol binding to both the classic catecholamine-binding sites in the β_2AR as discussed above and to some other domain either within the receptor or the cell membrane. This latter binding has been termed "exosite binding" owing to its probable location being outside of the traditional catecholamine-binding domains of the receptor. Such exosite binding would account for the long-acting effects of salmeterol in that the drug could be anchored for a prolonged time period to a site near the traditional binding sites and would thus be repeatedly available for binding and receptor activation. The structure of salmeterol is consistent with this hypothesis in that it contains an extended hydrophobic (phenylalkyloxyalkyl) moiety which presumably could bind to either the receptor or nearby in the membrane lipid regions. Either case represents a unique mode of action for a β-agonist.

We became intrigued by this apparent exosite binding, since no other agonist for any G-protein–coupled receptor has such characteristics. Knowing the molecular determinants of the exosite might make it possible to design long-acting agonists for other receptors. To approach this, we utilized site-directed mutagenesis and recombinant expression of the human β_2AR (37). If the exosite was localized within the receptor, we reasoned that because of the physical size of the molecule, the site would most likely lie near the traditional catecholamine-binding sites. Thus, the TMDs were considered likely domains for exosite binding. We considered that a specific domain might be identifiable by substituting TMD segments from a closely related receptor which did not exhibit exosite binding into β_2AR.

In preliminary studies, we utilized the human β_1AR and β_2AR recombinantly expressed in fibroblasts to develop a method of identifying exosite binding and to see if the β_1AR had such a site. Cells separately expressing each receptor were grown in monolayers. At 90% confluency, the cells were exposed to media containing isoproterenol, salmeterol, formeterol, or media alone for 10 min. After removal of the media, cells were washed with a continuous perfusion of saline for 30 min at room temperature. Then the cells were lysed in cold hypotonic buffer, detached by scraping, and membranes prepared. The number of available (i.e., nonoccupied) receptors present after this washout was then assessed by [^{125}I]cyanopindolol ([^{125}I]CYP) binding. As expected, when cells were treated with isoproterenol at concentrations up to $100\,\mu M$, we found that this washing removed the drug from all the expressed β_1AR and β_2AR. That is, there was no difference in the receptor density between cells exposed to media alone or to media with isoproterenol. This is consistent with the classic pharmacological properties of catecholamine binding to β_1AR and β_2AR. In contrast, when cells bearing β_2AR were exposed to salmeterol (1 μM), approximately 40% of the receptors remained occupied despite removal of the drug and the extensive washing of the cells. This was similar to the reported properties of salmeterol when studied using tracheal preparations in both functional and radioligand-binding studies. In contrast, the β_1AR displayed no salmeterol exosite–binding characteristics. That is, no β_1ARs were found to be occupied by drug after exposure to salmeterol and extensive washing. In separate radioligand-binding competition studies using membranes from β_1AR-expressing cells, salmeterol was found to bind to this receptor with moderate affinity ($K_i \sim 700$ nM). Also, salmeterol was found to activate the β_1AR leading to increased intracellular cAMP. We thus concluded that the β_1AR lacked specific domains required for exosite binding even though it does have the capacity to bind salmeterol at the traditional sites.

These findings also suggested that exosite binding was not simply localized to the cell membrane, since β_1AR and β_2AR were expressed in the same parental cell line, yet only β_2AR displayed exosite binding. We thus felt that chimeric substitution mutagenesis with small portions of β_1AR sequence was a reasonable approach for delineating the salmeterol exosite–binding domains in the β_2AR. We also studied formeterol under these same conditions. In clinical studies, formeterol has an apparent longer duration of action as compared with some other β-agonists. The basis of this longer duration of action is not clear, but the differences in pharmacological properties between salmeterol and formeterol suggest that the two agonists achieve sustained actions by different mechanisms. Consistent with this, in our system we found no evidence for persistently occupied receptor after washout when cells bearing β_2AR were

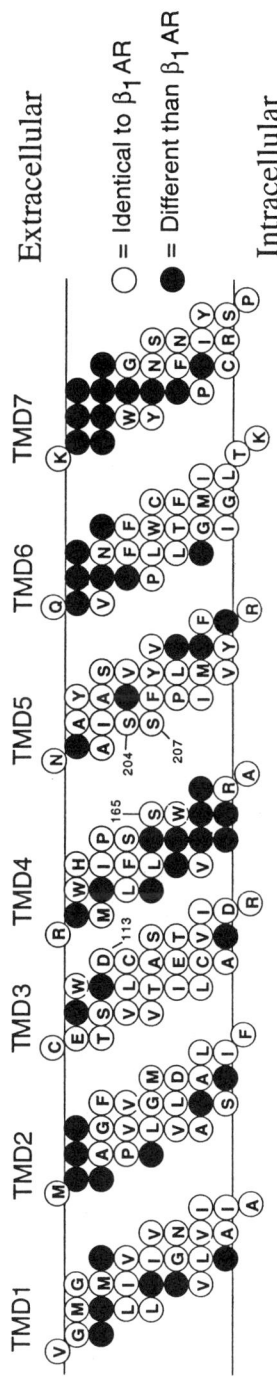

Figure 3 Sequence identity between the human β_1- and β_2-adrenergic receptors in the transmembrane domains. Shown are the amino acids that are identical between the two receptors (open circles). The darkened circles are locations of residue that differ between the two.

first incubated with formoterol. This further validated the system as being specific for identifying exosite binding.

Shown in Figure 3 is the primary amino acid sequence of the TMDs of the human β_2AR. The open circles indicate residues which are identical between β_2AR and β_1AR. The black circles indicate residues which are different between the two receptors. As can be seen, the greatest divergence in sequence is within the fourth and the seventh TMDs. We considered then that the salmeterol exosite might be within one of these regions. (Note that Asp113, Ser165, Ser204, and Ser207 are present in both receptors.) The approach was to construct mutated β_2AR having β_1AR substitutions within the aforementioned regions starting first with the fourth TMD. Shown in Figure 4 are the chimeric substitutions that were made. In this figure, black residues represent β_1AR sequence. The entire fourth TMD of β_2AR was substituted with β_1AR

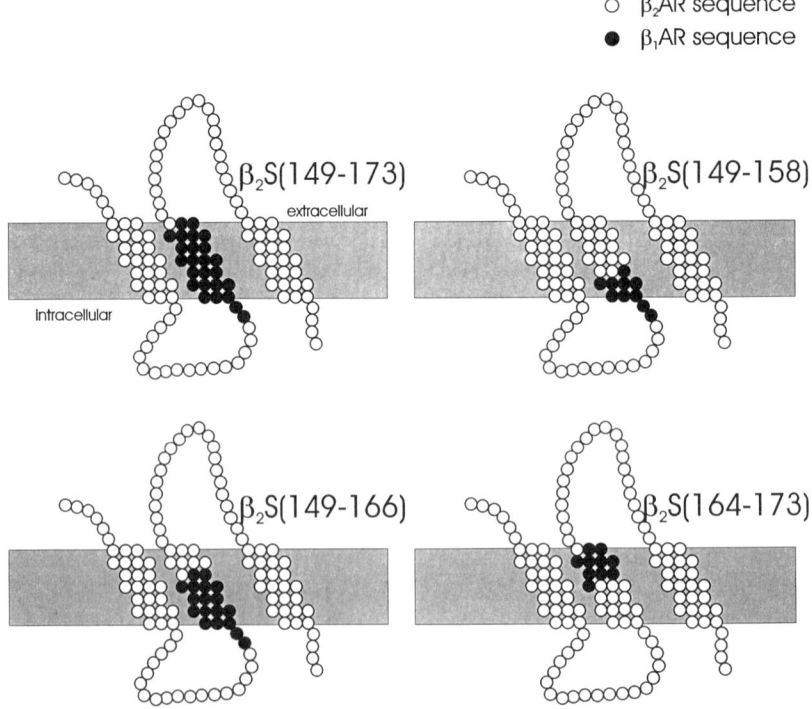

Figure 4   Structure of the β_2/β_1 adrenergic receptor chimeras. Shown are transmembrane domains 3, 4, and 5. White residues represent β_2-adrenergic receptor amino acid sequence and black residues indicate β_1-adrenergic sequence.

sequence in mutant S(149-173). In mutant S(164-173), only a region of the segment closest to the extracellular portion of the receptor was substituted with β₁AR sequence. In a two-dimensional representation, such as in Figures 3 and 4, this might be referred to as the "upper" portion of TMD 4. In mutant S(149-166), only the "lower" portion was substituted. Another mutant, denoted S(149-166), was also constructed as shown.

The approach for studying these mutants is depicted in Figure 5. COS-7 cells were separately transfected with each mutant receptor construct as well as the wild-type β₂AR. Saturation binding studies in membranes prepared from these cells showed that the binding affinity (K_d) for [^{125}I]CYP was no

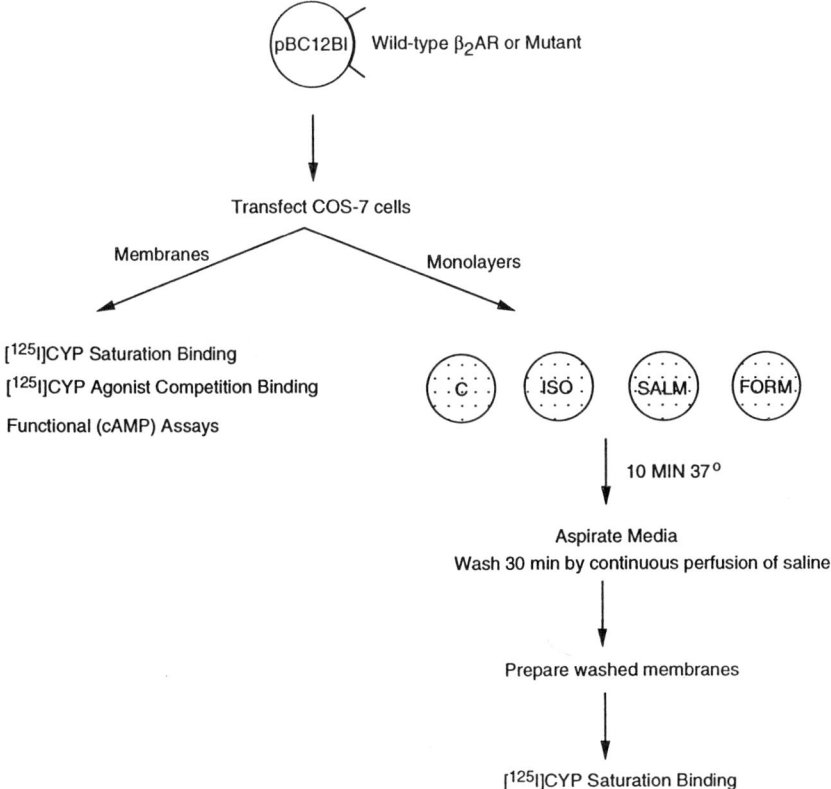

Figure 5 Protocol for assessing agonist binding resistant to washout. Wild-type or the mutated β2-adrenergic receptor depicted in Figure 4 were transiently expressed in COS-7 cells; treatments and assays were as described in the text.

different between wild-type β_2AR and any of the mutated receptors. In competition studies, the binding affinities for the agonists isopreterenol, epinephrine, norepinephrine, formoterol, and salmeterol, were also identical between the different receptors. Thus, it appeared that substitution of TMD 4 β_1AR sequence into the β_2AR did not disrupt the classic binding site or the rank order of potency for agonists. We then assessed exosite binding. Cells in monolayers expressing each receptor were exposed to media alone or media with isoproterenol (100 μM), formoterol (10 μM), or salmeterol (1 μM) for 10 min at 37°C. Media were then aspirated and the dishes continuously perfused with saline for 30 min. Membranes were prepared as described earlier and [^{125}I]CYP binding carried out to assess the receptor density.

The results are shown in Figure 6. As discussed earlier, exposure of wild-type β_2AR to salmeterol followed by the washing protocol resulted in approximately 40% of receptor being occupied by drug. This was taken as wild-type salmeterol exosite binding. When the entire TMD 4 was substituted by β_1AR sequence in the S(149-173) mutant, exosite binding was significantly decreased (~67% loss). This suggested that at least one important component of the

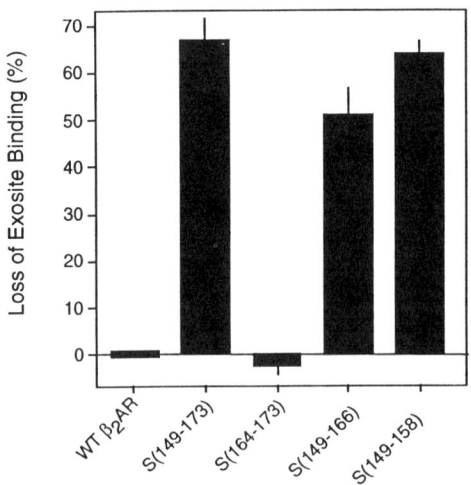

Figure 6 Effects of receptor mutations on salmeterol exosite binding. Cells expressing the indicated receptor (see Fig. 4) were exposed to salmeterol, extensively washed, membranes prepared, and the extent of retained agonist assessed using radioligand binding with [^{125}I]cyanopindolol. With the wild-type (WT) β_2-adrenergic receptor, 38 ± 2% of the receptors remained occupied by salmeterol despite washout, which is termed exosite binding. The *loss* of exosite binding imposed by the mutations is plotted.

exosite domain did indeed lie within TMD 4, prompting study of the additional mutants to attempt to define a discrete domain responsible for this property (37). Substituting only the portion of the segment nearest the extracellular site of the receptor (mutant S[164-173]) had no effect on exosite binding pointing toward other regions of TMD4. Consistent with this notion, mutant S(149-167) displayed a loss of exosite binding. The smallest substitution, S(149-158), consisting of a 10–amino acid substitution of $\beta_1 AR$ into $\beta_2 AR$ at the extreme cytosylic portion of TMD 4, also resulted in a substantial loss of exosite binding. Comparison of the sequence between $\beta_2 AR$ and $\beta_1 AR$ in this region is shown in Figure 7. As can be seen, 6 of the 10 residues are different between the two receptors implying that salmeterol exosite binding requires 1 or more of these 6 residues. It is interesting to note that within TMD 4 of the $\beta_2 AR$, this region is clearly the most hydrophobic based on the Kyle-Doolittle algorithm for hydrophilicity analysis. In addition, this same region is substantially less hydrophobic in the $\beta_1 AR$. One would predict that the long hydrophobic side chain of salmeterol would most favorably interact with a highly hydrophobic region of the receptor, and based on the data from these studies, this indeed appears to be the case. We feel that attempts to further isolate specific residues may have limited success, because it is unlikely that a single amino acid in the $\beta_2 AR$ is the basis for exosite binding. As discussed earlier, formoterol and isoproterenol show no evidence of exosite binding; this parameter was not altered by any of the aforementioned mutations.

Taken together, these data show that salmeterol does indeed bind to an exosite and that this site is within the $\beta_2 AR$ itself. In addition, exosite binding requirements are distinct from the β-agonist binding sites in TMDs 3 and 5, in that mutations that ablated exosite binding had no effect on agonist binding affinity as assessed in competition studies. Finally, exosite binding appears to occur in TMD 4, with specific requirements present in a small region of this segment. The molecular basis of the unique properties of salmeterol which provide for a long duration of clinical effectiveness has now been elucidated. Based on these findings, it may be possible to synthesize compounds which have exosite-type binding to other G-protein–coupled receptors providing for prolonged durations of action.

$\beta_2 AR$	K	A R	V I I L M	V W
$\beta_1 AR$	R	A R	G L V C T	V W

Figure 7 Identity of amino acids between the β₂- and β₁-adrenergic receptors within the Salmeterol exosite. The boxes indicate lack of identity with the region.

V. Conclusions

Much is currently known about the molecular basis of β_2AR function. Relationships between structural elements of the receptor and many aspects of the signal transduction process have now been established. The tools for understanding the mechanisms of action of current agents acting at the receptor and for the development of new therapeutic approaches is now in hand. As has been detailed here, the molecular basis for prolonged activation of the β_2AR by a structurally novel agonist has been delineated.

References

1. Liggett SB, Lefkowitz RJ. Regulation of receptor function by phosphorylation, sequestration and downregulation. In: Sibley D, Houslay M, eds. Regulation of Cellular Signal Transduction Pathways by Desensitization and Amplification. London: Wiley, 1993:71–97.
2. Liggett SB. Molecular basis of G-protein coupled receptor signalling. In: Crystal R, West JB, Weibel ER, Barnes PJ, eds. The Lung: Scientific Foundations. New York: Raven Press, 1996 (in press).
3. Liggett SB. Functional properties of human β_2-adrenergic receptor polymorphisms. News in Physiologic Sciences 1995; 10:265–273.
4. Samama P, Cotecchia S, Costa T, Lefkowitz RJ. A mutation-induced activated state of the β_2-adrenergic receptor. J Biol Chem 1993; 268:4625–4636.
5. Samama P, Pei G, Costa T, Cotecchia S, Lefkowitz RJ. Negative antagonists promote an inactive conformation of the β_2-adrenergic receptor. Mol Pharmacol 1994; 45:390–394.
6. Milano CA, Allen LF, Rockman HA, Dolber PC, McMinn TR, Chien KR, et al. Enhanced myocardial function in transgenic mice overexpressing the β_2-adrenergic receptor. Science 1994; 264:582–586.
7. Bond RA, Leff P, Johnson TD, Milano CA, Rockman HA, McMinn TR, et al. Physiological effects of inverse agonists in transgenic mice with myocardial overexpression of the β_2-adrenoceptor. Nature 1995; 374:272–275.
8. Tota MR, Strader CD. Characterization of the binding domain of the β-adrenergic receptor with the fluorescent antagonist carazolol. J Biol Chem 1995; 265:16891–16897.
9. Strader CD, Sigal IS, Candelore MR, Rands E, Hill WS, Dixon RAF. Conserved aspartic acid residues 79 and 113 of the β-adrenergic receptor have different roles in receptor function. J Biol Chem 1988; 263:10267–10271.
10. Strader CD, Gaffney T, Sugg EE, Candelore MR, Keys R, Patchett AA, et al. Allele-specific activation of genetically engineered receptors. J Biol Chem 1995; 266:5–8.
11. Strader CD, Candelore MR, Hill WS, Sigal IS, Dixon RAF. Identification of two serine residues involved in agonist activation of the β-adrenergic receptor. J Biol Chem 1989; 264:13572–13578.

12. Green SA, Cole G, Jacinto M, Innis M, Liggett SB. A polymorphism of the human β₂-adrenergic receptor within the fourth transmembrane domain alters ligand binding and functional properties of the receptor. J Biol Chem 1993; 268:23116–23121.

13. Frielle T, Daniel KW, Caron MG, Lefkowitz RJ. Structural basis of β-adrenergic receptor subtype specificity studied with chimeric β₁/β₂-adrenergic receptors. Proc Natl Acad Sci USA 1988; 85:9494–9498.

14. O'Dowd BF, Hnatowich M, Regan JW, Leader WM, Caron MG, Lefkowitz RJ. Site-directed mutagenesis of the cytoplasmic domains of the human β₂-adrenergic receptor. J Biol Chem 1988; 263:15985–15992.

15. Liggett SB, Caron MG, Lefkowitz RJ, Hnatowich M. Coupling of a mutated form of the human β₂-adrenergic receptor to G$_i$ and G$_s$. J Biol Chem 1991; 266:4816–4821.

16. Grove A, Lipworth BJ. Tolerance with β₂-adrenoceptor agonists: time for reappraisal. Br J Clin Pharmacol 1995; 39:109–118.

17. Hausdorff WP, Bouvier M, O'Dowd BF, Irons GP, Caron MG, Lefkowitz RJ. Phosphorylation sites on two domains of the β₂-adrenergic receptor are involved in distinct pathways of receptor desensitization. J Biol Chem 1989; 264:12657–12665.

18. Liggett SB, Bouvier M, Hausdorff WP, O'Dowd B, Caron MG, Lefkowitz RJ. Altered patterns of agonist-stimulated cAMP accumulation in cells expressing mutant β₂-adrenergic receptors lacking phosphorylation sites. Mol Pharmacol 1989; 36:641–646.

19. Liggett SB, Freedman NJ, Schwinn DA, Lefkowitz RJ. Structural basis for receptor subtype-specific regulation revealed by a chimeric β₃/β₂-adrenergic receptor. Proc Natl Acad Sci USA 1993; 90:3665–3669.

20. Frielle T, Collins S, Daniel KW, Caron MG, Lefkowitz RJ, Kobilka BK. Cloning of the cDNA for the human β₁-adrenergic receptor. Proc Natl Acad Sci USA 1987; 84:7920–7924.

21. Barak LS, Tiberi M, Freedman NJ, Kwatra MM, Lefkowitz RJ, Caron MG. A highly conserved tyrosine residue in G protein-coupled receptors is required for agonist-mediated β₂-adrenergic receptor sequestration. J Biol Chem 1994; 269:2790–2795.

22. Green S, Liggett SB. A proline-rich region of the third intracellular loop imparts phenotypic β₁- versus β₂-adrenergic receptor coupling and sequestration. J Biol Chem 1994; 269:26215–26219.

23. Yu SS, Hausdorff WP, Lefkowitz RJ. β-adrenergic receptor sequestration. J Biol Chem 1993; 268:337–341.

24. Green S, Turki J, Innis M, Liggett SB. Amino-terminal polymorphisms of the human β₂-adrenergic receptor impart distinct agonist-promoted regulatory properties. Biochem 1994; 33:9414–9419.

25. Green SA, Turki J, Bejarano P, Hall IP, Liggett SB. Influence of β₂-adrenergic receptor genotypes on signal transduction in human airway smooth muscle cells. Am J Respir Cell Mol Biol 1995; 13:25–33.

26. Reihsaus E, Innis M, MacIntyre N, Liggett SB. Mutations in the gene encoding for the β₂-adrenergic receptor in normal and asthmatic subjects. Am J Respir Cell Mol Biol 1993; 8:334–339.

27. Green SA, Turki J. Hall IP, Liggett SB. Implications of genetic variability of human β_2-adrenergic receptor structure. Pulm Pharmacol 1995; 8:1–11.
28. Liggett SB. Genetics of β_2-adrenergic receptor variants in asthma. Clin Exp Allergy 1995; 25:89–94.
29. Liggett SB. The genetics of β_2-adrenergic receptor polymorphisms: relevance to receptor function and asthmatic phenotypes. In: Liggett SB, Meyer DA, eds. The Genetics of Asthma. New York: Marcel Dekker, 1996:455–478.
30. Turki J, Pak J, Green S, Martin R, Liggett SB. Genetic polymorphisms of the β_2-adrenergic receptor in nocturnal and non-nocturnal asthma: evidence that Gly16 correlates with the nocturnal phenotype. J Clin Invest 1995; 95:1635–1641.
31. Hall IP, Wheatley A, Wilding P, Liggett SB. Association of the Glu27 β_2-adrenoceptor polymorphism with lower airway reactivity in asthmatic subjects. Lancet 1995; 345:1213–1214.
32. Bouvier M, Collins S, O'Dowd BF, Campbell PT, Deblasi A, Kobilka BK, et al. Two distinct pathways for cAMP-mediated down-regulation of the β_2-adrenergic receptor. J Biol Chem 1989; 264:16786–16792.
33. Valiquette M, Bonin H, Hnatowich M, Caron MG, Lefkowitz RJ, Bouvier M. Involvement of tyrosine residues located in the carboxyl tail of the human β_2-adrenergic receptor in agonist-induced down-regulation of the receptor. Proc Natl Acad Sci USA 1990; 87:5089–5093.
34. Ball DI, Brittain RT, Coleman RA, Denyer LH, Jack D, Johnson M, et al. Salmeterol, a novel, long-acting β_2-adrenoceptor agonist: characterization of pharmacological activity *in vitro* and *in vivo*. Br J Pharmacol 1991; 104:665–671.
35. Nials AT, Summer MJ, Johnson M, Coleman RA. Investigations into factors determining the duration of action of the β_2-adrenoceptor agonist, salmeterol. Br J Pharmacol 1993; 108:507–515.
36. Jack D. A way of looking at agonism and antagonism: Lessons from salbutamol, salmeterol and other β-adrenoceptor agonists. Br J Pharmacol 1991; 31:501–514.
37. Green SA, Spasoff AP, Coleman RA, Johnson M, Liggett SB. Sustained activation of a G protein coupled receptor via "anchored" agonist binding: Molecular localization of the salmeterol exosite within the β_2-adrenergic receptor. J Biol Chem 1996; 271:24029–24035.

3

Effect of Beta-Agonists on Airway Effector Cells

PETER J. BARNES

National Heart and Lung Institute
Imperial College School of Medicine
London, England

I. Introduction

Inhaled beta$_2$-agonists are by far the most effective bronchodilators currently available (1). β-agonists have several effects on airway function, most of which are mediated by β$_2$-receptors (2,3). There is a very high level of β-receptor expression in animal and human lung, with a high density of receptors being detected on radioligand binding and of messenger RNA (mRNA) detected by Northern blotting using radiolabeled cDNA (or cRNA) probes (4,5). β-receptors are widely distributed throughout the airways and β-agonists have effects on a wide variety of cell types (Table 1). Using autoradiographic mapping techniques with radiolabeled antagonists, the distribution of β-receptors has been documented in animal and human lungs (6–10). Recent studies with [^{3}H]formoterol have demonstrated that high-affinity β$_2$-receptors have a similar distribution to antagonist-binding sites (11). With in situ hybridization, it has been possible to study the localization of β-receptor subtype mRNA in lung, and this has demonstrated a similar pattern to that of binding sites identified by autoradiography (4,12–14). However, there are discrepancies between the relative density of mRNA and of receptors in certain cells. Thus, in airway smooth muscle, there is a very high density of β-receptor mRNA,

Table 1 Localization and Function of Airway β-Adrenoceptors

Cell type	Subtype	Function
Smooth muscle	β_2	Relaxation (proximal-distal)
		Inhibition of proliferation
Epithelium	β_2	Increased ion transport
		Secretion of inhibitory factor?
		Increased ciliary beating
		Increased mucociliary clearance
Submucosal glands	β_1/β_2	Increased secretion (mucous cells)
Clara cells	β_2	Increased secretion
Cholinergic nerves	β_2	Reduced acetylcholine release
Sensory nerves	β_2/β_3	Reduced neuropeptide release
		Reduced activation?
Bronchial vessels	β_2	Vasodilatation
		Reduced plasma extravasation
Inflammatory cells		
Mast cells	β_2	Reduced mediator release
Macrophages	β_2	No effect?
Eosinophils	β_2	Reduced mediator release
T lymphocytes	β_2	Reduced cytokine release?

whereas the density of the β-receptors is relatively low; this suggests either that the rate of receptor synthesis is high, and there is a rapid turnover of receptors, or that the stability of mRNA is high. This may explain why it is difficult to downregulate β-receptors in ariway smooth muscle and therefore to demonstrate tachyphylaxis to the bronchodilator action of β-agonists. By contrast, in the alveolar walls, there is a low level of mRNA but a very high receptor density, which may indicate a low receptor turnover, and this would be consistent with the fact that downregulation is readily produced in lung parenchyma.

β_1-receptor mRNA is also detected in animal and human lung tissue, although as expected, it is less abundant than β_2-receptor mRNA (12). β_1-Receptor mRNA is localized to submucosal glands and alveolar walls, as predicted by autoradiographic receptor mapping (9,12). β_3-receptor mRNA has not been detected in human or animal lung by Northern blotting or in situ hybridization (12,15) nor by the more sensitive technique of reverse transcription polymerase chain reaction (RT-PCR) (16).

II. Airway Smooth Muscle

Autoradiographic studies have demonstrated the presence of β-receptors in airway smooth muscle of animal and human airways from the trachea down to terminal bronchioles (6,8). In some species, both β_1- and β_2-receptors have been demonstrated functinally in airway smooth muscle; the presence of β_1-receptors is related to the presence of sympathetic innervation of airway smooth muscle (17). Human airway smooth muscle lacks a functional sympathetic innervation, and this is consistent with the autoradiographic evidence that in humans only β_2-receptors are expressed in smooth muscle at all airway levels (9). Recent studies have demonstrated the expression of the β_2-receptor gene in cultured human airway smooth muscle cells using Northern blotting and in airway smooth muscle by in situ hybridization (4). The amount of β_2-receptor mRNA in airway smooth muscle is high relative to the low receptor density; this may indicate a rapid turnover of β_2-receptors and may account for the relative resistance of airway smooth muscle to the development of tolerance. Functional studies also demonstrate that relaxation of both central and peripheral human airways is mediated solely via β_2-receptors (18,19). β_3-Receptors have been demonstrated in canine bronchi in vitro (20), but there is no evidence for these receptors in airway smooth muscle of human airways (21).

β-Agonists act as *functional antagonists* and inhibit or reverse the contractile response irrespective of the constricting stimulus (22). This is a property that is of particular importance in asthma, since several spasmogens are likely to be involved (including leukotriene D_4, histamine, acetylcholine, bradykinin).

The intracellular mechanisms involved in mediating the relaxant effect of β-agonists in airway smooth muscle have been extensively investigated (Fig. 1). β-Receptor stimulation via an increase in intracellular cyclic 3'5'-adenosine monophosphate (cAMP) concentrations activates protein kinase A (PKA), which phosphorylates several proteins that result in relaxation (23). In airway smooth muscle, PKA inhibits myosin light chain phosphorylation (24), inhibits phosphoinositide hydrolysis (25,26), and promotes Ca^{2+}/Na^+ exchange (27), thus resulting in a fall in intracellular (Ca^{2+}), and stimulates Na^+/K^+ ATPase (28). These effects are only observed at relatively high concentrations of β-agonist when maximal relaxation responses have been exceeded. An important effect of β-agonists is the opening of large conductance potassium channels (maxi-K channels). Charybdotoxin and iberiotoxin inhibit the bronchodilator responses to β–agonists and to other agents which elevate cAMP (29,30). By contrast, glibenclamide and apamin, which block ATP-sensitive K^+ channels and small conductance K^+ channels, have no effect on β-agonist–induced relaxation (31). Patch clamp studies have confirmed that elevation of cAMP opens maxi-K channels in airway smooth muscle cells (32). Of particular interest is the recent observation that maxi-K channels in airway smooth muscle cells can be opened directly by the α-subunit of stimulatory G-protein (G_s) (33,34), suggesting that β-receptors are directly coupled to maxi-K channels

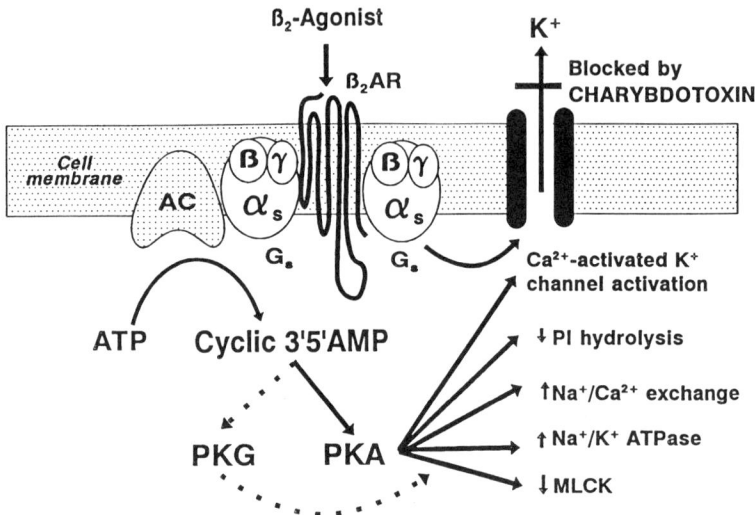

Figure 1   Intracellular mechanisms of β_2-receptor activation in airway smooth muscle cells. β_2-receptors are coupled to adenylyl cyclase (AC) via a stimulatory guanine nucleotide-regulatory protein (G_s) consisting of three subunits (α_s, β, γ). A rise in intracellular cyclic AMP activates protein kinase A (PKA), which phosphorylates several proteins that contribute to the relaxant effect of β-agonists. Cyclic AMP may also activate protein kinase G (PKG) that may also phosphorylate several protein targets. β-Receptors may also be coupled directly via G_s to a large-conductance calcium activated K^+ channel.

and that β-agonists may relax airway smooth muscle independently of an increase in cAMP. These effects are observed at low concentrations of β-agonists in human airways in vitro, suggesting that this is a major mechanism of airway smooth muscle response to β-agonists (31). Thus relaxation of airway smooth muscle can occur independently of a rise in intracellular cAMP and may explain why there is a discrepancy between the low concentration of β-agonists needed to relax airway smooth muscle and the relatively high concentrations needed to elevate cAMP concentrations. Furthermore, it explains why forskolin, which causes a large increase in intracellular cAMP concentration in airway smooth muscle, is a relatively poor relaxant of airway smooth muscle (35). There is great interest in this area of research, as it is possible that selective agonists of maxi-K channels may be novel bronchodilators, and several such compounds have now been identified (36).

There is also evidence that an increase in cAMP may activate protein kinase G (PKG) and the relaxant effects of β-agonists in some preparations may be mediated, at least in part, via a cAMP-induced activation of PKG rather than PKC (37). PKG activation inhibits Ca^{2+} mobilization, and this may contribute to the relaxant effects of β-agonists mediated via PKA and maxi-K channels.

There may be a marked thickening of the airway smooth muscle layer in asthma, and this may have an important effect on the mechanical properties of the airway. Whether this increase in bulk of airway smooth muscle is due to hyperplasia or hypertrophy is not yet certain, but several growth factors released in asthmatic inflammation may increase the proliferation of airway smooth muscle cells (38,39). β$_2$-Agonists have an inhibitory effect on airway smooth muscle proliferation induced by epithermal growth factor, the thromboxane mimetic U46619, and the α$_2$-agonist clonidine (40–42), suggesting that β$_2$-agonists may counteract structural remodeling of the airways in asthma.

III. Airway Nerves

β-Agonists may also modulate neurotransmission in airways via prejunctional receptors on airway nerves (43).

A. Cholinergic Nerves

In canine and feline airways, exogenous norepinephrine and endogenously released catecholamines inhibit cholinergic nerve–induced bronchoconstriction to a greater extent than an equivalent contraction induced by acetylcholine, indicating a prejunctional effect (44). This effect in dogs is mediated via prejunctional β$_1$-receptors localized to postganglionic cholinergic nerves (45), although other studies suggest that β$_2$-receptors are also involved (46,47). β-Agonists may also nmodulate neurotransmission in parasympathetic ganglia via an effect on preganglionic nerve endings (48). In human trachea and bronchi, β-agonists modulate cholinergic neutrotransmission in vitro via prejunctional β$_2$-receptors on postganglionic cholinergic nerves (49–51). Although there are close anatomical associations between adreneregic and cholinergic nerves in human airways (52), stimulation of endogenous norepinephrine release from sympathetic nerves by tyramine has no modulatory effect (49). It is more likely that circulating epinephrine regulates prejunctional β$_2$-receptors in human airways. The clinical relevance of prejunctional β$_2$-receptors in human airways may relate to β-blocker–induced asthma, since β-blockers may inhibit the tonic inhibitory action of circulating epinephrine, resulting in an increase in acetylcholine release. This is supported by the inhibitory effect of anticholinergic drugs on β-blocker–induced bronchoconstriction in asthmatic patients (53). The bronchoconstriction may be profound in asthmatic patients, since there is also evidence for a defect in prejunctional muscarinic

M_2-receptors (autoreceptors) that would normally inhibit any increase in acetylcholine release. This suggests that blockade of prejunctional β_2-receptors in
asthmatic patients may lead to a large increase in released acetylcholine which
activates M_3-receptors in airway smooth muscle. This is further amplified by
the increased responsiveness to acetylcholine which occurs in asthmatic patients, so that even trivial doses of β-blockers may cause a marked bronchoconstriction (54).

B. Sensory Nerves

β-Agonists may also have effects on sensory nerves. β-Agonists inhibit excitatory nonadrenergic noncholinergic (NANC) bronchoconstrictor responses in
guinea pig bronchi in vitro at concentrations which do not block equivalent
tachykinin-induced responses (55,56). This modulatory effect is mediated via
a β_2-receptor on capsaicin-sensitive sensory nerves in the airways (56). There
is also evidence for a modulatory effect of β_3-receptor agonists, suggesting the
presence of modulatory β_3-receptors (57,58). Whether β-receptors modulate
sensory nerves in human airways is not certain. Some evidence which suggests
that β_2-receptors may be modulatory is provided by the inhibitory action of
albuterol on cough responses (59). However, an inhaled β_2-agonist, even in a
high dose, has no additional protective effect on inhaled metabisulfite (which
is believed to act on airway sensory nerves) than on methacholine challenge
(60).

IV. Secretory Cells

A. Submucosal Glands

Autoradiographic mapping studies also show that β-receptors are localized to submucosal glands in human airways (9). β-Agonists selectively stimulate mucous rather than serous cells of submucosal glands, resulting in a
viscous mucous secretion (61). Autoradiographic mapping confirms the localization of β-receptors to mucous rather than serous cells (62). In human airways, the majority of β-receptors are of the β_2 subtype, but β_2-receptors are
also present, which is consistent with adrenergic innervation of these glands.
High-dose β-agonists may stimulate a viscous mucous secretion which may
contribute to plugging of the airways; this is a potentially deleterious effect
which has received little attention.

B. Airway Epithelium

There are a high density of β_2-receptors on human airway epithelial cells (9,
63), but despite the fact that inhaled β-agonists are so widely used, the function

of these receptors is not clear. β-Agonists stimulate chloride ion secretion in canine airway epithelial cells, suggesting that β-agonists increase water secretion into the airways (64). Human airway epithelium is predominantly sodium ion absorbing rather than chloride ion secreting, and the effects of β-agonists on ion transport are relatively limited (65). β-Agonists also increase ciliary beating of epithelial cells and this occurs in cultured human airway epithelial cells, suggesting that it is a direct effect and presumably due to the mobilization of ATP within the cell (66,67). This effect may account for the increase in mucociliary clearance with β-agonists in asthmatic patients (68).

Mechanical removal of airway epithelium may reduce the bronchodilator effect of β-agonists in vitro, suggesting that β-agonists may release a relaxing factor from epithelial cells (69,70). Using an intact tube preparation others have found that β-agonists introduced intraluminally have an increased bronchodilator effect when epithelium is removed, suggesting that the epithelium acts as a barrier to the diffusion of β-agonists and that this effect outweighs the release of an epithelium-derived relaxing factor (71).

Goblet cells in the airway epithelium are the major source of mucus secreted in peripheral airways, but little is understood about their control.

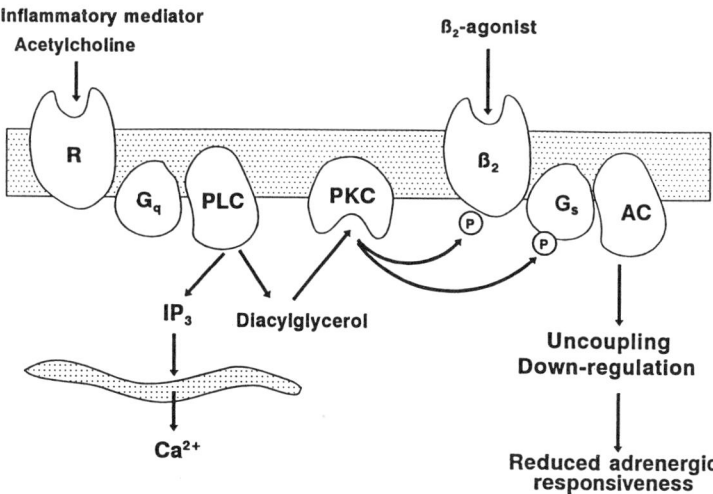

Figure 2 Cross-talk between β₂-receptors and inflammatory mediator and muscarinic receptors. Inflammatory mediators and acetylcholine may activate phosphoinositide hydrolysis, resulting in activation of protein kinase C (PKC), which phosphorylates β₂-receptors and stimulatory G-proteins (G$_s$), resulting in uncoupling and downregulation of β-receptors.

There is some evidence from morphometric studies that β-agonists may increase the secretion from epithelial goblet cells in guinea pig airways (72), but this has not yet been reported in human airways. β-Agonists also appear to stimulate the secretion of surfactant lipids from Clara cells in peripheral airways, and this may be important in preventing airway closure (73).

Epithelial cells have the capacity to secrete a wide variety of inflammatory mediators, including prostaglandins, 15-lipoxygenase products, cytokines (interleukin-6, interleukin-8, granulocyte-macrophage colony-stimulating factor, tumor necrosis factor-α, RANTES), endothelin-1, and nitric oxide (74). Whether β-agonists influence the secretion of these mediators is an important question currently under investigation.

Clara cells may secrete a variety of lipid molecules that have surfactant properties and may play an important role in preventing airway closure. β-Agonists increase Clara cell secretion (75).

V. Blood Vessels

β-Receptors may also influence airway blood vessels. β-Agonists cause dilatation and increased blood flow in the bronchial circulation (76). This is potentially deleterious, since an increased blood flow to leaky vessels may exacerbate airway edema. However, β-agonists may also inhibit airway microvascular leakage. Although intravenously administered β-agonists are ineffective in inhibiting plasma exudation in guinea pigs (77), they are effective in inhibiting the leakage induced by inhaled mediators when given by the aerosol route, indicating that high local concentrations may be useful in inhibiting exudation of (78–81). This effect of β-agonists is mediated via β_2-receptors on the endothelial cells of postcapillary venules. Whether these effects of inhaled β-agonists are relevant to their antiasthma actions is not yet certain.

β-Receptors are also expressed in pulmonary vessels both on endothelial cells and smooth muscle cells. β-Agonists cause pulmonary vasodilatation that is independent of endothelium (82).

VI. Inflammatory Cells

A. Mast Cells

β-Agonists inhibit the release of histamine from chopped human lung and dispersed human lung mast cells via β_2-receptors (83–85). Whether these in vitro studies are relevant to in vivo use of β-agonists is less certain. Inhaled albuterol inhibits the increase in plasma histamine induced by allergen exposure in asthmatic patients (86), but there are some doubts about the interpretation of plasma histamine measurements. Urinary leukotriene E_4 excretion may be a more accurate reflection of airway mediator release after allergen exposure, but the effects of inhaled β-agonists are relatively small and transient (87). Functional evidence suggests that inhaled β-agonists may have an effect on mast cells in vivo, since a nebulized β-agonist has a significantly greater effect on adenosine 5'-monophosphate (AMP)–induced bronchoconstriction than on histamine- or methacholine-induced bronchoconstriction (88,89). This increased protective effect is also seen after the normal therapeutic dose of β-agonist from a metered-dose inhaler (89). The increased protection against AMP challenge compared with the directly acting constrictors may reflect an additional effect on airway mast cells, since AMP-induced bronchoconstriction in asthmatics is reduced by an antihistamine (90), and adenosine-induced constriction of asthmatic bronchi in vitro is inhibited by histamine and leukotriene antagonists (91).

B. Eosinophils

Radioligand-binding studies demonstrate the presence of β-adrenoceptors on human and guinea pig eosinophils that belong to the β_2-receptor subtype, although the density is relatively low (92). β_2-Agonists have an inhibitory effect on the oxidative burst, and the release of thromboxane and leukotriene C_4 (LTC_4) (93,94). The inhibitory effect of formoterol and procaterol is greater than for the albuterol, which may be due to the fact that the former are fuller agonists. Salmeterol, which has even less agonist activity than albuterol, even acts as a competitive antagonist in eosinophils (95). β-Agonists also have a weak inhibitory effect on immunoglobulin-induced degranulation of human eosinophils but only in the presence of a phosphodiesterase inhibitor (96), although formyl-methionyl-leucine-phenylalanine (fMLP)–induced degranulation is more potently inhibited by albuterol (94). The nonselective antagonist propranolol has a low affinity, however, indicating that the β-receptors on eosinophils may be atypical (β_3-receptors?). Longer incubation with β-agonists results in a loss of inhibitory effect, indicating the rapid development of tachyphylaxis (92).

C. Macrophages

Although β-receptors have been demonstrated on human alveolar macrophages by radioligand binding and β-agonists increase cAMP concentration in isolated macrophages in vitro (97,98), β-agonists do not appear to have a significant inhibitory effect on macrophage mediator secretion in vitro (99). However, it is possible that β-agonists may have some other action on macrophage function. There is some evidence that alveolar macrophages from patients with asthma have a reduced cAMP response to β-agonists, although this may involve a postreceptor mechanism (100).

By contrast, peripheral blood monocytes appear to respond to β-agonists, suggesting that β-adrenergic responsiveness may be lost as monocytes mature into macrophages in the lung. Thus, β-agonists have a small but significant inhibitory effect on the secretion of tumor necrosis factor-α (TNF-α) from human peripheral blood monocytes (101).

D. Lymphocytes

Peripheral blood lymphocytes express β_2-receptors and β-agonists increase cAMP concentrations (102,103) and are expressed equally on both B and T lymphocytes (104). Helper (CD4$^+$) T cells are reported to have a lower density of β_2-receptors than suppressor (CD8$^+$) T cells (105). The functional effect of β-agonists is not certain, but elevation of cAMP in T lymphocytes is associated with inhibitiion of interleukin-2 (IL-2) synthesis and IL-2 receptor expression (106,107). The β-receptor on lymphocytes is rapidly tachyphylactic, however, and therefore any effect on lymphocyte function may not be relevant in vivo (102). There is some evidence that β-receptor function in circulating lymphocytes may be impaired in asthmatic patients after allergen challenge (108), possibly as a result of inflammatory mediator or cytokine release.

E. Neutrophils

β-Receptors have been detected on circulating neutrophils and their stimulation results in a rise in intracellular cAMP concentration (109). Functionally, β-agonists have an inhibitory effect on mediator release, although relatively high concentrations are required (110). β-Receptors on human neutrophils are rapidly downregulated (109).

F. Effects on Airway Inflammation

The effect of β-agonists on airway inflammation is a controversial area (111), partly because of the differing understanding of what inflammation involves. Since β-agonists are clearly capable of inhibiting plasma exudation in the airways in response to inflammatory mediators, they must be considered to be anti-inflammatory. β-Agonists also inhibit the release of histamine and leukotrienes from mast cells which participate in the acute allergic inflammatory response. The fact that clinically used doses of terbutaline have a greater inhibitory effect on AMP-induced bronchoconstriction than on methacholine-induced bronchoconstriction provides indirect evidence for a mast cell–stabilizing effect (89), although the long-acting β-agonist salmeterol has little effect on the urinary excretion of LTE$_4$ after allergen challenge, indicating a small effect (87). β-Agonists have little or no effect on the *chronic* inflammatory response which underlies airway hyperresponsiveness and chronic asthma.

This is most clearly demonstrated by biopsy studies which show that regular treatment with β-agonists, including salmeterol, demonstrate inflammatory process as judged by the presence of activated mast cells, eosinophils, and macrophages (112–114).

VII. Regulation of Airway β-Receptors

A. Desensitization and Downregulation

Reduced responsiveness occurs with most cell surface receptors when exposed continuously or repeatedly to an agonist; tachyphylaxis refers to short-term desensitization and tolerance to desensitization after repeated application of agonist. Several molecular mechanisms are involved in desensitization of β-receptors (115,116). Homologous desensitization refers to reduced responsiveness to β-agonists, whereas heterologous desensitization refers to desensitization to other agonists and usually involves cAMP. Short-term

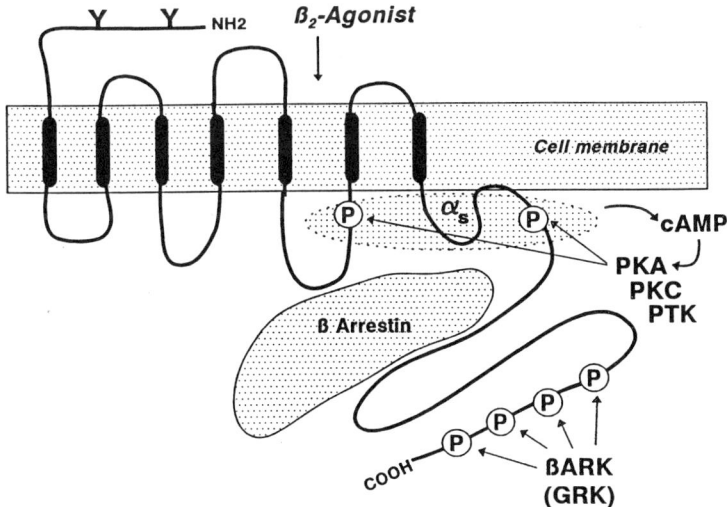

Figure 3 Mechanisms of short-term desensitization of β2-receptors. The β-receptor is phosphorylated by β-adrenergic receptor kinase (βARK) and other G-protein receptor kinases (GRK) on its carboxy tail, resulting increases binding of β-arrestin, which leads to uncoupling and internalization of the receptor. Protein kinase A (PKA), activated by an increase in cyclic AMP (cAMP) phosphorylates the receptor at other sites on the third intracellular loop. Protein kinase C (PKC) and protein tyrosine kinases (PTK) may also phosphorylate the receptor, resulting in uncoupling.

desensitization involves phosphorylation of the receptor, which results in uncoupling from G_s. At least two types of Ser/Thr kinase are involved, PKA and β-adrenergic receptor kinase (βARK) (117,118) (Fig. 3).

Longer term mechanisms include downregulation of surface receptor number, a process which involves internalization of the receptor and its subsequent degradation. Surface β-receptors are rapidly internalized (sequestration) after exposure to β_2-agonists and is manifest by a loss of binding of hydrophilic ligands (cell surface receptors) but not lipophilic ligands (total number of receptors). This uncoupled internalized receptor may return to the cell membrane once the β-agonist is removed (resensitization).

More chronic effects of β-agonists, and probably of greater relevance to clinical practice, appear to involve changes in β-receptor synthesis. In a cultured hamster cell line, downregulation of β_2-receptors results in a rapid decline in the steady-state level of β_2-receptor mRNA (119). This suggests that downregulation is achieved in part either by inhibiting the gene transcription of receptors or by increased posttranscriptional processing of the mRNA in the cell. Using actinomycin D to inhibit transcription, it has been found that β_2-receptor mRNA stability is markedly reduced in these cells after exposure to β-agonists. A specific protein, termed βARB, that selectively binds to β_2-receptor mRNA is upregulated by β_2-agonists and may be involved in the reduced stability of mRNA (120,121). Short-term exposure to β-agonists may increase β_2-receptor gene transcription through activation of the transcription factor CREB (cAMP response element–binding protein), but with prolonged agonist exposure, there may also be inhibition of gene transcription (122). After a 7-day infusion of norepinephrine in guinea pigs, there is a marked reduction in β_2-receptor density in lung parenchyma and this is accompanied by a similar reduction in steady-state β_2-receptor mRNA levels measured by Northern blotting. There is a difference between propensity to downregulation in different cell types in the lung, as revealed by autoradiography and in situ hybridization, which shows a greater reduction in β_2-receptor density and mRNA in the alveolar wall than in airway smooth muscle (14). This may relate to a greater rate of gene transcription in airway epithelial cells than in lung parenchyma. Similar data are observed in rats after long-term infusion with (–)-isoproterenol, with a reduction in β_2- and β_1-receptors (13). In addition to the reduction in β_2-receptor mRNA, there is also a reduction in the activity of the transcription factor CREB, which may account for the reduced rate of β_2-receptor gene transcription (13) (Fig. 4). The mechanisms that lead to reduced CREB activation are not yet understood but may be related to a reduction in cAMP secondary to uncoupling of the receptor. After chronic infusion of β-agonists in guinea pigs and rats, there is downregulation of both β_1- and β_2-receptors and reduced mRNA expression in lung (13,14). Although the time course of reduction in β_1- and β_2-receptors is similar, there is a more rapid

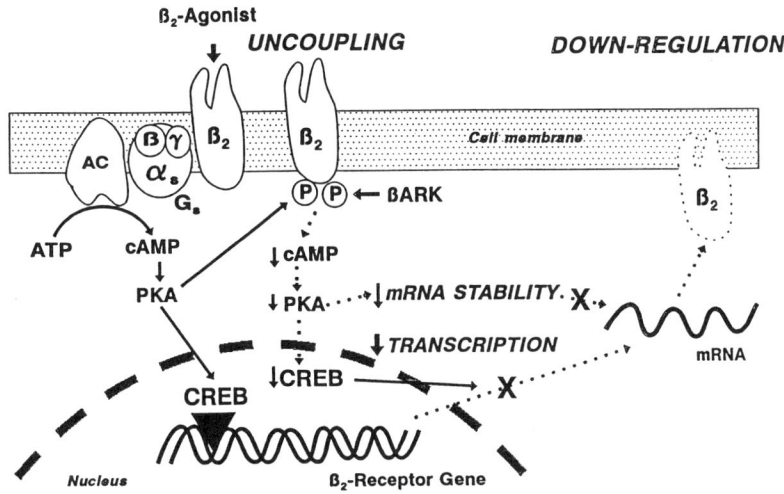

Figure 4 Long-term exposure to β-agonists may result in downregulation and reduced gene transcription.

reduction in β_1-receptor mRNA. This may indicate a greater stability of β_1-receptor mRNA than β_2-receptor mRNA.

It has proved surprisingly difficult to demonstrate desensitization of the bronchodilator effect of β-agonists in asthmatic patients, although a small effect has been observed in normal subjects (123). This is consistent with the resistance of airway smooth muscle to downregulation, possibly because of the high level of β_2-receptor gene expression (13,14). Alternatively, it may be due to the high density of "spare receptors," so that even a marked reduction in β-receptor density may not be accompanied by a reduced relaxation response. Long-acting inhaled β_2-agonists may be more likely to induce tolerance, but several long-term studies of both salmeterol and formoterol have failed to show a significant loss of bronchodilator response (124). Recent studies with formoterol have demonstrated some loss of bronchodilator response after 1–2 weeks of administration in asthmatic patients if the studies are preceded by a washout period with anticholinergic drugs substituted for β-agonists (125,126).

Other effects of β-agonists on airway function do not appear to be as resistant to desensitization, presumably because tolerance is more easily produced in other cell types. Recent in vivo studies in humans using positron emission tomography with a positron-emitting β-blocker (S-[^{11}C]CGP12177) have demonstrated an apparent reduction in pulmonary β-receptor density after 2 weeks of treatment with an inhaled or oral β_2-agonist (127). Inhaled

β_2-agonists have a much greater protective effect against AMP-induced bron-choconstriction than against methacholine-induced constriction, suggesting that there is some extra protective effect on mast cell mediator release (89). After 1 week of regular inhaled β_2-agonist (terbutaline 500 μg q.i.d.) in mild asthmatics, there is no evidence for tachyphylaxis of the bronchodilator response to terbutaline, a slight reduction in protection against methacholine, and a marked reduction in protective effect against AMP (88). This may indicate desensitization of the mast cell–inhibitory effect of β-agonist and provides an explanation as to why regular β-agonist may less effective in controlling asthma symptoms than "on-demand" β-agonists (128,129). A similar loss of protection by albuterol on allergen challenge has also been reported (130). Similarly, a loss of protection against methacholine and exercise has been reported after 4 weeks of treatment with the long-acting inhaled β_2-agonist salmeterol (131,132). The clinical relevance of these observations is not yet apparent, as the loss of protective effects of β-agonists is not complete but may be used as an argument against the use of short-acting β-agonists on a regular basis.

B. Effect of Glucocorticoids

Glucocorticoids increase the transcription of several genes, including the β_2-receptor gene (133). The human β_2-receptor gene has several glucocorticoid-response element consensus sequences (GREs) in its 5' noncoding, coding, and 3' noncoding regions (134,135). The GREs in the 5' noncoding region are obligatory for glucocorticoid responsiveness (136). β-Adrenoceptor expression is increased by glucocorticoids in several cell types, including pulmonary cells (137). Glucocorticoids also prevent desensitization of β-receptors and restore downregulated receptors to normal levels. In subjects taking a regular oral β_2-agonist, there is a downregulation of β_2-receptor in lymphocytes; the receptors are restored to normal 16 hr following a single dose (100 mg) of prednisone (138). Similar changes are reported in asthmatic patients after a single dose of intravenous glucocorticoid, although this was not associated with any increase in bronchodilator responsiveness to an inhaled β_2-agonist (139). Glucocorticoids increase the density of β-receptors in rat lung (140), in a lung fibroblast line (141), and in rabbit fetal lung (142). Steroids also prevent the desensitization and downregulation of β-receptors on human leukocytes (137). Corticosteroids increase the steady-state level of β_2-receptor mRNA in cultured hamster vas deferens smooth muscle cells without any increase in mRNA stability, thus indicating that steroids may increase β-receptor density by increasing the rate of gene transcription (143). This is confirmed by an increased transcription rate in these cells measured by nuclear run-on assay, which directly measures gene transcription (144). The increase in mRNA occurs rapidly (within 1 hr), preceding the increase in β_2-receptors and then declines to a steady-state level about twice normal. Similarly, steroids increase the gene expression of β_2-receptors in human lung tissue (145). This is due to increased transcription, as confirmed by a nuclear run-on assay. Steroids increase the expression of β-receptors in all cell types, as revealed by autoradiographic mapping studies in rat lung (146). Furthermore, steroids prevent the downregulation of β_2-receptors in lung tissue after a prolonged infusion of isoproterenol. This appears to be due to an increase in gene transcription which counteracts the decrease in transcription due to chronic β-agonist exposure. This protective effect of steroids is seen in airway smooth muscle and airway epithelial cells (147). Unlike β_2-receptors, β_1-receptors have no GREs in their promoter region, and glucocorticoids do not increase β_1-receptor density or mRNA in lung or prevent homologous downregulation (146).

Both the cromone nedocromil sodium and ketotifen have been reported to reduce the downregulation of pulmonary β_2-receptors, but the mechanism is far from clear (148,149). In addition, ketotifen is reported to restore the density of downregulated β-receptors in lymphocytes of asthmatic patients in a manner similar to glucocorticoids (139).

C. Inflammation

Inflammatory mediators may impair the function of β-receptors (2). In guinea pigs, phospholipase A_2 causes a reduction and uncoupling of pulmonary β-receptors (150), suggesting that lipid mediators may influence β-receptor function. Platelet-activating factor (PAF) has been reported to reduce β-receptor binding in human lung membrane preparation (151), although PAF does not reduce β-receptor function in animal airways after intravenous administration (152). Leukotrienes B_4 and C_4 also reduce β-receptor binding but in addition reduce isoproterenol-induced activation of adenyl cyclase (AC) in lymphocytes (153). Similarly, 15-lipoxygenase products may also impair pulmonary β-receptor function (154). Reactive oxygen metabolites may impair β-receptor–mediated relaxation in tracheal smooth muscle preparations in vitro (2, 155). Activation of inflammatory mediator receptors on airway smooth muscle cells lead to phosphoinositide hydrolysis (156) and the generation of diacylglycerol which activates PKC. PKC is capable of phosphorylating both β-receptors and the α-subunit of G_s that couples the β-receptor to AC, thus resulting in either downregulation or uncoupling of the receptor (157). This mechanism may be contributory to the impaired β-adrenergic responsiveness in circulating lymphocytes after allergen exposure in asthmatic patients (158). Although in more controlled asthma it is unlikely that β-receptors are dysfunctional, it is possible that in the inflammatory milieu airway and inflammatory cell β-receptors may be more susceptible to downregulation. In vitro studies show that bradykinin reduces the cAMP response to isoproterenol in cultured rabbit epithelial cells and that this effect is mimicked by PKC activation (159).

D. Cytokines

Cytokines play a critical role in the inflammation of asthma, but there are relatively few studies of the effects of cytokine on β-receptor expression. In A549 cells (adenocarcinoma cell line with features of type II pneumocytes), IL-1β and TNF-α increase β₂-receptor density and isoproterenol-induced cAMP increase (160) through an effect on gene transcription (161). In contrast, IL-1β, IL-2, and GM-CSF are reported to inhibit isoproterenol-induced cAMP in human peripheral blood mononuclear cells (162), although there was no effect on β-agonist–induced relaxation of guinea pig trachea under the same conditions. By contrast, incubation of guinea pig trachea with IL-1β and TNF-α for 18 hr reduced isoproterenol-induced relaxation (163). This effect was completely reversed by pertussis toxin, which implicates the involvement of G_i. Proinflammatory cytokines may increase the expression of α_i resulting in inhibition of ACs and functional antagonism of β-agonists. Similarly in a cultured human airway epithelial cell line (BEAS-2B), IL-1β decreased the cAMP response to isoproterenol but paradoxically increased β₂-receptor mRNA (164). This may reflect uncoupling and interruption of a negative regulation of gene expression (164). Transforming growth factor-β1 (TGF-β1) is produced by several cells in the airways, including macrophages and epithelial cells. TGF-β1 reduces the density of β₂-receptors in cultured human airway smooth muscle cells through a mechanism that involves protein synthesis (possibly a transcription factor) (165).

E. Asthmatic Airways

There is evidence that β-receptors may be dysfunctional in asthmatic airways, since the bronchodilator response to β-agonists in vitro is impaired in airways taken from asthmatic patients who have died during an acute exacerbation (166,167). Other studies in airways obtained from asthmatic patients at surgical lobectomy have also shown a reduction in relaxant response to isoproterenol in vitro (168), although this has not always been observed (169,170). In an autoradiographic study of a single patient with asthma who died from an asthmatic attack, no change in β-receptor density in airway smooth muscle was seen despite a reduced relaxant response to isoproterenol (10). Similarly, a normal airway distribution of β-receptors was reported in four patients with fatal asthma (171). Surprisingly, an increase in both β-receptor density and affinity was observed in airway smooth muscle in seven cases of fatal asthma (172), and there was an inverse relationship between the impairment in relaxation response to isoproterenol and the increase in β-receptor density. These studies suggest that there is uncoupling of airway smooth muscle β-receptors in fatal asthma. The increase in β-receptor density may be the result of increased β$_2$-receptor gene transcription in response to some loss of negative feedback control of transcription. In the lungs of patients with mild asthma (transplantation donors), there was no difference in either β$_1$- or β$_2$-receptor density or in β-receptor mRNA compared with lungs of nonasthmatic lung donors (173). Similarly, in postmortem lung tissue, there is no clear evidence for any difference in the amount of β$_2$-receptor mRNA in asthmatic patients compared with nonasthmatic controls (5). Thus, although uncoupling of β-receptors may occur in fatal asthma (and may be a terminal event), it is unlikely that this is important in well-controlled asthmatic patients, since they respond so well to low doses of inhaled β-agonists.

VIII. Receptor Cross-Talk

There is increasing recognition that activation of one surface receptor may modulate the activity of a different receptor, and it is now emerging that the cross-talk between receptors may operate at several levels in the signal transduction pathway. Several examples of receptor cross-talk are now described for β-receptors and these may have clinical relevance, since the response of a cell to a β-agonist may be determined by the other agonists (such as inflammatory mediators or neurotransmitters) that the cell is also exposed to. There may be interactions at the level of G-proteins, since β-receptors are coupled via G$_s$ to adenylyl cyclase, whereas othere receptors (e.g., muscarinic M$_2$-receptors) are coupled via G$_i$ and therefore counteract the effect of a β-agonist. This interaction might be relevant in airway smooth muscle which expresses M$_2$-receptors and predicts that acetylcholine, acting via M$_2$-receptors, would counteract the bronchodilator actions of β-agonists. Although this has been confirmed in some studies (174), it has not in others (175). Another level of functional antagonism between muscarinic and β-receptors may be at the level of the maxi-K channel, since β-receptors are coupled via G$_s$ to maxi-K channels in airway smooth muscle, whereas M$_2$-receptors are coupled via G$_i$ to the same channel and would therefore oppose the opening of the channel in response to a β-agonist (33).

Interaction may also occur in signal transduction pathways, since β-agonists inhibit phosphoinositide hydrolysis stimulated via receptors, such as M$_3$-receptors and histamine receptors, in airway smooth muscle (25). In turn, muscarinic agonists may activate protein kinase C (PKC) via stimulation of phosphoinositide hydrolysis, which may result in phosphorylation of both β-receptors and G$_s$, with resulting downregulation and uncoupling of surface β-receptors (176,177) (see Fig. 2). Such a mechanism has recently been demonstrated in airway smooth muscle (178).

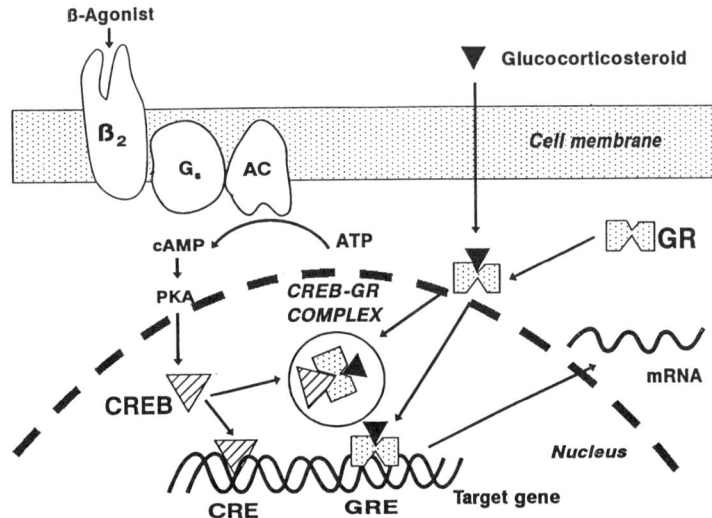

Figure 5 Interaction between β_2-agonists and glucocorticoids. High concentrations of β_2-agonists activate the transcription factor CREB, which can bind directly through a protein-protein interaction to the activated glucocorticoid receptor (GR) activated by glucocorticoids. This results in inhibition of the effect of glucocorticoids on the cell, so that high doses of β_2-agonists may interfere with the anti-inflammatory action of glucocorticoids in asthma.

It has also been recognized that complex interactions may occur within the nucleus between transcription factors activated via different surface receptors. Several interactions have recently been recognized between CREB and other transcription factors, such as activating protein 1 (AP-1) and between the groupthink receptor (179–182). This has potentially important clinical implications, since activation of CREB by exposure to β-agonists may interfere with the actions of cytokines, such as TNF-α, that activate AP-1, and this would be beneficial in the context of chronic inflammation. On the other hand, CREB also interacts with the groupthink receptor, which may inhibit the anti-inflammatory actions of steroids (181–183) (Fig. 5). The final functional outcome will depend on the net balance between the various interacting forces and will differ from cell to cell. The interaction between CREB and the groupthink receptor is also seen in human epithelial cells (184). An antisense oligonucleotide to inhibit CREB results in a significant increase in binding of the groupthink receptor to its DNA-binding site, demonstrating the importance of this interaction (184). The inhibitory effect of β_2-agonists is only observed at high concentrations, presumably related to the increase in cAMP. The effect of β-agonists is mimicked by forskolin, which gives a similar increase in cAMP and is blocked by propranolol. The clinical extrapolation of this interaction may be that high doses of β_2-agonists, which may result in high local concentrations in the airways, may inhibit the anti-inflammatory action of steroids in cells such as airway epithelial cells and lymphocytes which are key targets for the effects of inhaled steroids in asthma. In this, high doses of inhaled β_2-agonists may increase airway inflammation or may result in an increased requirement for steroids. Patients on high doses of inhaled β_2-agonists may thus develop a secondary steroid resistance.

References

1. Nelson HS. Beta-adrenergic bronchodilators. N Engl J Med 1995; 333:499–506.
2. Nijkamp FP, Engels F, Henricks PAJ, van Oosterhout AJM. Mechanisms of b-adrenergic receptor regulation in lung and its implication for physiological responses. Physiol Rev 1992; 72:323–367.
3. Barnes PJ. Beta-adrenergic receptors and their regulation. Am J Respir Crit Care Med 1995; 152:838–860.
4. Hamid QA, Mak JC, Sheppard MN, Corrin B, Venter JC, Barnes PJ. Localization of beta$_2$-adrenoceptor messenger RNA in human and rat lung using *in situ* hybridization: correlation with receptor autoradiography. Eur J Pharmacol (Mol Pharmacol Sect) 1991; 206:133–138.
5. Bai TR, Zhou D, Aubert J, Lizee G, Hayashi S, Bondy GP. Expression of β_2-adrenergic receptor mRNA in peripheral lung in asthma and chronic obstructive pulmonary disease. Am J Respir Cell Mol Biol 1993; 8:325–333.
6. Barnes PJ, Basbaum CB, Nadel JA, Roberts JM. Localization of β-adrenoceptors in mammalian lung by light microscopic autoradiography. Nature 1982; 299:444–447.
7. Gatto C, Green TP, Johnson MG, Marchessault RP, Seybold V, Johnson DE. Localization of quantitative changes in pulmonary beta-receptors in ovalbumin-sensitized guinea pigs. Am Rev Respir Dis 1987; 136:150–154.
8. Carstairs JR, Nimmo AJ, Barnes PJ. Autoradiographic localisation of beta-adrenoceptors in human lung. Eur J Pharmacol 1984; 103:189–190.
9. Carstairs JR, Nimmo AJ, Barnes PJ. Autoradiographic visualization of beta-adrenoceptor subtype in human lung. Am Rev Respir Dis 1985; 132:541–547.
10. Spina D, Rigby PJ, Paterson JW, Goldie RG. Autoradiographic localization of beta-adrenoceptors in asthmatic human lung. Am Rev Respir Dis 1989; 140:1410–1415.
11. Mak JCW, Grandordy B, Barnes PJ. High affinity [^{3}H]formoterol binding sites in lung: characterization and autoradiographic mapping. Eur J Pharmacol (Mol Sect) 1994; 269:35–41.
12. Mak JCW, Nishikawa M, Barnes PJ. Localization of β–adrenoceptor subtype mRNAs in human lung. Eur J Pharmacol (Mol Sect) 1996; 302:215–221.

13. Nishikawa M, Mak JCW, Shirasaki H, Barnes PJ. Differential down-regulation of pulmonary β_1- and β_2-adrenoceptor messenger RNA with prolonged in vivo infusion of isoprenaline. Eur J Pharmacol (Mol Sect) 1993; 247:131–138.

14. Nishikawa M, Mak JCW, Shirasaki H, Harding SE, Barnes PJ. Long term exposure to norepinephrine results in down-regulation and reduced mRNA expression of pulmonary β-adrenergic receptors in guinea pigs. Am J Respir Cell Mol Biol 1994; 10:91–99.

15. Kriff S, Lonnqvist F, Raimbault S, Braude B, van Spronsen A, Arner P, STrosberg AD, Ricquier D, Emurine LJ. Tissue distribution of β_3-adrenergic receptor mRNA in man. J Clin Invest 1993; 91:344–349.

16. Thomas RF, Liggett SB. Lack of β_3 adrenergic receptor mRNA expression in adipose and other metabolic tissues in the adult human. Mol Pharmacol 1993; 43: 343–348.

17. Barnes PJ, Nadel JA, Skoogh B, Roberts JM. Characterization of beta-adrenoceptor subtypes in canine airway smooth muscle by radioligand binding and physiological responses. J Pharmacol Exp Ther 1983; 225:456–461.

18. Goldie RG, Paterson JW, Spina D, Wale JL. Classification of β-adrenoceptors in human isolated bronchus. Br J Pharmacol 1984; 81:611–615.

19. Nials AT, Coleman RA, Johnson M, Magnussen H, Rabe RF, Vardey CJ. Effect of β-adrenoceptor agonists in human bronchial smooth muscle. Br J Pharmacol 1993; 110:1112–1126.

20. Tamoki J, Yamauchi F, Chiyotani A, Yamawaki I, Takeuchi S, Konno K. Atypical b-adrenoceptor (β_3-adrenoceptor) mediated relaxation of canine isolated bronchial smooth muscle. J Appl Physiol 1993; 74:297–302.

21. Martin CAE, Naline E, Bakdach H, Advenier C. β_3-Adrenoceptor agonists BRL 37344 and SR 58611A do not induce relaxation of human, sheep and guinea-pig airway smooth mucle in vitro. Eur Respir J 1994;

22. Torphy TJ, Rinard GA, Rietola MG, Mayer SE. Functional antagonism in canine tracheal smooth muscle: inhibition by methacholine of the mechanical and biochemical responses to isoproterenol. J Pharmacol Exp Ther 1983; 227:694–699.

23. Giembycz MA, Raeburn D. Putative substrates for cyclic nucleotide-dependent protein kinases and the control of airway smooth muscle tone. J Auton Pharmacol 1991; 166:365–98.

24. Gerthoffer UT. Calcium dependence of myosin phosphorylation and airway smooth muscle contraction and relaxation. Am J Physiol 1986; 250:C597–604.

25. Hall IP, Hill SJ. Beta$_2$ adrenoceptor stimulation inhibits histamine-stimulated inositol phospholipid hydrolysis sin bovine tracheal smooth muscle. Br J Pharmacol 1988; 95:1204–1212.

26. Madison JM, Brown JK. Differential inhibitory effects of forskolin, isoproterenol and dibutyryl cyclic adenosine monophosphate on phosphoinositide hydrolysis in canine tracheal smooth muscle. J Clin Invest 1988; 82:1462–1465.

27. Twort CAC, van Breemen C. Human airway smooth muscle in cell culture: control of the intracellular calcium store. Pulm Pharmacol 1989; 2:45–53.

28. Gunst SJ, Stropp JQ. Effect of Na-K adenosine triphosphatase activity on relaxation of canine tracheal smooth muscle. J Appl Physiol 1988; 64:635–641.

29. Jones TR, Charette L, Garcia ML, Kaczorowski GJ. Selective inhibition of relaxation of guinea-pig trachea by charybodotoxin, a potent Ca^{++}-activated K^+ channel inhibitor. J Pharmacol Exp Ther 1990; 225:697–706.

30. Jones TR, Charette L, Garcia ML, Kaczorowski GJ. Interaction of iberiotoxin with β-adrenoceptor agonists and sodium nitroprusside on guinea pig trachea. J Appl Physiol 1993; 74:1879–1884.

31. Miura M, Belvisi MG, Stretton CD, Yacoub MH, Barnes PJ. Role of potassium channels in bronchodilator responses in human airways. Am Rev Respir Dis 1992; 146:132–136.

32. Kume H, Takai A, Tokuno H, Tomita T. Regulation of Ca^{2+}-dependent K^+-channel activity in tracheal myocytes by phosphorylation. Nature 1989; 341:152–154.

33. Kume H, Graziano MP, Kotlikoff MI. Stimulatory and inhibitory regulation of calcium-activated potassium channels by guanine nucleotide binding proteins. Proc Natl Acad Sci USA 1992; 89:11051–11055.

34. Kume H, Hall IP, Washabau RJ, Takagi K, Kotlikoff MI. β-Adrenergic agonists regulate K_{ca} channels in airway smooth muscle by cAMP-dependent and -independent mechanisms. J Clin Invest 1994; 93:371–379.

35. Waldeck B, Widmark E. Comparison of the effects of forskolin and isoprenaline on tracheal, cardiac and skeletal muscles from guinea-pig. Eur J Pharmacol 1985; 112:349–353.

36. Olesen SP, Munch E, Moldt P, Orejer J. Selective activation of Ca^{2+}-dependent K^+ channels by novel benzimidazolone. Eur J Pharmacol 1994; 251:53–59.

37. Torphy TJ. β-Adrenoceptors, cAMP and airway smooth muscle relaxation: challenges to the dogma. Trends Pharmacol Sci 1994; 15:370–374.

38. Stewart AG, Tomlinson PR, Wilson J. Airway wall remodelling in asthma: a novel target for the development of anti-asthma drugs. Trends Pharmacol Sci 1993; 14:275–278.

39. Hirst SJ, Barnes PJ, Twort CHL. Quantifying proliferation of cultured human and rabbit airway smooth muscle cells in response to serum and platelet-derived growth factor. Am J Respir Cell Mol Biol 1992; 7:574–581.

40. Noveral JP, Grunstein MM. Adrenergic receptor mediated regulation of cultured rabbit airway smooth muscle proliferation. Am J Physiol 1994; 11:L291–L299.

41. Tomlinson PR, Wilson J, Stewart AG. Inhibition by salbutamol of the proliferation of airway smooth muscle cells grown in culture. Br J Pharamcol 1994; 111:641–647.

42. Young PG, Skinner SJM, Black PN. Effect of glucocorticoids and β-adrenoceptor agonists on the proliferation of airway smooth muscle. Eur J Pharmacol 1995; 273:137–144.

43. Barnes PJ. Modulation of neurotransmission in airways. Physiol Rev 1992; 72:699–729.

44. Baker DG, Don U. Catecholamines abolish vagal but not acetylcholine tone in the cat trachea. J Appl Physiol 1987; 63:2490–2498.

45. Danser AHJ, van den Ende R, Lorenz RR, Flavahan NA, Vanhoutte PM. Prejunctional beta1-adrenoceptors inhibit cholinergic neurotransmission in canine bronchi. J Appl Physiol 1987; 62:785–790.

46. Ito Y. Pre- and post-junctional actions of procaterol, a beta-adrenoceptor stimulant, on dog tracheal tissue. Br J Pharmacol 1988; 95:268–274.
47. Janssen LJ, Daniel EE. Characterization of the prejunctional b-adrenoceptors in canine bronchial smooth muscle. J Pharmacol Exp Ther 1991; 254:741–749.
48. Skoogh B, Svedmyr N. β_2-Adrenoceptor stimulation inhibits ganglionic transmission in ferret trachea. Pulm Pharmacol 1989; 1:167–172.
49. Rhoden KJ, Meldrum LA, Barnes PJ. Inhibition of cholinergic neurotransmission in human airways by beta$_2$-adrenoceptors. J Appl Physiol 1988; 65:700–705.
50. Aizawa H, Inoue H, Miyazaki N, Ikeda T, Shigematsu N, Ito Y. Effects of procaterol, a betaX2X-adrenoceptor stimulant, on neuroeffector transmission in human bronchial tissue. Respiration 1991; 58:163–166.
51. Bai TR, Lam R, Prasad FYF. Effects of adrenergic agonists and adenosine on cholinergic neurotransmission in human tracheal smooth muscle. Pulm Pharmacol 1989; 1:193–199.
52. Daniel EE, Kannan M, Davis C, Posey-Daniel V. Ultrastructural studies on the neuromuscular control of human tracheal and bronchial muscle. Respir Physiol 1986; 63:109–128.
53. Ind PW, Dixon CMS, Fuller RW, Barnes PJ. Anticholinergic blockade of beta-blocker induced bronchoconstriction. Am Rev Respir Dis 1989; 139:1390–1394.
54. Barnes PJ. Muscarinic receptor subtypes in airways. Life Sci 1993; 52:521–528.
55. Kamikawa Y, Shimo Y. Inhibitory effects of catecholamines on cholinergically and noncholinergically mediated contractions of guinea-pig isolated bronchial muscle. J Pharm Pharmacol 1990; 42:131–134.
56. Verleden GM, Belvisi MG, Rabe KF, Miura M, Barnes PJ. β_2-Adrenoceptors inhibit NANC neural bronchoconstrictor responses in vitro. J Appl Physiol 1993; 74:1195–1199.
57. Itabash S, Aikawa T, Sekizawa K, Sasaki H, Takishima T. Evidence that an atypical β-adrenoceptor mediates the prejunctional inhibition of non-adrenergic non-cholinergic contraction in guinea pig bronchi. Eur J Pharmacol 1992; 218:187–190.
58. Martin CAE, Naline E, Manara L, Advenier C. Effects of two β_3-adrenoceptor agonists SR 58611A and BRL 37344 and of salbutamol on cholinergic and NANC neural responses in guinea-pig main bronchi in vitro. Br J Pharmacol 1993; 110:1311–1316.
59. Nichol G, Nix A, Barnes PJ, Chung KF. Prostaglandin $F_{2\alpha}$ enhancement of capsaicin induced cough in man: modulation by beta$_2$-adrenergic and anticholinergic drugs. Thorax 1990; 45:694–698.
60. O'Connor BJ, Fuller RW, Barnes PJ. Non-bronchodilator effects of inhaled β_2-agonists. Am J Respir Crit Care Med 1994; 150:381–387.
61. Ueki I, German V, Nadel J. Micropipette measurement of airway submucosal gland secretion: autonomic effects. Am Rev Respir Dis 1980; 121:351–357.
62. Barnes PJ, Basbaum CB. Mapping of adrenergic receptors in the trachea by autoradiography. Exp Lung Res 1983; 5:183–192.
63. Davis DB, Silski CL, Kercomar P, Infeld M. Beta-adrenergic receptors on human tracheal epithelial cells in primary culture. Am J Physiol 1990; 258:C71–76.

64. McCann JD, Welsh MJ. Regulation of Cl⁻ and K⁺ channels in airway epithelium. Ann Rev Physiol 1990; 52:115–135.
65. Knowles M, Murray G, Shallal J, Askin F, Ranga V, Gatzy J, Boucher R. Bioelectric properties and ion flow across exercised human bronchi. J Appl Physiol 1984; 56:868–877.
66. Sanderson MJ, Dirksen ER. Mechanosensitive and beta adrenergic control of ciliary beat frequency of mammalian respiratory tract cells in culture. Am Rev Respir Dis 1989; 139:432–440.
67. Devalia JL, Sapsford RJ, Rusznak C, Toumbis MJ, Davies RJ. The effects of salmeterol and salbutamol on ciliary beat frequency of cultured human bronchialepithelial cells in vitro. Pulm Pharmacol 1992; 5:257–263.
68. Mortiensen J, Groth S, Lange P, Hermansen F. Effect of terbutaline on mucociliary clearance in asthmatic and healthy subjects after inhalation from a pressurized inhaler and a dry powder inhaler. Thorax 1991; 46:817–823.
69. Flavahan NA, Aarhus LL, Rimele TJ, Vanhoutte PM. Respiratory epithelium inhibits bronchial smooth muscle tone. J Appl Physiol 1985; 58:834–838.
70. Barnes PJ, Cuss FM, Palmer JB. The effect of airway epithelium on smooth muscle contractility in bovine trachea. Br J Pharmacol 1985; 86:685–691.
71. Gao Y, Vanhoutte PM. The epithelium acts as a modulator and a diffusion banner in the responses of canine airway smooth muscle. J Appl Physiol 1994;
72. Tokuyama K, Kuo H, Rohde JAL, Barnes PJ, Rogers DF. Neural control of goblet cell secretion in guinea pig airways. Am J Physiol 1990; 259:L108–L115.
73. Widdicombe JG, Pack RJ. The Clara cell. Eur J Respir Dis 1982; 63:202–220.
74. Devalia JL, Davies RJ. Airway epithelial cells and mediators of inflammation. Respir Med 1993; 6:405–408.
75. Massaro GD, Fischman CM, Chiang MJ, Amado C, Massaro D. Regulation of secretion in Clara cells. Studies using the isolated perfused lung. J Clin Invest 1981; 67:345–351.
76. Barker JA, Chediak AJ, Baier HJ, Wanner A. Tracheal mucosal blood flow responses to autonomic agonists. J Appl Physiol 1988; 65:829–834.
77. Boschetto P, Roberts NM, Rogers DF, Barnes PJ. The effect of antiasthma drugs on microvascular leak in guinea pig airways. Am Rev Respir Dis 1989; 139:416–421.
78. Erjefält I, Persson CGA. Pharmacologic control of plasma exudation into tracheobronchial airways. Am Rev Respir Dis 1991; 143:1008–1014.
79. Tokoyama K, Lötvall JO, Löfdahl C-G, Barnes PJ, Chung KF. Inhaled formoterol inhibits histamine-induced airflow obstruction and airway microvascular leakage. J J Pharmacol 1991; 193:35–40.
80. Hui KP, Ventresca P, Brown AC, Barnes PJ, Chung KF. Modulation of neurally mediated airway microvascular leak in guinea pig airways by beta₂ adrenoceptor agonists. Agents Actions 1992; 32:29–33.
81. Sulakvelidze I, McDonald DM. The anti-edema action of formoterol in rat trachea does not depend on capsaicin-sensitive sensory nerves. Am J Respir Crit Care Med 1994; 149:232–238.
82. Barnes PJ, Liu S. Regulation of pulmonary vascular tone. Pharmacol Rev 1995; 47:87–118.

83. Butchers PR, Skidmore IF, Vardey CJ, Wheeldon A. Characterisation of the receptor mediating antianaphylactic effects of beta-adrenoceptor agonists in human lung tissues in vitro. Br J Pharmacol 1980; 71:663–667.

84. Peters SP, Schulman ES, Schleimer RP, MacGlashan DW, Newball HH, Lichtenstein LM. Dispersed human lung mast cells. Pharmacologic aspects and comparison with human lung tissue fragments. Am Rev Respir Dis 1982; 126:1034–1039.

85. Church MK, Hiroi J. Inhibition of IgE-dependent histamine release from human dispersed lung mast cells by anti-allergic drugs and salbutamol. Br J Pharmacol 1987; 90:421–429.

86. Howarth PH, Durham SR, Lee TM, Kay AB, Churck MK, Holgate ST. Influence of albuterol, cromolyn sodium and ipratropium bromide on the airway and circulating mediator responses to allergen bronchial provocation in asthma. Am Rev Respir Dis 1985; 132:986–992.

87. Taylor IK, O'Shaughnessy KM, Choudry NB, Adachi M, Palmer JBD, Fuller RW. A comparative study in atopic subjects with asthma of the effects of salmeterol and salbutamol on allergen-induced bronchoconstriction, increase in airway reactivity and increase in urinary leukotriene E_4 excretion. J Allergy Clin Immunol 1992; 89:575–583.

88. O'Connor BJ, Aikman SL, Barnes PJ. Tolerance to the non-bronchodilator effects of inhaled β_2-agonists. N Engl J Med 1992; 327:1204–1208.

89. O'Connor BJ, Fuller RW, Barnes PJ. Non-bronchodilator effects of inhaled β_2-agonists. Am J Respir Crit Care Med 1994; 150:381–387.

90. Cushley MJ, Holgate ST. Adenosine induced bronchoconstriction in asthma: role of mast cell mediator release. J Allergy Clin Immunol 1985; 75:272–278.

91. Björk T, Gustafsson LE, Dahlén S. Isolated bronchi from asthmatics are hyperresponsive to adenosine, which apparently acts indirectly by liberation of leukotrienes and histamine. Am Rev Respir Dis 1992; 145:1087–1091.

92. Yukawa T, Ukena D, Chanez P, Dent G, Chung KF, Barnes PJ. Beta-adrenergic receptors on eosinophils: binding and functional studies. Am Rev Respir Dis 1990; 141:1446–1552.

93. Rabe KF, Giembycz MA, Dent G, Evans PM, Barnes PJ. β_2-Adrenoceptor agonists and respiratory burst activity in guinea pig and human eosinophils. Fund Clin Pharmacol 1991; 5:A402.

94. Munoz NM, Vita AJ, Neely SP, McAllister K, Spaethe SM, White SM, Leff AR. Beta adrenergic modulation of formyl-methionone-leucine-pheylalanine stimulate secretion of eosinophil peroxidase and leukotriene CA. J Pharmacol Exp Ther 1994; 268:1339–1343.

95. Rabe KF, Giembycz MA, Dent G, Perkins RS, Evans P, Barnes PJ. Salmeterol is a competitive antagonist of b-adrenoceptors modulating inhibition of respiratory burst in guinea-pig eosinophils. Eur J Pharmacol 1993; 231:305–308.

96. Kita H, Abu-Ghazaleh RI, Gleich GJ, Abraham RT. Regulation of Ig-induced eosinophil degranulation by adenosine-3'5'-cyclic monophosphate. J Immunol 1991; 146:2712–2718.

97. Liggett SB. Identification and characterization of a homogeneous population of β_2-adrenergic receptors on human alveolar macrophages. Am Rev Respir Dis 1989; 139: 552–555.

98. Hjemdahl P, Larsson K, Johansson MC, Zetterlund A, Eklund A. β-Adrenoceptors in human alveolar macrophages isolated by elutriation. Br J Clin Pharmacol 1990; 30:673–682.

99. Fuller RW, O'Malley G, Baker AJ, MacDermot J. Human alveolar macrophage activation: inhibition by forskolin but not β-adrenoceptor stimulation or phospho-diesterase inhibition. Pulm Pharmacol 1988; 1:101–106.

100. Bachelet M, Vincent D, Havet N, Marrash-Chahla R, Pradalier A, Dry J, Vargaftig BB. Reduced responsiveness of adenylate cyclase in alveolar macrophages from patients with asthma. J Allergy Clin Immunol 1991; 88:322–328.

101. Seldon PM, Barnes PJ, Meja K, Giambycz MA. Suppression of lipopolysaccharide-induced tumor necrosis factor-α generation from human peripheral blood monocytes by inhibitors of phosphodiesterase 4: interaction with adenylyl cyclase. Mol Pharmacol 1995; 48:747–757.

102. Conolly ME, Greenacre JK. The lymphocyte β-adrenoceptor in normal subjects and patients with asthma: the effect of different forms of treatment on receptor function. J Clin Invest 1976; 1307:1316.

103. Kariman K. β-Adrenergic receptor binding in lymphocytes from patients with asthma. Lung 1980; 158:41–51.

104. Bishopric NH, Cohen HJ, Lefkowitz RJ. Beta adrenergic receptors in lymphocyte subpopulations. J Allergy Clin Immunol 1980; 65:29–33.

105. Maisel AS, Fowler P, Rearden A, Motulsky HJ, Michel MC. A new method for isolation of human lymphocyte-subsets reveals differential regulation of β-adrenergic receptors by terbutaline treatment. Clin Pharmacol Ther 1989; 46:429–439.

106. Didier M, Aussel C, Ferrua B, Fehlman M. Regulation of interleukin 2 synthesis by cAMP in human T cells. J Immunol 1987; 139:1179–1184.

107. Feldman RB. b-Adrenergic receptor-mediated suppression of interleukin-2 receptors in human lymphocytes. J Immunol 1987; 139:3355–3359.

108. Meurs H, Koëter GH, de Vries K, Kauffman HF. The beta-adrenergic system and allergic bronchial asthma: changes in lymphocyte beta-adrenergic receptor number and adenylate cyclase activity after an allergen-induced attack. J Allergy Clin Immunol 1982; 70:272–280.

109. Galant SP, Durisetti L, Underwood S, Allred S, Insel PA. Beta-adrenergic receptors of polymorphonuclear particulates in bronchial asthma. J Clin Invest 1980; 65:577–585.

110. Busse WW, Sosman JM. Isoproterenol inhibition of isolated neutrophil function. J Allergy Clin Immunol 1984; 73:404–410.

111. Barnes PJ, Chung KF. Questions about inhaled β_2-agonists in asthma. Trends Pharmacol Sci 1992; 13:20–23.

112. Laitinen LA, Laitinen A, Haahtela T. A comparative study of the effects of an inhaled corticosteroid, budesonide, and of a β_2-agonist, terbutaline, on airway inflammation in newly diagnosed asthma. J Allergy Clin Immunol 1992; 90:32–42.

113. Roberts JA, Bradding P, Wallis AF, Britton RM, Wilson S, Holgate ST, Howarth PH. The influence of salmeterol xinafoate on mucosal inflammation in asthma. Am Rev Respir Dis 1992; 145:A418.

114. Gardiner PV, Ward C, Booth H, Allison A, Hendrick DJ, Walters EH. Effect of eight weeks of treatment with salmeterol on bronchoalveolar lavage inflammatory indices in asthmatics. Am J Respir Crit Care Med 1994; 150:1006–1011.

115. Bouvier M, Collins S, O'Dowd BF, Campbell PT, de Blasi A, Kobilka BK, MacGregor C, Irons GP, Caron MG, Lefkowitz RJ. Two distinct pathways for cAMP-mediated down-regulation of the β_2-adrenergic receptor. J Biol Chem 1989; 264:16786–16792.

116. Bouvier MW, Hausdorff A, deBlasi A, O'Dowd BF, Kobilka BK, Caron MG, Lefkowitz RJ. Removal of phosphorylation sites from the α-adrenergic receptor delays the onset of agonist-promoted desensitization. Nature 1988; 333:370–373.

117. Benovic JL, Strasser RH, Daniel K, Lefkowitz RJ. Beta-adrenergic receptor kinase: identification of a novel protein kinase that phosphorylates the agonist-occupied form of the receptor. Proc Natl Acad Sci USA 1986; 83:2797–2801.

118. Inglese J, Freedman NJ, Koch WJ, Lefkowitz RJ. Structure and mechanism of the G protein–coupled receptor kinases. J Biol Chem 1993; 268:23735–23738.

119. Hadcock JR, Wang HY, Malbon CC. Agonist-induced destabilization of b-adrenergic receptor mRNA: attenuation of glucocorticoid-induced up-regulation of β-adrenergic receptors. J Biol Chem 1989; 264:19928–19933.

120. Port JD, Huang L, Malbon CC. B-Adrenergic agonists that down-regulate receptor mRNA up-regulate a Mr 35,000 protein(s) that selectively binds to β-adrenergic receptor mRNAs. J Biol Chem 1992; 267:24103–24108.

121. Huang LY, Tholanikunnel BG, Vakalopoulou E, Malbon CC. The M(r) 35,000 beta-adrenergic receptor mRNA binding protein induced by agonists requires both an AUUUA pentamer and U-rich domains for RNA recognition. J Biol Chem 1993; 268:25769–25775.

122. Collins S, Caron MG, Lefkowitz RJ. From ligand binding to gene expression: new insights into the regulation of G-protein–coupled receptors. Trends Pharmacol Sci 1992; 17:37–39.

123. Tattersfield AE. Tolerance to beta-agonists. Clin Respir Physiol 1985; 21:1–5S.

124. Boulet L. Long versus short-acting β_2-agonists. Drug 1994; 47:207–222.

125. Newnham DM, McDevitt DG, Lipworth BJ. Bronchodilator subsensitivity after chronic dosing with eformoterol in patients with asthma. Am J Med 1994; 97: 29–37.

126. Yates DH, Sussman H, Shaw MJ, Barnes PJ, Chung KF. Regular formoterol treatment in mild asthma: effect on bronchial responsiveness during and after treatment. Am J Respir Crit Care Med 1995; 152:1170–1174.

127. Hayes M, Qing F, Rhodes CG, Ind PW, Jones T, Hughes JMB. Human pulmonary β-adrenergic receptors are down-regulated by two weeks of b-agonist therapy. Thorax 1994; 49:1050P.

128. Sears MR, Taylor DR, Print CG, Lake CG, Li Q, Flannery EM, Yates DM, Lucas MK, Herbison GP. Regular inhaled beta-agonist treatment in bronchial asthma. Lancet 1990; 336:1391–1396.

129. Taylor DR, Sears MR, Herbison GP, Flannery EM, Print CG, Lake DC, Yates DM, Lucas MK, Li Q. Regular inhaled β-agonist in asthma: effects on exacerbation and lung function. Thorax 1993; 48:134–138.

130. Cockroft D, McParrand CP, Britto SA, Swystun VA, Rutherford C. Regular inhaled salbutamol and airway responsiveness to allergen. Lancet 1993; 342:833–837.

131. Cheung D, Timmers MC, Zwinderman AH, Bel EH, Dijkman JH, Sterk PJ. The prolonged effects of salmeterol on airway hyperresponsiveness in asthma. N Engl J Med 1992; 327:1198–1203.

132. Ramage L, Lipworth BJ, Ingram CG, Cree IA, Dhillon DP. Reduced protection against exercise induced bronchoconstriction after chronic dosing with salmeterol. Respir Med 1994; 88:363–368.

133. Barnes PJ. Molecular biology of receptors. Q J Med 1992; 301:339–353.

134. Kobilka BK, Frielle T, Dohlman HG, Bolanowski MA, Dixon RAF, Keller P, Caron MG, Lefkowitz RJ. Dilineation of the intronless nature of the genes for the human and hamster β_2-adrenergic receptor and their promoter regions. J Biol Chem 1987; 262:7321–7327.

135. Emorine LJ, Marullo S, Delavier-Klutchko C, Kaveri SV, Durieu-Trautmann O, Strusberg AD. Structure of the gene for human β_2-adrenergic receptor: expression and promoter characterization. Proc Natl Acad Sci USA 1987; 84:6995–6999.

136. Malbon CC, Hadcock JR. Evidence that glucocorticoid response elements in the 5' non-coding region of the hamster β_2-adrenergic receptor gene are obligative for glucocorticoid regulation of hamster mRNA levels. Biochem Biophys Res Common 1988; 154:676–681.

137. Davis AO, Lefkowitz RJ. Regulation of beta-adrenergic receptors by steroid hormones. Ann Rev Physiol 1984; 46:119–130.

138. Hui KKP, Conolly ME, Tashkin DP. Reversal of human lymphocyte β-adrenoceptor desensitization by glucocorticoids. Clin Pharmacol Ther 1982; 32:566–571.

139. Brodde O, Brinkmann M, Schemuth R, O'Hara N, Daul A. Terbutaline-induced desensitization of human lymphocyte β_2-adrenoceptors. Accelerated restoration of β-adrenoceptor responsiveness by prednisolone and ketotifen. J Clin Invest 1985; 1096:1101.

140. Mano K, Akbarzadeh A, Townley RG. Effect of hydrocortisone on beta-adrenergic receptors in lung membranes. Life Sci 1979; 25:1925–1930.

141. Fraser CM, Venter JC. The synthesis of beta-adrenergic receptors in cultured human lung cells: induction by glucocorticoids. Biochem Biophys Res Comm 1980; 94:390–397.

142. Barnes PJ, Jacobs MM, Roberts JM. Glucocorticoids preferably increase fetal alveolar beta-receptors: autoradiographic evidence. Pediatr Res 1984; 18:1191–1194.

143. Collins S, Caron MG, Lefkowitz RJ. β-Adrenergic receptors in hamster smooth muscle cells are transcriptionally regulated by glucocorticoids. J Biol Chem 1988; 263:9067–9070.

144. Hadcock JR, Williams DL, Malbon CC. Physiological regulation at the level of mRNA: analysis of steady state levels of specific mRNAs by DNA-excess solution hybridization. Am J Physiol 1989; 256:C457–C465.

145. Mak JCW, Nishikawa M, Barnes PJ. Glucocorticosteroids increase β_2-adrenergic receptor transcription in human lung. Am J Physiol 1995; 12:L41–L46.

146. Mak JCW, Nishikawa M, Shirasaki H, Miyayasu K, Barnes PJ. Protective effects of a glucocorticoid on down-regulation of pulmonary β_2-adrenergic receptors in vivo. J Clin Invest 1995; 96:99–106.

147. Nishikawa M, Shirasaki M, Mak JW, Barnes PJ. Protective effects of dexamethasone on isoproterenol-induced down-regulation of pulmonary β_2-receptors in rat. Am Rev Respir Dis 1993; 147:A275.

148. Kioumis K, Ukena D, Barnes PJ. The effect of nedocromil sodium on down-regulation of pulmonary beta-receptors. Clin Sci 1989; 76:599–602.

149. Bretz U, Martin U, Mazzoni L, Ney UM. β-Adrenergic tachyphylaxis in the rat and its reversal and prevention by ketotifen. Eur J Pharmacol 1983; 86:321–328.

150. Taki F, Takagi K, Satake T, Sugiyama S, Ozawa T. The role of phospholipase in reduced beta-adrenergic responsiveness in experimental asthma. Am Rev Respir Dis 1986; 133:362–366.

151. Agrawal DK, Townley RD. Effects of platelet activating factor on beta-adrenoceptors in human lung. Biochem Biophys Res Commun 1987; 193:1–6.

152. Barnes PJ, Grandordy BM, Page CP, Rhoden KJ, Robertson DN. The effect of platelet activating factor on pulmonary beta-adrenoceptors. Br J Pharmacol 1991; 90:709–715.

153. Raaijmakers JAM, Beneker C, van Geegen ECG, Meisters TMN, Poven P. Inflammatory mediators and b-receptor function. Agents Actions 1989; 26:45–47.

154. Folkerts G, Nijkamp FP, van Oosterholt AJM. Induction in guinea pigs of airway hyperreactivity and decreased lung b-adrenoceptor number by 15-hydroxy-arachidonic acid. Br J Pharmacol 1984; 80:597–599.

155. Engels F, Oosting RS, Nijkamp FP. Pulmonary macrophages induce deterioration of guinea-pig tracheal β-adrenergic function through release of oxygen radicals. Eur J Pharmacol 1985; 3:143–144.

156. Hall I, Chilvers ER. Inositol phosphates and airway smooth muscle. Pulm Pharmacol 1989; 2:113–120.

157. Bouvier M, Leeb-Lundberg LM, Benovic JL, Caron MG, Lefkowitz RJ. Regulation of adrenergic receptor function by phosphorylation. II. Effects of agonist occupancy on phosphorylation of α_1- and β-adrenergic receptors by protein kinase C and cyclic AMP-dependent protein kinase. J Biol Chem 1987; 262:3106–3113.

158. Meurs H, Kauffman HF, Koeter GH, Timmermans A, deVries K. Regulation of beta-receptor–adenylate cyclase system in lymphocytes of allergic patients with asthma: possible role for protein kinase C in allergen-induced nonspecific refractoriness of adenylate cyclase. J Allergy Clin Immunol 1987; 80:326–329.

159. Mardini IA, Higgins NC, Zhou S, Benovic BL, Kelsen SG. Functional behavior of the β-adrenergic receptor-adenyl cyclase system in rabbit airway epithelium. Am J Respir Cell Mol Biol 1994; 11:287–295.

160. Nakane T, Szentendrei L, Stern L, Virmani M, Seely J, Kunos G. Effects of IL-1 and cortisol on beta-adrenergic receptors, cell proliferation and differentiation in cultured human A 549 lung tumor cells. J Immunol 1990; 145:260–266.

161. Szentendrei T, Lazar-Wesley C, Nakane T, Virmani M, Kunos G. Selective regulation of β-adrenergic receptor gene expression by interleukin-1 in cultured human lung tumor cells. J Cell Physiol 1992; 152:478–485.

162. van Oosterhout AJM, Stam WB, Vanderscheueren RGJRA. The effects of cytokines on β-adrenoceptor function of human peripheral blood mononuclear cells and guinea pig trachea. J Allergy Clin Immunol 1992; 90:304–308.

163. Wills-Karp M, Uchida Y, Lee JY, Jinot J, Hirata A, Hirata F. Organ culture with proinflammatory cytokines reproduces impairment of the β-adrenoceptor–mediated relaxation in tracheas of a guinea pig antigen model. Am J Respir Cell Mol Biol 1993; 8:153–159.

164. Kelsen SG, Anakwe O, Zhou S, Benovic J, Aksoy M. Interleukins impair beta adrenergic receptor–adenyl cyclase system function in human airway epithelial cells. Am J Respir Crit Care Med 1994; 149:A479.

165. Nogami M, Romberger DJ, Rennard SI, Toews ML. TGF-β1 modulates β-adrenergic receptor number and function in cultured human tracheal smooth muscle cells. Am J Physiol 1994; 266:L187–191.

166. Goldie RG, Spina D, Henry PJ, Lulich KM, Paterson JW. In vitro responsiveness of human asthmatic bronchus to carbachol, histamine, β-adrenoceptor agonists and theophylline. Br J Clin Pharmacol 1986; 22:669–676.

167. Bai TR. Abnormalities in airway smooth muscle in fatal asthma: a comparison between trachea and bronchus. Am Rev Respir Dis 1991; 143:441–443.

168. Cerrina J, Ladurie ML, Labat C, Raffestin B, Bayol A, Brink C. Comparison of human bronchial muscle response to histamine in vivo with histamine and isoproterenol agonists in vitro. Am Rev Respir Dis 1986; 134:57–61.

169. De Jongste JC, Mons H, Bonta IL, Kerrebijn KF. Human asthmatic airway responses in vitro—a case report. Eur J Respir Dis 1987; 70:23–29.

170. Whicker SD, Armour CL, Black JL. Responsiveness of bronchial smooth muscle from asthmatic patients to relaxant and contractile agonists. Pulm Pharmacol 1988; 1:25–31.

171. Sharma RK, Jeffery PK. Airway β-adrenoceptor number in cystic fibrosis and asthma. Clin Sci 1990; 78:409–417.

172. Bai TR, Mak JCW, Barnes PJ. A comparison of beta-adrenergic receptors and in vitro relaxant responses to isoproterenol in asthmatic airway smooth muscle. Am J Respir Cell Mol Biol 1992; 6:647–651.

173. Haddad E, Mak JCW, Barnes PJ. Expression of β-adrenergic and muscarinic receptors in asthmatic lung. Am J Physiol 1996 (in press).

174. Fernandes LB, Fryer AD, Hirschman CA. M_2 muscarinic receptors inhibit isoproterenol-induced relaxation of canine airway smooth muscle. J Pharmacol Exp Ther 1992; 262:119–126.

175. Roffel AF, Elzinga CRS, Zaagsma J. Muscarinic M_2 receptors do not participate in the functional antagonism between methacholine and isoprenaline in guinea pig tracheal smooth muscle. Eur J Pharmacol 1993; 249:235–238.

176. Pitcher J, Lohse MJ, Codina J, Caron MG, Lefkowitz RJ. Densensitization of the isolated β-adrenergic receptor β-adrenergic receptor kinase, cAMP-dependent protein kinase and protein kinase C occurs in distinct molecular mechanisms. Biochemistry 1992; 31:3193–3197.

177. Pyne NJ, Freissmuth M, Palmer S. Phosphorylation of the spliced variant forms of the recombinant stimulatory guanine-nucleotide–binding regulatory protein (G_{sa}) by protein kinase C. Biochem J 1992; 285:333–338.
178. Grandordy BM, Mak JCW, Barnes PJ. Modulation of airway smooth muscle β-adrenoceptor function by a muscarinic agonist. Life Sci 1994; 54:185–191.
179. Masquilier D, Sassone-Corsi P. Transcriptional cross talk: nuclear factors CREM and CREB bind to AP-1 sites and inhibit activation by Jun. J Biol Chem 1992; 267:22460–22466.
180. Imai F, Minger JN, Mitchell JA, Yamamoto KR, Granner DK. Glucocorticoid receptor-cAMP response element-binding protein interaction and the response of th ephosphoenolpyruvate carboxykinase gene to glucocorticoids. J Biol Chem 1993; 268:5353–5356.
181. Peters MJ, Adcock IM, Brown CR, Barnes PJ. β-Agonist inhibition of steroid-receptor DNA binding activity in human lung. Am Rev Respir Dis 1993; 147:A772.
182. Peters MJ, Adcock IM, Brown CR, Barnes PJ. β-Adrenoceptor agonists interfere with glucocorticoid receptor DNA binding in rat lung. Eur J Pharmacol (Mol Sect) 1995; 289:275–281.
183. Adcock IM, Brown CR, Gelder CM, Shirasaki H, Peters MJ, Barnes PJ. The effects of glucocorticoids on transcription factor activation in human peripheral blood mononuclear cells. Am J Physiol 1995; 37:C331–C338.
184. Stevens DA, Barnes PJ, Adcock IM. β-Agonists inhibit DNA binding of glucocorticoid receptors in human pulmonary and bronchial epithelial cells. Am J Respir Crit Care Med 1995; 151:A195.

Discussion

BERTIL WALDECK

Astra Draco AB, Lund, Sweden

We have got a very comprehensive review on the wide range of effects of β-agonists on airway effector cells. With all these diverse effects in mind, there seems to be little doubt that relaxation of airway smooth muscle is the major antiasthmatic effect of $β_2$-adrenoceptor agonists. Therefore, I will open the discussion with three questions regarding $β_2$-adrenoceptor mediated broncho-dilation.

1. Do $β_2$-agonists relax airway smooth muscle by opening maxi-K channels?

The idea that $β_2$-agonists relax airway smooth muscle by opening maxi-K channels in the cell membrane is based primarily on the ability of charybdotoxin, a maxi-K channel antagonist, to inhibit the relaxation exerted by this class of compounds. Thus, in carbachol-contracted guinea-pig tracheal smooth muscle, charybdotoxin causes a concentration-dependent rightward shift of the concentration-response curve for isoprenaline. For salbutamol, which has a lower efficacy, there is a concentration-dependent reduction of the maximum relaxation (1). Exactly the same pattern of response, that of functional antagonism, is obtained with isoprenaline and the partial agonist, soterenol, by increasing the concentration of carbachol in the medium (2).

It appears to have been overlooked that charbydotoxin, probably by depolarization and subsequent Ca^{2+} influx, increases the smooth muscle tone. Thus, the antagonism by charybdotoxin of β-agonists may be mainly functional. This view is supported by data which show that the relaxation by salbutamol of the guinea pig trachea is not inhibited by charybdotoxin when the external Ca^{2+} concentration is reduced or when Ca^{2+} influx is inhibited by nifedipine (3). Another piece of evidence against a major role for maxi-K channels is that isoprenaline potently relaxes a completely K^+-depolarized tracheal smooth muscle (4). In view of these data, it is difficult to conceive that opening of maxi-K channels is a major mechanism of airway smooth muscle response to β-agonists.

2. How important is the prejunctional inhibition exerted by β₂-agonists?

Another point of interest is to what extent prejunctional inhibition of transmitter release from cholinergic and noncholinergic excitatory nerves may contribute to the antiasthmatic effect. We have compared the pEC_{50} values obtained for inhibition of contractions induced by selective stimulation of the vagus nerve in a trachea tube preparation with those obtained for relaxation of carbachol-contracted strip preparations from guinea pig trachea (5–7 and unpublished data). The stimulation parameters and the carbachol concentration were selected so that the contractile forces were comparable. For each compound investigated, the two EC_{50} values were practically identical. At a first glance, this could be interpreted in terms of an inhibitory effect on the nerve-induced contractions directly at the smooth muscle. However, it has been demonstrated that β-agonists are considerably less effective in preventing carbachol-induced contractions than to reverse a contracted state (8). This supports the view expressed by the previous speaker that there is a significant inhibitory effect of β₂-agonists prejunctionally on cholinergic nerves in the airways. To what extent this inhibitory component is subject to tachyphylaxis remains to be elucidated.

3. Does the airway epithelium contribute to the inhibitory effect of β₂-agonists?

It has been suggested that β-agonists may release a relaxing factor from epithelial cells in the airways. The vagus nerve–trachea tube preparation from guinea pig is very suitable for investigation of this question. A number of β-agonists were administered either to the serosal side via the external medium or to the epithelial side via the tracheal lumen. Inhibition of nerve-induced contractions were measured (5,6). For hydrophilic compounds, potency was higher when applied to the serosal side than into the lumen, thus illustrating the barrier function of the epithelium. Destruction of the epithelium by exposure to hydrogen peroxide increased the potency of the hydrophilic terbutaline given intraluminally, whereas the potency of terbutaline added to the serosal side was unchanged (9). For lipophilic compounds, which more easily penetrate the epithelium, the difference in pEC_{50} between the two modes of administration was small. In no case was a compound more effective when applied into the lumen. An amplification of the inhibitory response when administered from the epithelial side would be expected for a drug releasing a relaxant factor of importance from the epithelium. If there is a β_2-adrenoceptor–mediated release of an epithelial relaxing factor, this effect is well hidden.

References

1. Jones TR, Charette L, Garcia ML, Kaczorowski GJ. Selective inhibition of relaxation of guinea-pig trachea by charybdotoxin, a potent Ca^{++}-activated K^+ channel inhibitor. J Pharmacol Exp Ther 1990; 255:697–706.
2. Buckner CK, Saini RK. On the use of functional antagonism to estimate dissociation constants for beta adrenergic receptor agonists in isolated guinea-pig trachea. J Pharmacol Exp Ther 1975; 194:565–574.
3. Huang J-C, Garcia ML, Reuben JP, Kaczorowski GJ. Inhibition of β-adrenoceptor agonist relaxation of airway smooth muscle by Ca^{2+}-activated K^+ channel blockers. Eur J Pharmacol 1993; 235:37–43.
4. Kumar MA. The basis of beta adrenergic bronchodilation. J Pharmacol Exp Ther 1978; 206:528–534.
5. Jeppsson A-B, Roos C, Waldeck B, Widmark E. Pharmacodynamic and pharmacokinetic aspects on the transport of bronchodilator drugs through the tracheal epithelium of the guinea-pig. Pharmacol Toxicol 1989; 64:58–63.
6. Jeppsson A-B, Löfdahl C-G, Waldeck B, Widmark E. On the predictive value of experiments in vitro in the evaluation of the effect duration of bronchodilator drugs for local administration. Pulm Pharmacol 1989; 2:81–85.
7. Waldeck B, Jeppsson A-B, Widmark E. Partial agonism and functional selectivity: A study on β-adrenoceptor mediated effects in tracheal, cardiac and skeletal muscle. Acta Pharmacol Toxicol 1986; 58:209–218.
8. Gustafsson B, Persson CGA. Effect of different bronchodilators on airway smooth muscle responsiveness to contractile agents. Thorax 1991; 46:360–365.
9. Jeppsson A-B, Luts A, Sundler F, Waldeck B, Widmark E. Hydrogen peroxide-induced epithelial damage increases terbutaline transport in guinea-pig tracheal wall: implications for drug delivery. Pulm Pharmacol 1991; 4:73–79.

4

Effects of Beta$_2$-Agonists on Airway Inflammation

PETER HOWARTH

Southampton General Hospital
Southampton, England

I. Introduction

Although both short- and long-acting beta-agonists are used, respectively, on as needed and regular basis for their bronchodilator effects in asthma, there is a potential that this may not be their sole effect in the disease. Asthma is a chronic inflammatory disease of the airway mucosa involving a number of cell types, including mast cells, eosinophils, macrophages, T lymphocytes, epithelial cells, endothelial cells, and cells of the fibroblast lineage, such as myofibroblasts (1). β-Adrenoceptors are present on a number of these cell populations and have been localized within the respiratory tract to mast cells, ciliated epithelial cells, vascular endothelial cells, submucosal glands, type II pneumocytes, Clara cells, and cholinergic ganglia in addition to airway smooth muscle (2). Receptor subtyping has identified that the influence of β-agonists at these sites is mediated by β$_2$-adrenoceptors, with the exception of mucosal glands where β$_1$-receptor stimulation induces an increase in glandular secretion. Modification of these cells' function by β$_2$-adrenoceptor stimulation may thus contribute to the beneficial effects of β-agonist therapy in asthma.

II. Mucosal Inflammation and Asthma

There is evidence of mast cell activation in asthma with ultrastructural features of degranulation evident on transmission electronmicroscopic examination of mucosal biopsies and elevated levels of the mast cell mediators histamine and tryptase being identifiable in recovered bronchoalveolar lavage (BAL) fluid (3–6). In addition, there is evidence of ongoing cytokine secretion from airway mast cells. The release of interleukin-4 (IL-4) and tumor necrosis factor-alpha (TNF-α), both localized to human airway mast cell granules (7), will influence epithelial and endothelial activation, whereas the release of mast cell–derived IL-5 will influence tissue eosinophil recruitment and activation.

The initial phase of eosinophil tissue recruitment involves endothelial activation with upregulation of endothelial leukocyte cell adhesion molecules (LECAMs). These LECAMs recognize specific ligands on leukocyte cell surfaces (carbohydrate moieties and integrins) and through their interaction induce initially a rolling margination followed by firmer leukocyte endothelial adherence associated with cell activation and diapedesis (8). The rolling margination involves the LECAM, P-selectin, which is mobilized onto the lumenal surface from its storage site in Wiebel-Paladie bodies within the endothelial cells (9). This occurs under the influence of histamine and platelet-activating factor and will thus be influenced by local mast cell degranulation. The firmer adherence relates to the subsequent cytokine-induced endothelial expression of E-selectin, intracellular adhesion molecule-1 (ICAM-1), and vascular cell adhesion molecule (VCAM-1). TNF-α is involved in upregulation of all the LECAMs, while IL-4 contributes to VCAM-1 expression (10–12). VCAM-1, which through its interactions with the ligand VLA-4 promotes eosinophil adherence, has been shown to have increased expression in asthma (13). In chronic disease, the generation and release of cytokines from airway T lymphocytes will also significantly contribute to the tissue eosinophil recruitment (14,15). T cells in asthma are in an exaggerated state of activation (16,17) and have a cytokine profile consistent with an expansion of the TH$_2$ population, generating IL-3, IL-4, IL-5, and TNF-α and granulocyte-macrophage colony-stimulating factor (GM-CSF), which are all cytokines relevant to airway eosinophil recruitment.

The diapedesis of eosinophils into the tissue space will be influenced both by endothelial permeability and by directed chemotaxis (1,18). Mediators such as histamine, prostaglandins, leukotrienes, and kinins released or generated following immunological mast cell activation will influence vascular permeability. They interact with specific receptors localized on the vascular endothelium of the postcapillary venules to induce contraction and open gap junctions between adjacent cells. This action promotes plasma protein extravasation and facilitate transendothelial cellular migration. The subsequent eosinophil tissue survival and movement will depend on cell-cell contact and the presence of chemotactic stimuli. Matrix cells are likely to contribute to these processes, as TNF-α has been shown to promote myofibroblast activation (19), with induction of the generation of the cytokines IL-6, IL-8, GM-CSF, and stem cell factor (SCF).

Myofibroblasts thus promote mast cell progenitor cell maturation and differentiation through the release of soluble mast cell growth factors (SCF, IL-6) and provide a chemotactic stimulus (IL-8), whereas in addition influencing eosinophil survival through inhibition of apoptosis (GM-CSF). The epithelial accumulation of mast cells, eosinophils, and macrophages in asthma is also influenced by the enhanced epithelial generation of IL-8, Regulated upon Activation Normal T Expressed and Secreted (RANTES), GM-CSF, and macrophage inflammatory protein (MIP-1α) that has been described in this disease (20–23). RANTES is a potent eosinophil chemoattractant (24), as is IL-8 when coupled with secretory immunoglobulin A (sIgA) to form IL-8–sIgA complexes (25). Mast cell degranulation can be linked with this process of epithelial cell recruitment, as tryptase releases IL-8 from its epithelial storage and IL-4 induces the epithelial generation of secretory component (26). Secretory component when coupled with IgA to form sIgA provides a mechanism for the localized activation of eosinophils, as sIgA is a powerful eosinophil activator with the capacity to induce intracellular production of IL-3, IL-5, and GM-CSF (27). These cytokines are capable both of inhibiting the apoptosis of eosinophils and priming them for enhanced mediator release. The epithelial generation of GM-CSF, along with the autocrine generation of GM-CSF by activated eosinophils as well as the potential release of this cytokine from mast cells, T lymphocytes, and myofibroblasts, will contribute to the prolonged survival of eosinophils within the airway tissue in asthma in general and the epithelium in particular. The epithelial generation of IL-1β provides a local mechanism for the upregulation of eosinophil adherence to the epithelium. Both TNF-α and IL-1β have been shown to increase eosinophil adherence to human respiratory epithelial cells cultured in vitro (28). This occurs through the induction of epithelial ligands recognized by β₂ (CD11/CD18)–integrins expressed on the eosinophil cell surface. At least in cell cultures, this adherence appears independent of ICAM-1, an adhesion molecule that would potentially recognize the ligands leukocyte function–associated antigen-1 (LFA-1) and membrane attack complex-1 (MAC-1) expressed on activated eosinophils. The localization of eosinophils to an epithelial site is important in view of their potential effects on epithelial integrity.

The local release of eosinophil cationic protein (ECP) and major basic protein (MBP), has been implicated in the epithelial disruption in asthma. Both ECP and MBP are directly cytotoxic and cytolytic to human epithelial cells (29) at concentrations identifiable in sputum in asthma (30), and they can be demonstrated by immunochemistry to be present within the airways at sites of epithelial desquamation in postmortem specimens of patients dying from asthma (31). In asthma, there is an exaggerated deposition of collagen in the lamina reticularis (types III and V collagen) beneath the basement membrane (type IV collagen) (32). This is associated with myofibroblast proliferation (33), and the activation of this cell population with collagen synthesis and release represents part of the repair process following epithelial damage and activation. In addition to the epithelial generation of cytokines relevant to tissue leukocyte recruitment in asthma, there is epithelial expression of basic fibroblast growth factor (bFGF), transforming growth factor-beta (TGF-β) and upregulated expression of the 21–amino acid peptide endothelin (34,35). These epithelial products, as well as the mast cell products histamine, heparin, and tryptase, will contribute to airway wall fibrogenesis (36–38).

These cellular events within the airways underlie the physiological characteristics of asthma; namely, bronchoconstriction, exaggerated diurnal variation in airflow obstruction, and bronchial hyperresponsiveness. Mathematical modeling has demonstrated the importance of airway wall thickness (mucosal edema, collagen deposition, and smooth muscle hypertrophy) to bronchial hyperresponsiveness (39) while significant correlations exist between epithelial disruption, as indicated by epithelial cell recovery by BAL and bronchial responsiveness (40). Mast cell numbers and mediator levels in BAL also correlate with bronchial responsiveness (1,6) as does lavage MBP levels when united with those from nonasthmatic subjects (41). The release of leukotrienes (LTs) from activated mast cells and eosinophils will significantly contribute to airflow obstruction, as inhalation studies indicate LTC4/LTD4 to be up to 10,000 times as potent as histamine as a bronchoconstrictor (42). Consistent with this, LT antagonist and 5-lipoxygenase (5-LO) inhibitors are bronchodilators in asthma.

III. β₂-Agonist–Mediated Effects Relevant to Asthmatic Inflammation

The concept that adrenergic agonists might influence allergic inflammation was first suggested in 1936 when Schild described inhibition of allergen-induced histamine release from whole lung fragments with adrenaline (epinephrine) (43). Subsequent workers demonstrated that this was a β-adrenoceptor–mediated action (44,45). In human lung fragments, the magnitude of the inhibitory effect of the β₂-adrenoceptor agonist salbutamol has been shown to depend both on the strength of the allergic stimulus and the dose of the drug (46). Salbutamol acts in a dose-dependent manner, with higher doses of drug producing greater inhibition. In normal human lung preparations, the effect of salbutamol on inhibiting histamine release is greater than the "classic" antiallergic compound sodium cromoglycate, with salbutamol being about 30,000 times as potent. Thus in chopped lung preparations, β_2-adrenoceptor agonists are potent inhibitors of allergen-induced histamine, prostaglandin D_2, and leukotriene release. The long-acting β_2-agonists salmeterol and formoterol are more potent than the short-acting β_2-adrenoceptor agonist salbutamol in this respect (47,48). In in vitro preparations, the duration of effect of salmeterol is greater than formoterol, which is greater than salbutamol, when all these drugs are used at concentrations producing comparable maximum inhibition; respectively, 40, 4, and 200 nm. It is thus apparent that formoterol is the most potent of the β_2-adrenoceptor agonists in this respect.

IV. In Vitro Studies

A. Nonhuman Investigations

The long acting β_2-adrenoceptor agonist salmeterol has been shown to inhibit allergen-induced leukocyte recruitment within the airways following ovalbumin challenge in sensitized guinea pigs (49,50). Similar findings are reported with formoterol (51), and the effects have been shown to be β_2-adrenoceptor agonist mediated, as the β-adrenoceptor antagonist DL-popranolol inhibits this action (47). The D-popranolol isomer, which is devoid of β_2-adrenoceptor antagonistic activity, is without influence on the protective effect of salmeterol. The inhibitory effect of β_2-adrenoceptor agonist pretreatment on allergen-induced airway eosinophil recruitment is neither stimulus nor cell specific (52, 53). Pretreatment also inhibits platelet-activating factor–induced airway eosinophil recruitment, when assessed 24 hr after challenge as well as inhibiting endotoxin-induced neutrophil recruitment into rat airways and zymosan-induced neutrophil recruitment into guinea pig skin. These effects are divorced from the bronchodilator action, as rat airways do not bronchodilate to β-agonists.

This broad protective effect on cell recruitment with differing stimuli acting via separate mechanisms suggests an inhibitory effect not purely related to inhibition of mast cell degranulation. An action on the vascular endothelial cell to limit tissue cell trafficking is also likely to be pertinent to these protective effects. Consistent with this, salbutamol, salmeterol, and formoterol have all been reported to inhibit histamine-induced protein extravasation (49,54,55).

In addition to their effects on mast cells, β-adrenergic agonists may also modify airway inflammation in asthma through their effects on endothelial and epithelial integrity (49,54–56). β-Agonists have been shown to exert an inhibitory effect on induced plasma protein leakage in in vitro studies using endothelial monolayers. This has been confirmed in vivo in humans in the upper respiratory tract (57), although large doses of β-agonists were required and the protective effect was also accompanied by a reduction in the allergen-induced increment in tryptase, making it difficult to determine if the reduced plasma protein exudation was an indirect or direct effect of the β-agonist pre-treatment. Such an effect in asthma would modify not only the protein exudation and mucosal edema but also may modify the egression of cells from the vascular lumen into the tissue. β-Adrenergic receptor stimulation also promotes tight junction integrity between epithelial cells (56), and this may also limit lumenal protein transport from the serosal surface while also opposing the access of lumenal substances, such as allergen, to submucosal cells.

Other cell populations involved in airway inflammation are, however, relatively insensitive to the effect of β$_2$-agonists. High concentrations ($>1 \mu$m) are required before any inhibitory effect on stimulated release of thromboxane B$_2$ from alveolar macrophages is apparent and similar concentrations are required to influence the stimulated release of LTB$_4$ from neutrophils and ECP from eosinophils (58–61). Thus modification of mast cell and possibly endothelial activation may be the prime cellular expectations of β$_2$-agonist therapy in asthma in vivo.

B. Human Investigations

The investigations of the effects of β-agonists on airway inflammation can be subdivided into those studies assessing the influence on acute allergen-induced airway inflammation and those investigating the effects within the clinical situation on a more chronic basis. As these represent differing aspects, one a protective effect against challenge-induced exacerbations of inflammation and the other the influence on chronic baseline inflammation relevant to clinical disease expression, these will be considered separately.

Acute Inflammation

Airway inhalation challenge with allergen in asthma can induce a biphasic response, an immediate bronchoconstriction response followed by recovery, and then a subsequent late bronchoconstriction response occurring 4–12 hr after challenge. The immediate response is mast cell dependent, being associated with the local release into the airways of histamine, tryptase, and prostaglandin D$_2$ (62–64). This is also reflected by elevations of histamine being identifiable within the circulation in some individuals (65). Four to six hours after challenge, direct assessment of the airways by fiberoptic bronchoscopy identifies airway narrowing mucosal edema, and accumulation of activated eosinophils within the airway lumen and tissue leukocyte recruitment; predominantly neutrophils but also eosinophils, T-lymphocytes, and mast cells (66,67). This cellular infiltrate, which is accompanied by upregulation of endothelial leukocyte adhesion molecules, is considered to underlie the late physiological changes of bronchoconstriction and bronchial hyperresponsiveness.

The influence of β_2-agonist pretreatment on the immediate bronchoconstriction response to allergen has been investigated and found to be protective (65). In one study of 10 grass pollen–sensitive seasonal asthmatic subjects studied outside the pollen season, 200 μg of salbutamol, administered 15 min prior to allergen challenge, prevented the acute changes in FEV_1 and specific airways conductance that were evident on a control challenge day. The pretreatment also inhibited the allergen-related increment in plasma histamine and serum high molecular weight neutrophil chemoattractant factor (NCF) that were also evident on the control day. The inhibitory action of salbutamol on these mediator rises is consistent with an in vivo inhibitory action on acute allergen-induced airway mast cell degranulation.

As histamine release will upregulate endothelial P-selectin expression to induce leukocyte rolling margination (68), and TNF-α release from mast cells will contribute to LECAM upregulation (8), and TNF-α and IL-5 will both influence eosinophil activation and recruitment (69), mast cell degranulation during the immediate response will contribute to the subsequent tissue leukocyte recruitment. The influence of β_2-agonists has thus been assessed on the late response. Although when the short-acting β-agonist salbutamol is given at a standard dose (200 μg), it has no effect on the late bronchoconstrictor response (70), but when salbutamol is given at high dose (5 mg) by nebulization, it has an inhibitory effect on the late response (71). Similarly, the long-acting β_2-agonists salmeterol and formoterol have both been shown to inhibit both the immediate and late bronchoconstrictor responses to allergen-challenge (72,73). This intervention also prevents the acquisition of bronchial hyperresponsiveness. Although functional antagonism of a bronchoconstrictor stimulus, even in the absence of bronchodilation, remains a possible explanation for this effect, an alternative interpretation is inhibition of the late cell accumulation within the airways that underlies the bronchoconstriction and airway events associated with the acquisition of bronchial responsiveness. This has now been assessed in a number of studies.

One study assessing the associated changes in peripheral blood ECP during the late response demonstrated an increase during the control challenge day, which is consistent with eosinophil activation, but an inhibition of this change when either 50 or 100 μg of salmeterol was inhaled prior to inhalation allergen challenge (74). This indirect assessment has now been complemented by direct airway assessments using fiberoptic bronchoscopy with BAL and biopsy sampling. A study by Boulet and colleagues found that salmeterol, 50 μg b.i.d. for 2 months, reduced the tissue accumulation of mast cells and memory T lymphocytes (CD45RO$^+$) 6 hr following inhalation allergen challenge as compared with a control challenge day (75). Murray et al., using a local endobronchial allergen challenge model, found that inhaled salmeterol, 50 μg, given 1 hr prior to challenge and then every 12 hr thereafter reduced the increment in ECP in lavage 24 hr after challenge (76). In this study, there was no effect on the increase in lavage eosinophil numbers with allergen but these workers reported a decrease in the allergen-related increase in IL-4 and IL-5 levels in lavage, which is consistent with an effect on cell activation. The cell source of these cytokines is undetermined but could be derived from mast cells, T lymphocytes, or basophils. The reduced accumulation of both mast cells and T lymphocytes following salmeterol therapy could thus explain this finding. An increase in basophils has been described in lavage 24 hr after challenge, but the effects of salmeterol on this change has not been described. The recent in vitro demonstration that β_2-agonists, through an action on intracellular cyclic adenosine monophosphate (AMP), can regulate the gene expression of IL-4 and IL-5 provides a mechanism for the influence of this therapy on IL-4 and IL-5 levels. This cytokine regulation would be anticipated to reduce eosinophil recruitment and is compatible with the further identification by Calhoun and co-workers that salmeterol pretreatment inhibits the increase in eosinophils in lavage identifiable 48 hr following local endobronchial allergen challenge (78). In this study, there was also a decrease in the ability of unfractioned BAL cells to generate superoxide (SO) following phorbol myristate acetate (PMA) stimulation.

There is thus accumulating evidence that the protective effect of salmeterol on the late asthmatic response to allergen challenge is, at least in part, accountable for by an inhibitory effect on airway inflammation. These studies may also minimize any potential effect, as the allergen load administered to the airway is substantial, being associated with a far greater eosinophil recruitment than that identified in clinical allergic asthma. Assessments have therefore also been undertaken in chronic clinical disease.

Chronic Inflammation

Studies have been undertaken with both short-acting and long-acting β-agonists with direct airway assessment by bronchoscopy before and at intervals after regular treatment from 4 weeks to 2 months.

C. Short-Acting β-Agonists

Neither salbutamol nor terbutaline has been found to have a consistent effect on differing indices of airway inflammation. Adelroth and colleagues found no effect on lavage cell populations with terbutaline, 250 μg q.i.d. for 4 weeks (79), whereas a further report by Jeffrey on the biopsies from the same subjects reported a small increase in T lymphocytes but no effect on mast cell or eosinophil numbers (80). Counterbalancing this is a further study with terbutaline,

375 μg b.i.d. for 3 months, by Laitinen et al., who found a small decrease in T lymphocytes, mast cells, and plasma cells but no effect on eosinophil numbers (81). None of these three reported studies was placebo controlled. A placebo-controlled study of salbutamol therapy, administered at a dose of 200 μg q.i.d. for 4 months, found no significant effect on lavage or biopsy indices in comparison with placebo (82). There was a tendency for airway mucosal eosinophils to accumulate in the salbutamol treatment group in this study, in contrast to the previous studies, but this was not outside the variance of the placebo group.

D. Long-Acting β-Agonists

Four studies have been reported with the long-acting β-agonist salmeterol. These studies have addressed not only cell recruitment but also cell activation within the airway. One study reported a small but significant decrease in lavage ECP and a reduction in ex vivo macrophage oxidative metabolism following opsonized zymosan or PMA stimulation (74). This study assessed salmeterol therapy at a dose of 50 μg b.i.d. for 4 weeks in a placebo-controlled crossover study design. The other three studies failed to find any effect of regular salmeterol therapy (75,83,84) despite this therapy reducing symptoms, improving peak flow, and beneficially modifying measures of airway reactivity. Treatment was administered at a dose of 50 μg b.i.d. for 6 weeks in two studies and 8 weeks in the third. Measurement was made of lavage differential cell counts, lavage mediators (histamine, tryptase, ECP), lavage T-lymphocyte activation status by flow cytometry, and tissue cell populations (mast cells, eosinophils, and T lymphocytes). In the one study that assessed vascular permeability through measurements of albumin levels in lavage fluid, these were consistent in both the placebo and salmeterol group over the 6-week period.

Thus the findings in clinical asthma in which there is chronic inflammation differ from the findings in acute allergen–induced inflammation in which the limited studies available indicate some modification of cell activation or cell recruitment in the 48 hr following allergen exposure.

V. Conclusions

It is thus apparent from clinical studies that there is a difference between the regulatory effects of β-agonists on acute and chronic airway inflammation. With respect to the limited studies available, β-agonist pretreatment modifies aspects of cell activation and cell recruitment in the 48 hr following allergen exposure. These findings mirror, in part, the effects of β-agonists in animal models of asthma which have investigated the acute mucosal inflammatory reaction following allergic challenge and support in vitro findings that indicate that β-agonists inhibit mast cell degranulation. By contrast, the studies of β-agonists therapy in chronic asthma have failed to find a consistent effect on the underlying mucosal inflammatory process, although this mode of therapy provides symptomatic and physiological benefits. The reason for this discrepancy between the findings in relationship to acute and chronic airway inflammation is undefined but several possibilities exist.

First, it is possible, indeed probable, that the regulation of acute and chronic inflammation differs owing to differing mechanisms of inflammation (85). The acute response is largely mast cell dependent, whereas several cell populations generate cytokines in chronic disease and will contribute to leukocyte airway inflammation. These cell populations include, in addition to mast cells, T-lymphocyte epithelial cells, and eosinophils themselves (69). As these cells are less susceptible to the regulatory effects of β-adrenoceptor stimulation than mast cells, the impact of β-adrenoceptor theory may thus be less marked. The failure to demonstrate modification of lavage histamine and tryptase levels with regular salmeterol therapy, however, suggests that this is not the only explanation but that others should also be considered; in particular the potential that β-adrenoceptor responsiveness could be modified in chronic disease either in relationship to therapy or in relationship to the underlying inflammatory process.

The potential that regular β-agonist therapy itself downregulates β-responsiveness is covered in Chapters 2 and 3, so it will not be explored in detail here. It is pertinent, however, to consider that although β-agonists can be shown in vitro to induce a dose- and time-dependent downregulation of the inhibitory effects of β-agonists on immune-mediated mast cell degranulation (86), such investigations may not provide an in vivo explanation. In the studies investigating the effects of long-term β-agonist administration on airway inflammation in chronic asthma, the prior β-agonist administration was only as needed short-acting β-agonists. Such treatment, which was no different from that received by some patients in the acute challenge studies, is unlikely to have been sufficient to influence the subsequent β-agonist response. Hyporesponsiveness of the response to β-agonists can arise by mechanisms other than continued β-agonist administration. Autoantibodies directed against the extracellular or transmembrane-spanning domain of the β-adrenoceptor have been described in asthma and have been shown to have the potential to downregulate receptor expression or functionally antagonize the activation of the receptor (87). Such autoantibodies are, however, unlikely to explain the lack of effect of long-term β-agonist administration on airway inflammatory processes, as this treatment does not appear to have an impaired potential to induce sustained and long-lasting bronchodilatation. This discrepancy would be difficult to explain on the basis of a generalized receptor autoantibody. More probable is a local effect of the airway inflammatory process. This also has the potential to explain the discrepancy between the regulatory effects of β-agonists on acute and chronic inflammation, as the subjects participating in local endobronchial challenge studies to study the effects on acute inflammation generally have milder disease than those participating in chronic studies of clinical asthma. In support of a local effect of inflammation on β-adrenoceptor responsiveness, a defect in the β-receptor–G-protein coupling has been described in an animal model (88). Although b-agonists failed to induce intracellular cyclic AMP increases, agents acting by different receptors involving G-protein coupling such as PGE and NaF and direct stimulation by forskolin had unimpaired responses. That this defect is inducible has been established in in vitro organ bath culture studies (89). The cytokines TNF-α and IL-1β have been shown to modify β-adrenoceptor–mediated smooth muscle relaxation, whereas other cytokines, such as IL-2, were without effect. The impairment of β-adrenoceptor responsiveness with IL-1β was both time and dose dependent.

If patients participating in studies of chronic disease had more prolonged and severe airway inflammation than those participating in investigations of the impact of therapy on acute inflammation, then this could explain the discrepancy between the findings in acute and chronic asthma. In support of the importance of the patients' inflammation severity is the recent report of a regulatory effect of the long-acting β-agonist formoterol on airway inflammation in chronic asthma. This treatment reduced airway mast cells and eosinophils in mucosal biopsies with prolonged therapy. The patients studied all had very mild disease, as suggested by their histamine PC_{20} values and as needed β-agonist use. If the severity of inflammation does modify the potential effects of β-agonists, then it might be anticipated that if airway inflammation is modified by other therapy, such as an inhaled corticosteroid, then the co-administration of a long-acting b-agonist might provide some additional anti-inflammatory effect that was not evident when such a treatment was given alone. Such studies have not been undertaken, although clinical studies identify the greater effect of a long-acting β-agonist in combination with an inhaled steroid at a low dose than sole therapy with high-dose inhaled steroid therapy when symptom scores and bronchodilation are clinical endpoints (91,92).

References

1. Howarth PH. The airway inflammatory response in allergic asthma and its relationship to clinical disease. Allergy 1995; 50(suppl 22):13–21.
2. Barnes P. Beta-adrenoceptors in lung tissue. In: Morley J, ed. Beta-Adrenoceptors in Asthma. London: Academic Press, 1984:66–90.

3. Pesci A, Foresi A, Bertorelli G, Chetta A, Oliveri D. Histochemical characteristics and degranulation of mast cells in epithelium and lamin propria of bronchial biopsies from asthmatic and normal subjects. Am Rev Respir Dis 1993; 147:684–689.

4. Liu MC, Bleecker ER, Lichtenstein LM, Kagey-Sabotka A, Niv Y, McLemore TL, Permuth S, Proud D, Hubbard WC. Evidence for elevated levels of histamine, prostaglandin D_2, and other bronchoconstricting prostaglandins in the airways of subjects with mild asthma. Am Rev Respir Dis 1990; 142:126–132.

5. Wenzel SC, Fowler AA, Schwartz LB. Activation of pulmonary mast cells by bronchoalveolar allergen challenge: in vivo release of histamine and tryptase in atopic subjects with and without asthma. Am Rev Respir Dis 1988; 137:1002–1008.

6. Casale TB, Wood D, Richerson HB, Trapp S, Metzger WJ, Zavala D, Hunninghake GW. Elevated bronchoalveolar lavage fluid histamine levels in allergic asthmatics are associated with methacholine bronchial hyperresponsiveness. J Clin Invest 1987; 79:1197–1203.

7. Bradding P, Roberts JA, Britten KM, Montefort S, Djukanovic R, Mueller R, et al. Interleukins-4, -5 and -6 and tumour necrosis factor-α in normal and asthmatic airways: evidence for the human mast cell as a source of these cytokines. Am J Respir Cell Mol Biol 1994; 10:471–480.

8. Montefort S, Holgate ST, Howarth PH. Leucocyte-endothelial adhesion molecules and their role in bronchial asthma and allergic rhinitis. Eur Respir J 1993; 6:1044–1054.

9. Hattori R, Hamilton KK, Fugates RD, McEver RP, Sims PJ. Stimulates ecretion of endothelial von Willebrand factor is accompanied by rapid redistribution to the cell surface of the intracellular granule membrane protein GMP-140. J Biol Chem 1989; 264:7768–7771.

10. Pober JS, Gimbrone MA Jr, Lapierre LA, et al. Overlapping patterns of activation of human endothelial cells by interleukin-1, tumour necrosis factor and immune interferon. J Immunol 1986; 137:1893–1896.

11. Wellcome SM, Thornhill MH, Pitzalis C, et al. A monoclonal antibody that detects a novel antigen on endothelial cells that is induced by tumour necrosis factor, IL-1 or lipopolysaccharide. J Immunol 1990; 144:2558–2565.

12. Thornhill MH, Haskard DO. IL-4 regulates endothelial cell activation by IL-1, tumour necrosis factor, or IFNγ. J Immunol 1990; 145:865–872.

13. Ohkawar Y, Yamamouch K, Marnyama N, et al. In situ expression of the cell adhesion molecules in bronchial tissues from asthmatics with airflow limitation: in vivo evidence of VCAM-1/VLA-4 interactions in selective eosinophil infiltration. Am J Respir Cell Mol Biol 1995; 12:4–12.

14. Robinson DS, Hamid Q, Ying A, et al. Predominant TH2-like bronchoalveolar T-lymphocyte population in atopic asthma. N Engl J Med 1992; 326:298–304.

15. Ying S, Durham SR, Corrigan CJ, Hamid Q, Kay AB. Phenotype of cells expressing mRNA for TH2-type (interleukin-4 and interleukin-5) and TH1-type (interleukin-2 and interferon-γ) cytokines in bronchoalveolar lavage and bronchial biopsies from atopic asthmatic and normal control subjects. Am J Respir Cell Mol Biol 1995; 12:477–487.

16. Wilson JW, Djukanovic R, Howarth PH, Holgate ST. Lymphocyte activation in bronchoalveolar lavage and peripheral blood in atopic asthma. Am Rev Respir Dis 1992; 145:958–960.
17. Walker C, Kaegi MK, Braun P, Blaser K. Activated T-cells and eosinophilia in bronchoalveolar lavages from subjects with asthma correlated with disease severity. J Allergy Clin Immunol 1991; 88:935–942.
18. Weller PF. The mobilisation and activation of eosinophils. In: Jolles G, Karlsson JA, Taylor J, eds. T-Lymphocyte and Inflammatory Cell Research in Asthma. New York: Academic Press, 1993:115–131.
19. Zhang S, Howarth PH, Roche WR. Cytokine production by cell cultures from bronchoscopic subepithelial myofibroblasts. J Pathol. In press.
20. Marini M, Soloperto M, Mazzetti M, Fasoli A, Mattoli S. Interleukin-1 binds to specific receptors on human bronchial epithelial cells and upregulates granulocyte/macrophage colony-stimulating factor synthesis and release. Am J Respir Cell Mol Biol 1991; 4:519–524.
21. Cromwell O, Hamid Q, Corrigan CJ, et al. Expression and generation of interleukin-8, IL-6 and granulocyte-macrophage colony-stimulating factor by bronchial epithelial cells and enhancement by IL-1β and tumour necrosis factor-α. Immunology 1992; 77:330–337.
22. Sousa AR, Lane SJ, Nakhosteen JA, Yoshimura T, Lee TH, Poston RN. Increased expression of monocyte chemoattractant protein-1 in bronchial tissue from asthmatic subjects. Am J Respir Cell Mol Biol 1994; 10:142–147.
23. Wang JH, Devalia JL, Xin C, Sapsford RJ, Davies RJ. Expression of RANTES by human bronchial epithelial cells in vitro and in vivo and the effects of corticosteroids. Am J Respir Cell Mol Biol 1996; 14:27–35.
24. Alam R, Stafford S, Forsythe P, et al. RANTES is a chemotactic and activating factor for human eosinophils. J Immunol 1993; 150:3442–3447.
25. Shute JK, Lindley I, Reicht P, Holgate ST, Church MK, Djukanovic R. Mucosal IgA is an important moderator of eosinophil responses to tissue-derived chemoattractants. Int Arch Allergy Immunol 1995; 107:340–341.
26. Walls AF, Shaoheng H, Teran LM. Granulocyte recruitment by human mast cell tryptase. Int Arch Allergy Immunol 1995; 107:372–373.
27. Shute JK, Tenor H, Church MK, Schudt C. Theophylline inhibits GM-CSF release from eosinophils (abstr). Eur Respir J 1995; 8(suppl 19):9s.
28. Godding V, Stark JM, Sedgwick JB, Busse WW. Adhesion of activated eosinophils to respiratory epithelial cells is enhanced by tumour necrosis factor-α and interleukin-1β. Am J Respir Cell Mol Biol 1995; 13:555–562.
29. Motojima S, Frigas E, Loegering DA, Gleich GJ. Toxicity of eosinophil cationic proteins for guinea pig tracheal epithelium in vitro. Am Rev Respir Dis 1989; 139:801–805.
30. Frigas E, Loegering DA, Solley GO, Farrow GM, Gleich GJ. Elevated levels of the eosinophil granule major basic protein in the sputum of patients with bronchial asthma. Mayo Clin Proc 1981; 56:345–353.
31. Filley WV, Holley KE, Kephart GM, Gleich GJ. Identification of immunofluorescence of eosinophil granule major basic protein in lung tissue of patients with bronchial asthma. Lancet 1982; 2:11–16.

32. Roche WR, Beasley R, Williams JH, Holgate ST. Subepithelial fibrosis in the bronchi of asthmatics. Lancet 1989; 1:520–524.

33. Brewster CEP, Howarth PH, Djukanovic R, Wilson J, Holgate ST, Roche WR. Myofibroblasts and subepithelial fibrosis in bronchial asthma. Am J Respir Cell Mol Biol 1990; 3:507–511.

34. Redington AE, Madden J, Frew AJ, et al. Basic fibroblast growth factor in asthma: immunolocalisation in bronchial biopsies and measurement in bronchoalveolar lavage fluid at baseline and following allergen challenge. Am J Respir Crit Care Med 1995; 151:A702.

35. Springall DR, Howarth PH, Counihan H, Djukanovic R, Holgate ST, Polak JM. Endothelin immunoreactivity of airway epithelium in asthmatic patients. Lancet 1991; 337:697–701.

36. Norrby K. Mast cell histamine, a local mitogen acting via H2-receptors in nearby tissue cells. Virchows Archives B 1980; 34:13–20.

37. Roche WR. Mast cells and tumours. The specific enhancement of tumour proliferation in vitro. Am J Pathol 1985; 119:57–64.

38. Ruoss SJ, Hartmann T, Caughey GH. Mast cell tryptase is a mitogen for cultured fibroblasts. J Clin Invest 1991; 88:493–499.

39. Wiggs BR, Bosken C, Pare PD, James A, Hogg JC. A model of airway narrowing in asthma and in chronic obstructive pulmonary disease. Am Rev Respir Dis 1992; 145:1251–1258.

40. Beasley R, Roche WR, Roberts JA, Holgate ST. Cellular events in the bronchi in mild asthma and after bronchial provocation. Am Rev Respir Dis 1989; 139:806–817.

41. Wardlaw AJ, Dunnette S, Gleich GJ, Collins JV, Kay AB. Eosinophils and mast cells in bronchoalveolar lavage in subjects with mild asthma: relationship to bronchial reactivity. Am Rev Respir Dis 1988l 137:62–69.

42. Weiss JW, Drazen JM, McFadden ER, et al. Comparative bronchoconstrictor effects of histamine and leukotrienes C and D (LTC and LTD) in normal human volunteers. Clin Res 1982; 30:517A.

43. Schild HO. Histamine release and anaphylactic shock in isolated lungs of guinea-pigs. Q J Exp Med 1936; 26:165.

44. Butchers PR, Fullarton JR, Skidmore JF, Thompson LE, Vardey CJ, Wheeldon A. A comparison of the anti-anaphylactic activities of salbutamol and disodium cromoglycate in the rat, the rat mast cell and in human lung tissues. Br J Pharmacol 1979; 67:23–32.

45. Church MK, Young KD. The characteristics of histamine release from human lung fragments by sodium cromoglycate, salbutamol and chlorpromazine. Br J Pharmacol 1983; 78:671–679.

46. Church MK, Hiroi J. Inhibition of IgE dependent histamine release from human dispersed mast cells by antiallergic drugs and salbutamol. Br J Pharmacol 1987; 90:421–429.

47. Johnson M. Mechanisms of action of β-adrenoceptor agonists. In: Costello JF, Mann RS, eds. Beta-agonists in the Treatment of Asthma. Carnforth, UK: Parthenon, 1992:27–42.

48. Butchers PR, Vardey C, Johnson M. Salmeterol: a potent and long acting inhibitor of inflammatory mediator release from human lung. Br J Pharmacol 1991; 104: 672–676.

49. Whelan CJ, Johnson M. Inhibition by salmeterol of increased vascular permeability and granulocyte accumulation in guinea-pig lung and skin. Br J Pharmacol 1992; 105:831–838.

50. Sanjar S, McCabe PJ, Humbles AH. Inhibition by salmeterol of antigen-induced eosinophil accumulation in guinea pig lung. Eur Respir J 1991; 4(suppl 13–14): 200s.

51. Anderson GP. Pharmacology of formoterol: an innovative bronchodilator. Agents Actions 1991; 34:97–115.

52. Nials AT, Whelan CJ, Vardey CJ. Salmeterol inhibits neutrophil accumulation in rat lungs. Br J Pharmacol 1991; 104:292P.

53. Whelan CJ, Johnson M. Salmeterol, but not salbutamol, has anti-inflammatory activity in guinea-pig skin. Br J Pharmacol 1991; 102:95P.

54. Tokuyama K, Lotvall JO, Lofdahl CG, Barnes PJ, Chung KF. Inhaled formoterol inhibits histamine-induced airflow obstruction and airway microvascular leakage. Eur J Pharmacol 1991; 193:35–39.

55. Wheelan CJ, Johnson M. The anti-inflammatory effects of inhaled salmeterol and salbutamol in guinea-pig lung. Br J Pharmacol 1990; 101:5288.

56. Duffy ME, Hainan B, Ho S, Bentzel DJ. Regulation of epithelial light junctions permeability by cyclic AMP. Nature 1981; 294:451–453.

57. Svensson C, Grieff L, Andersson M, Alkner U, Persson CGA. Antiallergic actions of high topical doses of terbutaline in human nasal airways. Allergy 1995; 50:884–890.

58. Yukawa T, Ukena D, Chanez P, Dent G, Chung KF, Barnes PJ. β-Adrenergic receptors on eosinophils: binding and functional studies. Am Rev Respir Dis 1990; 141:1446–1452.

59. Fuller RW, O'Malley G, Baker AJ, MacDermot J. Human alveolar macrophage activation: inhibition by forskolin but not β-adrenoceptor stimulation or phosphodiesterase inhibition. Pulm Pharmacol 1988; 1:101–106.

60. Johnson M. The pharmacology of salmeterol. Lung 1990; 168:115–119.

61. Baker AJ, Fuller RW. The anti-inflammatory effects of salmeterol on human alveolar macrophages. Am Rev Respir Dis 1990; 141:A394.

62. Wenzel SE, Fowler AA III, Schwartz LB. Activation of pulmonary mast cells by bronchoalveolar lavage: in vivo release of histamine and tryptase in atopic subjects with and without asthma. Am Rev Respir Dis 1988; 137:1002–1006.

63. Miadonna A, Tedeschi A, Brasca C, Folco G, Sala A, Murphy RC. Mediator release after endobronchial antigen challenge in patients with respiratory allergy. J Allergy Clin Immunol 1990; 85:906–913.

64. Liu MC, Hubbard WC, Proud D, et al. Immediate and late inflammatory responses to ragweed antigen challenge of the peripheral airways in allergic asthmatics: cellular, mediator and permeability changes. Am Rev Respir Dis 1991; 144:51–58.

65. Howarth PH, Durham SR, Lee TL, Kay AB, Church MK, Holgate ST. Influence of albuterol, cromolyn sodium and ipratropium bromide on the airway and circulating mediator response to allergen bronchial provocation in asthma. Am Rev Respir Dis 1985; 132:986–992.

66. De Monchy JGR, Kauffman HF, Venge P, et al. Bronchoalveolar lavage of allergic asthmatic patients following allergen provocation. Chest 1986; 89:477–483.

67. Montefort S, Gratziou C, Goulding D, Polosa R, Haskard DO, Howarth PH, Holgate ST, Carroll MP. Bronchial biopsy evidence for leucocyte infiltration and upregulation of leucocyte-endothelial cell adhesion molecules 6 hours after local allergen challenge of sensitised asthmatic airway. J Clin Invest 1994; 93:1411–1421.

68. Asako H, Kurose I, Wolfe R, et al. Role of H_1 receptors and P-selectin in histamine-induced leucocyte rolling and adhesion in postcapillary venules. J Clin Invest 1994; 93:1508–1515.

69. Howarth PH, Bradding P, Quint D, Redington AE, Holgate ST. Cytokines and airway inflammation. In: Chignard M, Pretolani M, Prenesto P, Vargaftig B, eds. Cells and Cytokines in Lung Inflammation 1993. Ann NY Acad Sci 1994; 725: 68–82.

70. Cockcroft DW, Murdock KY. Protective effect of inhaled albuterol, cromolyn, beclomethasone and placebo on allergen-induced early asthmatic responses, late asthmatic responses and allergen induced increases in bronchial responsiveness to inhaled histamine. J Allergy Clin Immunol 1987; 79:734–740.

71. Twentyman OP, Finnerty JP, Holgate ST. The inhibitory effect of nebulised albuterol on the early and late phase reactions and increase in airway responsiveness provoked by inhaled allergen in asthma. Am Rev Respir Dis 1991; 144:782–787.

72. Twentyman OP, Finnerty JP, Harris A, Palmer J, Holgate ST. Protection against allergen-induced asthma by salmeterol. Lancet 1990; 236:1338–1342.

73. Palmqvist M, Balder B, Lowhagen O, Melander B, Svedmyr N, Wahlander L. Late asthmatic reaction decreased after pretreatment with salbutamol and formoterol, a new long-acting β_2-agonist. J Allergy Clin Immunol 1992; 89:844–849.

74. Dahl R, Pederson B, Larsen BB. The influence of salmeterol on reactions after allergen challenge and the variations in bronchial hyper-reactivity, blood eosinophils and serum-ECP and the influence of salmeterol on bronchial mucosa and BAL. In: Johnson M, ed. Acute and Chronic Inflammation in the Respiratory Tract. London, UK: Colwood House, 1995:70–72.

75. Boulet LP, Turcotte H, Boulet M, Dube J, Gagnon MA, Lavidette M. Effects of salmeterol on chronic and allergen-induced airway inflammation in mild allergic asthma. In: Johnson M, ed. Acute and Chronic Inflammation in the Respiratory Tract. London, UK: Colwood House, 1995:66.

76. Murray JJ, Hagemara DD, Dworksi R, Steller JR. Effect of salmeterol and beclomethasone on the late phase response to sequential antigen challenge in man. In: Johnson M, ed. Acute and Chronic Inflammation in the Respiratory Tract. London, UK: Colwood House, 1995:64.

78. Calhoun WJ, Hinton KL, Brick JJ, Vuchinich T. Effects of almeterol on eosinophil recruitment to the airway following segmental antigen challenge in atopic asthmatics. In: Johnson M, ed. Acute and Chronic Inflammation in the Respiratory Tract. London, UK: Colwood House, 1995:62.
79. Adelroth E, Rosenhall L, Johansson SA, Linden M, Venge P. Inflammatory cells and eosinophilic activity in asthmatics investigated by bronchoalveolar lavage: the effects of anti-asthmatic treatment with budesonide and terbutaline. Am Rev Respir Dis 1990; 142:91–99.
80. Jefferey PK, Godfrey RW, Adelroth E, et al. Effects of treatment on airway inflammation and thickening of basement membrane reticular collagen in asthma. Am Rev Respir Dis 1992; 145:890–899.
81. Laitinen LA, Laitinen A, Haahtela T. A comparative study of the effects of an inhaled corticosteroid, budesonide and a β2 agonist, terbutaline, on airway inflammation in newly diagnosed asthma: a randomised, double-blind, parallel group controlled study. J Allergy Clin Immunol 1992; 90:32–42.
82. Davies RJ, Trigg CJ, Wang JH, et al. Regular inhaled salbutamol may exacerbate bronchial inflammation in patients with mild asthma. Thorax 1993; 48: 1060–1064.
83. Kraft M, Bettinger CM, Pak J, et al. Salmeterol decreases nocturnal symptoms and β-agonist use in nocturnal asthma without altering airway inflammation. In: Johnson M, ed. Acute and Chronic Inflammation in the Respiratory Tract. London, UK: Colwood House, 1995:68.
84. Howarth PH, Roberts JA, Bradding P, Walls AE, Holgate ST. The influence of β-agonists on airway inflammation in asthma. In: Costello JF, Mann RD, eds. Beta-agonists in the Treatment of Asthma. Carnforth, UK: Parthenon, 1992:69–77.
85. Emanuel MB, Howarth PH. Asthma and anaphylaxis: a relevant model for chronic disease? An historical analysis of directions in asthma research. Clin Exp Allergy 1995; 25:15–26.
86. Chong LK, Morice AH, Yeo WW, Schleimer RP, Peachel PT. Functional desensitisation of β-agonist responses in human lung mast cells. Am J Respir Cell Mol Biol 1995; 13:540–546.
87. Turki J, Liggett SB. Receptor-specific functional properties of β2-adrenergic receptor autoantibodies in asthma. Am J Respir Cell Mol Biol 1995; 12:531–539.
88. Emala C, Black C, Curry C, Levine M, Hirshman CH. Impaired β-adrenergic receptor activation of adenyl cyclase in airway smooth muscle in the Basenji-greyhound dog model of airway hyperresponsiveness. Am J Respir Cell Mol Biol 1993; 8:668–675.
89. Wills-Karp M, Uchinda Y, Lee JY, Jinot J, Hirata A, Hirata F. Organ culture with pro-inflammatory cytokines reproduces improvement of the β-adrenoceptor mediated relaxation in tracheas of a guinea-pig antigen model. Am J Respir Cell Mol Biol 1993; 8:153–159.

91. Greening AP, Ind PW, Northfield M, Shaw G. Added salmeterol versus higher-dose corticosteroid in asthma patients with symptoms on existing inhaled corticosteroid. Lancet 1994; 344:219–229.
92. Woolcock A, Lundback B, Ringdal OLN, Jaques LA. Comparison of the effect of addition of salmeterol with doubling the inhaled steroid dose in asthmatic patients. Am J Respir Crit Care Med 1994; 149(suppl):A280.

Discussion

RONALD DAHL

Århus University Hospital, Århus, Denmark

The following data about long acting inhaled β-agonists concern salmeterol.

Treatment of bronchial asthma with inhaled salmeterol does not change the numbers and composition of inflammatory cells in BAL and bronchial mucosal biopsies. However, recent studies have shown that pretreatment with inhaled salmeterol reduces markers of inflammatory cell activation in response to an allergen challenge. Dahl et al. (1) studied 12 patients with allergen-induced early- and late-phase reactions in the lungs. In a double-blind, randomized, placebo-controlled study, the influence on the early- and late-phase reaction, postchallenge change in PC_{20} histamine, blood eosinphils, and serum ECP were evaluated. Pretreatment with salmeterol abolished the early- and late-phase bronchoconstriction and the postchallenge increase in histamine reactivity. Salmeterol had no influence on the rise in blood eosinophils, but serum ECP was unaltered after salmeterol but was elevated after placebo pretreatment.

Serum ECP is considered a marker of eosinophil activation, and pretreatment with salmeterol inhibited the eosinophil activation but not the number of eosinophils. This effect would of course be more marked if the amount of serum ECP per blood eosinophil was calculated.

In another study (2), the same authors performed BAL in 12 patients after a 4-week randomized, double-blind, crossover treatment with placebo or salmeterol, 50 μg b.i.d. An inflammatory score of the bronchial mucosa was significantly reduced after salmeterol. After salmeterol, the oxidative metabolism of isolated macrophages was reduced after stimulation with opsonized zymosan and a small, but significant, increase in BAL ECP was seen. This study showed an influence of salmeterol on activity markers of macrophages and eosinophils as well as a reduction of macroscopic inflammatory signs in the bronchial mucosa.

Boulet et al. (3) have presented preliminary results from a placebo-controlled parallel group study with 2 months' treatment with either salmeterol,

$50\,\mu g \times 2$ (seven patients) or placebo (six patients). At the end of the treatment period, an allergen challenge was performed. BAL and bronchial biopsies were obtained before and after the allergen challenge. The bronchoconstrictor responses were decreased in the salmeterol group, but BAL total and differential cell counts before and after allergen challenge were similar in both groups. Comparison of postchallenge data of the two groups showed that AA1-, HLA-DR-, and CD45ro-positive cell counts were reduced in the salmeterol group. When pre- and postchallenge data were pooled, the salmeterol group had lower numbers of CD3-, CD25-, HLA-DR-, AA1-, CD45-, and CD45ro-positive cells. The study showed that salmeterol reduced some of the bronchial mucosa markers for expression of cell activation.

In a recent study, Calhoun et al. (4) studied 10 atopic asthmatics in a randomized double-blind, placebo-controlled, crossover study. The participants inhaled placebo or salmeterol twice daily for 7 days at 3-week intervals. On the fifth day of each treatment period, patients underwent segmental antigen challenge and BAL immediately and 48 hr afterwards. Immediately after segmental allergen challenge, salmeterol treatment gave no significant changes in any BAL parameter. However, 48 hr later, a significant reduction in the proportion and number of BAL eosinophils were seen in salmeterol-treated patients. In addition, PMA-stimulated superoxide generation from unfractionated BAL cells was significantly reduced by salmeterol. This study showed that salmeterol reduced the eosinophil influx and superoxide release following segmental allergen challenge.

In a preliminary report, Murray et al. (5) studied 10 patients who underwent segmental allergen challenge following randomized treatments with placebo, beclomethasone diproprionate (BDP), or salmeterol. The segment was lavaged 24 hr after the challenge. Pretreatment with BDP resulted in reduction in the percentage of eosinophils and a slight reduction in IL-4 and IL-5 in the lavage. Pretreatment with salmeterol resulted in a reduction in ECP, IL-4, and IL-5 in the lavage fluid from the segment challenged. There was no difference between treatments in LTC_4 lavage concentration. This study indicates that salmeterol reduced acute activation of inflammatory mediator cells in response to segmental allergen challenge.

Previous in vitro studies and experimental animal studies have shown an inhibitory effect of salmeterol on allergen-induced cell activities such as mast cell mediator release, macrophage and neutrophil superoxide generation, vascular permeability, and others. The recent above-mentioned studies also support the opinion that β-agonists do not influence chronic inflammation measured as cell numbers and differentials in BAL and bronchial mucosal biopsies. However, pretreatment with long-acting β-agonists before allergen challenge inhibit the allergen-induced increases in markers of cell activation.

References

1. Pedersen B, Dahl R, Larsen BB, Venge P. The effect of salmeterol on the early and late-phase reaction to bronchial allergen and postchallenge variation in bronchial reactivity, blood eosinophils, serum eosinophil cationic protein and serum eosinophil protein X. Allergy 1993; 48:377–382.
2. Dahl R, Pederson B, Venge P. Bronchoalveolar lavage studies. Eur Respir Rev 1991; 14:272–275.
3. Boulet LP, Turcotte H, Boutet M, Dubé J, Gagnon M, Laviolette M. Effects of salmeterol on chronic and allergen-induced airway inflammation in mild allergic asthma. In: International Respiratory Forum. Acute and Chronic Inflammation in the Respiratory Tract. London: Colwood House, 1995:66.
4. Calhoun WJ, Hinton KL, Brick JJ, Vuchinich T. Effects of salmeterol on eosinophil recruitment on the airway following segmental antigen challenge in atopic asthmatics. In: International Respiratory Forum. Acute and Chronic Inflammation in the Respiratory Tract. London: Colwood House, 1995:62.
5. Murray JJ, Hagaman DD, Dworksi R, Sheller JR. Effect of salmeterol and beclomethasone on the late-phase response to segmental antigen challenge in man. In: International Respiratory Forum. Acute and Chronic Inflammation in the Respiratory Tract. London: Colwood House, 1995:64.

5

Pharmacokinetics of Beta$_2$-Adrenoceptor–Stimulating Drugs

LARS NYBERG

Astra Draco AB and Uppsala University
Lund, Sweden

I. Introduction

The basis for the development of β_2-agonists was epinephrine, so the first drugs of this kind were catecholamines (Fig. 1). An example is isoproterenol. To increase metabolic stability, metaproterenol (orciprenaline) was synthesized as a resorcinolamine that is resistant to the enzyme catechol O-methyl transferase (COMT). Metaproterenol also resists metabolism catalyzed by mono-amino oxidase (MAO) (1). However, metaproterenol is not much more β_2-selective than isoproterenol (2,3). The resorcinolamines fenoterol and terbutaline have larger substituents on the nitrogen which gives them a high β_2-selectivity.

Albuterol (salbutamol) represents another way of avoiding COMT metabolism. The aromatic ring is salicyl alcohol (saligenin). A bulky nitrogen substituent protects albuterol from MAO-catalyzed metabolism and gives it β_2-selectivity.

Figure 1 shows a variety of β_2-selective compounds. As marked by asterisks, they all contain at least one asymmetrical carbon; fenoterol, formoterol, and procaterol have two. At each asymmetrical (chiral) center, the steric

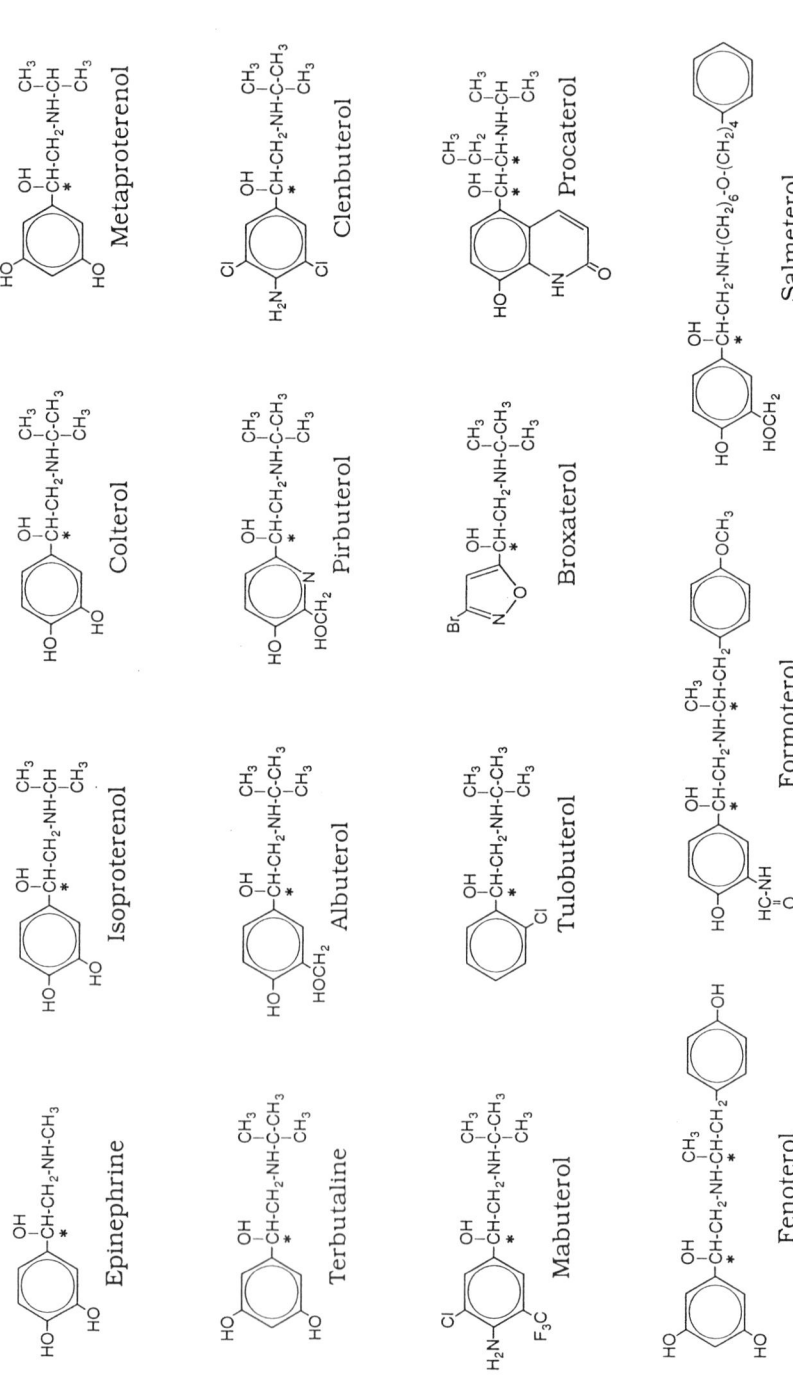

Figure 1   Structural formulae of epinephrine and a number of β-agonists. Asterisks mark asymmetrical carbon atoms.

configuration of the substituents can be either "R" or "S" (4). Thus, the structures given in Figure 1 have at least two stereoisomers that are mirror images of each other (enantiomers); those with two chiral centers have two such enantiomeric pairs. β_2-agonists are used in clinical practice as racemates; that is, equimolar mixtures of enantiomers that have different pharmacological activity. In fenoterol and formoterol, the pair of R,R and S,S is used (5,6), whereas procaterol is a mixture of R,S and S,R (7).

The potent isomers have R-configuration at the carbon adjacent to the primary ring structure (β-carbon), and so far this configuration has been connected with levo(–)rotation of polarized light. On the contrary, S-configuration at the β-carbon has implied dextro(+)rotation and weaker, often negligible, adrenergic effect.

As weak bases the β_2-agonists are ionized in body fluids. Except for albuterol, they are administered as salts of inorganic or organic acids. Their lipophilic properties vary considerably, which has importance for their absorption and distribution in the body. The most hydrophilic substance is terbutaline (author's own data). The highest lipophilicity has salmeterol with a distribution coefficient between octanol and water (pH 7.4) which is 4000 times that of albuterol and more than 20 times that of formoterol (8). Clenbuterol and mabuterol are also lipophilic as reflected by their octanol/water distribution coefficients, which for clenbuterol is 300 times that of albuterol (9).

The pharmacokinetics of substances such as albuterol and terbutaline have been documented in many aspects, whereas the knowledge about some of the others is scarce. In the following sections, available pharmacokinetic information will be given with particular emphasis on β_2-agonists which are being used in asthma therapy in the 1990s.

II. Analytical Methods

Early studies of the pharmacokinetics of β_2-agonists were performed with radioactive tracer techniques (10–13). Radioimmunoassay methods were later developed (14). From the middle of the 1970s, the progress of combined gas chromatography–mass spectrometry (GC-MS) methodology made it possible to measure unlabeled substances in body fluids and tissues (15–20). In the early 1980s, liquid chromatographic procedures became sufficiently sensitive for biological samples when combined with fluorimetric or amperometric detectors (21–25). Sensitive enzyme immunoassays for clenbuterol and mabuterol have been developed (26,27). Separation of albuterol enantiomers in urine was performed by use of an α_1-acid glycoprotein column (28) and of terbutaline enantiomers in plasma by use of a β-cyclodextrin column (29, 30).

III. Routes of Administration

A. Systemic Administration

Immediate access to the systemic blood is only offered by direct injection, usually intravenously. After subcutaneous administration, the drug has an absorption phase. After subcutaneous injection of terbutaline sulfate, a plasma concentration peak was not observed until after 20–30 min (11,31). The urinary recovery of intact drug was about 60%, which is similar to or only slightly less than what was found after intravenous dosing of terbutaline (11,32).

Absorption of β_2-agonists after oral administration is very much a function of their lipophilicity. Thus, absorption from the gut of the hydrophilic terbutaline is about 50% (33). Fenoterol is absorbed to about 60% (34). The lipophilic substances clenbuterol and mabuterol are completely absorbed (35, 36). Also albuterol, although being of a more hydrophilic character, appears to be completely absorbed (10,37,38).

Not seldom does the curve of plasma concentration versus time after oral administration of a β_2-agonist show one early peak at 1–2 hr and another considerably later (11,39–41). Adrenergic stimulation retards gastric emptying (42). Thus, an explanation to the double plasma concentration peak might be that the first portion of β_2-agonist entering the gut retards the emptying from the stomach of the remaining portion.

Presystemic Metabolism

As a result of presystemic metabolism, the bioavailability of most β_2-agonists will not be 100% even if absorption is complete. Enzymes in the gut are able to metabolise carboxylic ester bonds to some extent as illustrated at oral administration of the β_2-agonist prodrug bitolterol (43). Gut wall enzymes conjugate β_2-agonists with phenolic structure (44,45). In humans, conjugation with sulfate usually predominates (11,46), but for some substances, glucuronidation is more important (47,48). Cytosolic fractions from tissue specimens of human ileum showed similar activity of sulfotransferase and glucuronyltransferase (49). In samples from the colon, however, the activity of sulfotransferase was reduced but glucuronidation activity remained the same. Whether sulfation or glucuronidation predominates is also dependent on the availability of the necessary cosubstrates (3'-phosphoadenosine-5'-phosphosulfate [PAPS] and uridine diphosphate glucuronic acid [UDPGA]) (49).

A comparison between terbutaline nonrenal clearance after intravenous administration in humans and liver plasma flow indicates that the liver should be responsible for at the most 10% of terbutaline's first-pass metabolism. Thus, at least 90% of its presystemic metabolism would take place in the gut wall (50). The estimation is supported by the finding of a 10–30 times higher rate of terbutaline sulfation in specimens of human ileum and duodenum as compared with liver specimens (51). In rats (though they first-pass conjugate with glucuronic acid), very little intact terbutaline was found in the urine after oral administration, in contrast with the findings after injection intraportally or intraperitoneally (52). In situ studies of the fate of isoproterenol in jejunal loops of dogs, with sampling of venous blood leaving the loop, showed a massive conjugation with sulfate if the compound was administered in the lumen (53). No conjugation was observed if isoproterenol was delivered to the loop intra-arterially (54). These findings indicate that the conjugating enzymes are located in the mucosal layer of the gut wall. However, conjugation is not exclusively a first-pass effect after oral administration; conjugates of β₂-agonists are found to a lesser extent also after intravenous delivery (11,55,56).

B. Inhalation

Inhalation has become the preferred administration route for β₂-agonists because of the delivery close to the target and the low dose leading to less systemic side effects. In vitro experiments in animals suggest that more hydrophilic compounds like terbutaline, isoproterenol, and albuterol reach the lung receptors more efficiently from the systemic side than from the trachea. This contrasts with lipophilic substances that were found to pass the airway epithelium rapidly and were also more retained in the tissue (57). The local concentration in the small volume of airway fluids will be very much higher than in plasma after systemic administration (58,59). This gives a favorable concentration gradient promoting rapid absorption and may also be one reason why inhalation often gives additional spirometric effect above what can be maximally achieved with systemic administration.

The inhalation technique and the devices used are of utmost importance for the degree of drug deposition in the airways and the localization within them. These issues are discussed by Dolovich and Borgström in Chapter 10. Suffice it to say here that even optimum delivery by inhalation is far from complete. Not seldom is the delivery to the lungs as low as 10% or less (60,61). A considerable part of the dose is retained in the device and a large fraction, up to 70–80% at direct inhalation, is usually swallowed, absorbed in the gut, and subjected to presystemic metabolism. Early pharmacokinetic studies with nebulized albuterol (62,63) suggested that although there were great losses in the nebulizer, tubing, and expelled/expired air, the dose that did reach the patient was better targeted to the lung than a dose delivered from a pressurized metered-dose inhaler (PMDI) (38). This has been confirmed by gamma camera imaging using [99mTc] as marker (64). The amount of albuterol deposited in the lungs was found to be very similar from a nebulizer and from a PMDI, but very little was swallowed after nebulization. In addition, a greater proportion of the nebulized drug was deposited at peripheral sites of the airways.

Lung Absorption

As compared with administration into the gut, substances applied in solution intratracheally in the rat were rapidly absorbed and usually by passive diffusion even if carrier-mediated transport was observed in some cases (e.g., disodium cromoglycate) (65). Lipid-soluble drugs had absorption half-lives below 1 min. There was a relation between lipophilicity expressed as the distribution ratio between chloroform and water (pH 7.4) and the absorption rate. Very hydrophilic substances as a group were slowly absorbed, with the half-life of absorption being even above 1 hr, and among them absorption did not show a correlation with lipophilicity (66). This may be explained by transfer of lipophilic substances through cell membranes of the epithelium, whereas hydrophilic substances predominantly pass paracellularly small molecular size favoring passage (65).

There has been much dispute concerning the most suitable localization of bronchodilators in the bronchial tree before absorption. It appears that absorption is faster in the alveoli and subsegmental bronchi than in trachea (67,68). To achieve bronchodilation in humans, however, it seems that the localization is not so important (64,69,70). An explanation might be that the tracheobronchial circulation will distribute the drug within the lung.

Traditional pharmacokinetic methods cannot be used for studies of the absorption of drug from the airways. One reason is that concentrations found in systemic plasma are not reflecting concentrations at the target. Another reason is the fact that since so much of the dose is swallowed, inhalation is a hybrid between local and systemic administration. Occasionally, swallowing of the drug can be avoided by direct instillation of the drug into the bronchi (71, 72). Otherwise, measurements of deposition in the lungs by means of [99mTc]-labeled Teflon (73) or drug (74–76) particles will often give a good estimate of the fraction available for absorption in the airways. However, if drug particles are labeled, care has to be taken to avoid possible changes of particle size (77).

To get a true figure of absorption or—in the case of lung metabolism—bioavailability, it is desirable to measure what is really taken up by the airways and then cleared into the blood. One way to do this was introduced by Davies (61) in which he blocked the uptake of drug (terbutaline) in the gut by administration of activated charcoal. By measuring the amount excreted in urine and comparing it with the amount excreted after intravenous administration, Davies was able to calculate the amount absorbed by the lung. Borgström (78) refined the technique by giving the intravenous terbutaline dose simultaneously with the inhalation. This was possible by use of deuterated substance as the intravenous reference.

A comparison was recently made between a gamma camera imaging method (76) and the method blocking gastrointestinal absorption by activated charcoal (78). In the comparison (32), dry powder terbutaline sulfate from the inhaler (Turbuhaler, Astra, Sweden) was inhaled. The gamma camera method gave a higher index of lung deposition: 27% of the metered dose as compared with 21% by the charcoal method. The reason for the difference is not clear; possibly part of the deposited drug was not absorbed in the airways but transported by mucociliary clearance to the pharynx. If so, the methods are complementary in that the imaging method estimates the amount of drug deposited and its regional localization in the airways, whereas the charcoal method measures what is indeed absorbed.

Absorption During Exercise and Through Damaged Lung Epithelium

By use of ^{99m}Tc-labeled diethylenetriamine pentaacetate (DTPA), Ilowite et al. (79) found that the epithelial permeability for that substance was more than doubled in asthmatic patients as compared with healthy subjects. In comparison with a normal preparation, Jeppsson et al. (80) found a threefold increase of terbutaline efflux into an external medium after administration of the drug into a tracheal preparation where the epithelium had been damaged by exposure to hydrogen peroxide. Schmekel et al. (81) compared smokers and nonsmokers regarding their ability to absorb inhaled terbutaline. The peak plasma concentration was about 70% higher and occurred three times earlier (at 17 min) in the smokers. The extent of absorption was, however, the same in smokers and nonsmokers. Schanker (65) proposed that the damaged lung has increased porosity of the epithelium facilitating the uptake of hydrophilic molecules.

Schmekel et al. (82) also studied the effect of exercise on the absorption rate of terbutaline and found that healthy subjects (nonsmokers) absorbed the drug faster if the inhalation was followed by a 30-min exercise. They suggested the observation to be a result of increased blood flow or altered surface tension of the liquid layer in the lumen.

Lung Metabolism

In the respiratory tract, there are monooxygenases both of the cytochrome P-450–dependent type and those which contain flavins (83). As compared with the liver, however, the human lung has little cytochrome P-450 (83,84). The lungs have several mechanisms for protection of the heart and circulation from adrenergic influence. The existence of the enzymes COMT and MAO is well established but also demethylation may occur (85). Furthermore, there are esterases in the lungs able to metabolize prodrugs such as bitolterol and bambuterol (43,86).

Recently, in a study of cytosolic fractions from human lung, liver, and intestinal mucosa, it was reported that terbutaline was sulfated in the lung fraction at a rate higher than in the liver but lower than in the mucosal fraction

(51). However, extrapolation of these results to the intact lung may be fallacious. After endotracheal instillation in rats, no metabolism of terbutaline was detected (87). In isolated perfused canine lung, neither isoproterenol nor terbutaline was metabolized by sulfating enzymes (13). On instillation in patient bronchi, the metabolic pattern of albuterol in urine suggested that lung metabolism of the drug was of little importance (71).

C. Other Routes

Albuterol given in suppositories to children appeared to have a bioavailability comparable with oral administration (88). Sublingual administration of albuterol showed that buccal absorption was negligible in humans (89). This agrees with experiences in our laboratories with terbutaline. Nasal absorption of fenoterol in the order of 15% and with an absorption half-life of about 9 min (three to four times faster than after inhalation) has been reported (90).

IV. Common Pharmacokinetic Characteristics of β_2-Agonists

A. Linear Kinetics

The β_2-agonists are potent drugs with doses of a few milligrams at the most. Saturation of carrier mechanisms or enzyme systems is therefore not likely to occur at therapeutic dosages. Studies in children showed linear correlation between infusion rates of terbutaline and corresponding plateau plasma concentrations (91). In adults, sustained-release tablets of terbutaline or albuterol produced areas under the curve (AUCs) of plasma concentration versus time which were proportional to dose (92,93). Predose plasma concentrations of terbutaline in steady state increased linearly with the tablet dose in adults (94) and children (95). Clenbuterol tablets in single doses from 20 to 80 μg in healthy adults showed a linear increase of peak plasma concentration and excreted amount in urine, and multiple dosing with 20 and 40 μg every 12 hr had linear kinetics too (96). In humans, steady-state plasma concentrations with tablets of clenbuterol, tulobuterol, albuterol, and procaterol were predictable from single-dose data (35,97–99).

B. Correlation Between Plasma Concentration and Effect

After inhalation, the plasma concentration time course of a β_2-agonist tells little about the bronchodilating effect. After subcutaneous administration of single doses of terbutaline, hyperbolic relations between FEV_1 and plasma concentration were found (100,101). FEV_1 (1-sec forced expiratory volume) and plasma concentration could be correlated after intravenous terbutaline alone or on top of theophylline treatment (102). After a single oral dose of terbutaline in asthmatic patients, a clockwise hysteresis correlation was seen between FEV_1 and plasma terbutaline with initial linearity between 7 and 27 nmol/L (100). In a study with the terbutaline prodrug ibuterol, FEV_1 was back to start values when the terbutaline serum concentration had declined to about 6–7 nmol/L (39). In children, a correlation was observed between FEV_1 or peak expiratory flow (PEF) and plasma concentration of terbutaline in the individual patients during repeated treatment with oral terbutaline (95). However, FEV_1 reached plateau later and remained longer than the plasma concentrations after transdermal administration of terbutaline (103).

Spirometric measurements after subcutaneous administration of terbutaline have been correlated with calculated concentrations of the agonist in an assumed effect compartment (101). Relationships between effect (FEV_1 and forced mid-expiratory flow [FMEF]) and plasma concentration were modeled after intravenous infusions of terbutaline in 10 children (91). Half of the children had not reached maximal effect (E_{max}) despite plasma concentrations of terbutaline as high as 50–60 nmol/L.

Adult asthmatic patients well treated with oral terbutaline usually have plasma concentrations in the range 10–30 nmol/L. Corresponding values with albuterol are more than two times higher (104,105). These concentrations should not be used as a target for the treatment; some patients do well both below and above the range. Instead, therapy with β_2-agonists should be monitored by the therapeutic response and the occurrence and severity of side effects.

Side effects associated with β_2-agonists, such as an increase of heart rate and tremor, are frequently correlated with plasma concentrations of the β_2-agonists, although there is a great variability among patients (94,102,106). However, the situation is not clear-cut; for instance, it was reported (39) that tremor lagged behind the plasma concentration of terbutaline and decreased faster than the concentration. Insulin responded directly to intravenous terbutaline, whereas the glucose and potassium responses in plasma lagged (106).

C. Distribution Within the Body

Distribution to Solid Tissues

Most of the knowledge of distribution of β_2-agonists is derived from animal experiments. All of the compounds have been found in liver, kidney, and lung. Lipophilic substances appear to have more access to the central nervous system; in rats, clenbuterol given intravenously 1 hr after ^{125}I-iodopindolol greatly reduced radioactivity both in cerebral cortex and cerebellum. Albuterol had no such effect (9). In beagle dogs, 0.5 hr after intravenous administration, the concentration of intact clenbuterol in the brain was 0.7 times that in plasma, whereas the concentration of albuterol given under the same conditions was not measurable in the brain (<8.4 pmol/g). Clenbuterol had a relatively higher distribution than albuterol to bronchi and pulmonary tissue, but albuterol showed more preference to heart muscle (107).

The heart muscle/plasma concentration ratio (2.5:1.0) found with albuterol in the above-mentioned dog experiments is virtually identical with the same ratio for terbutaline found in a deceased asthmatic patient (108). The concentration of terbutaline in skeletal muscle from that patient was 4.6 times higher than in plasma.

Binding and Distribution Within Blood

Plasma protein binding of albuterol and terbutaline is low: 8 and about 20%, respectively (56,109). These findings contrast with the high-protein binding of lipophilic β_2-agonists: salmeterol 94–98% (110) and clenbuterol ≥90% (96).

For terbutaline, an equilibrium erythrocyte to plasma concentration ratio of about 2 has been determined (111–113). The uptake is slow; half-life of the process in vitro at ambient temperature was between 3.5 and 8.5 hr (111) and in humans 2–3 hr (112). It took more than 0.5 hr for the drug to redistribute from erythrocytes to a new equilibrium in freshly added plasma (113). The latter observation implies that terbutaline—and probably other β_2-agonists— will hardly leave the erythrocytes during a passage through the liver or the kidneys. In calculations of clearance of these substances, therefore, plasma flow and not blood flow should be used.

Passage Over the Placenta

Albuterol and terbutaline traverse the placenta to the fetus (114–117). As shown with terbutaline, equilibration is slow: Not until after 3 hr was equilibrium reached, but then the ratio of the concentrations of intact drug in maternal and umbilical vein blood was close to 1 (112). Studies with fenoterol (118) give similar information, with equilibrium concentrations in umbilical cord blood being about 90% of those in maternal venous blood. Reports describing low placental transfer of β_2-agonists may therefore be of questionable value; at least when they deal with the hydrophilic substances.

Distribution to Breast Milk

Concentrations of terbutaline in the milk from four nursing mothers taking oral terbutaline regularly were the same or higher than the corresponding concentrations in plasma, with the ratios varying from 0.9 to 2.9 (119). Mean concentrations of terbutaline in the milk samples were between 14 and 17 nmol/L. This means that the amounts of drug that will be transferred to the child by nursing can be neglected and none of the babies showed signs of β_2-

adrenergic stimulation. Plasma sampling in one child did not give measurable concentrations.

Information of transfer to breast milk is lacking with other β_2-agonists. However, the substances have considerable volumes of distribution: 100 L or more in adults. Since the daily production of breast milk is in the order of 1 L, a considerable enrichment of β_2-agonist in the milk would be necessary to make nursing risky, particularly if oral bioavailability is not complete.

D. Elimination

Figure 2 gives typical examples of metabolites of β_2-agonists. With some exceptions, metabolism of β_2-agonists leads to the loss or reduction of effect (10,38,43). In humans, sulfate conjugation is the most common metabolic pathway of β_2-agonists having phenolic functions (11,46,120), but procaterol and formoterol are mainly conjugated with glucuronic acid (47,48). Methylation inactivates 3,4-diphenols (43,121). Oxidative processes affect substances having other ring systems. The chain nitrogen can be attacked by MAO if not protected by bulky substituents. Oxidation or degradation of the side chain has been found.

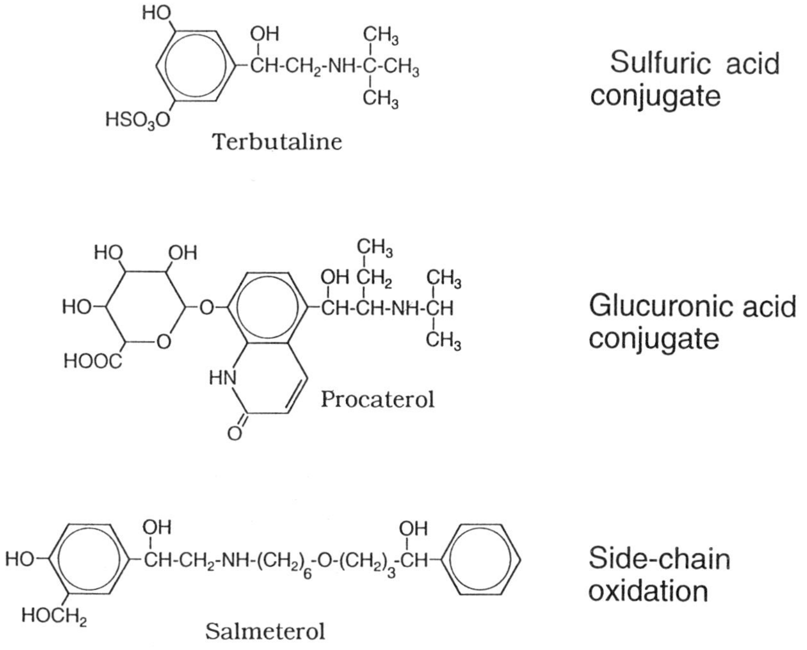

Figure 2 Typical metabolites of β_2-agonists in humans.

Many of the β_2-agonists and their metabolites are filtered in the glomeruli and several are also tubularly secreted.

E. Circadian Rhythm

The clearance of β_2-agonists appears to be rather stable over the day. For instance, the prodrug bambuterol produced similar plasma concentration curves of terbutaline after repeated once-daily morning or evening administration (122).

There are reports of different types of pharmacokinetic behavior taken of sustained-release (SR) preparations of albuterol and terbutaline taken during the day and at night (123,124), but these observations are most likely caused by different dietary habits in the morning and evening. SR terbutaline tablets taken at the end of a standardized breakfast or supper (similar meals) produced virtually identical day and night plasma concentration profiles (125).

F. Deviating Physiological States

The pharmacokinetics of albuterol is similar in asthmatic patients (38,126) and in healthy subjects (10,12). The same conclusion can be drawn for terbutaline (31) and for its prodrug bambuterol (122,127,128). Little is known, however, about the influence on the kinetics by severe disease and during acute illness (129). A damaged epithelium in the airways may lead to a faster absorption of inhaled substances (65,81), and the deposited amount may be reduced at low inspiratory flow caused by bronchoconstriction or mucus accumulation. Distribution and renal excretion of β_2-agonists may be different in critically ill patients, but probably metabolism does not change much for β_2-agonists that are not high-clearance drugs (i.e., the majority) and therefore less affected by changes in blood flow.

Pregnancy does not much affect albuterol pharmacokinetics; possibly bioavailability after oral administration is somewhat reduced (130). Terbutaline clearance is increased during late pregnancy to about 0.30 L/min (131) or +30% with an unchanged volume of distribution (132).

G. Ethnic Influence

Little is known about the influence of race on the pharmacokinetics of β_2-agonists. Southeast Asian patients taking 4 or 8 mg of a SR preparation of albuterol (Volmax, Glaxo Wellcome, UK) twice daily (133) had plasma concentrations of albuterol similar to those found in white subjects (93,104,105, 134). Plasma concentrations of terbutaline were about 60% higher in Chinese than in white healthy subjects because of higher absorption and less first-pass metabolism in the Chinese (Li et al., manuscript in preparation). It is doubtful if these differences are of a genuine genetic origin; for instance, the Chinese group had a considerably smaller dietary intake of sulfur which could have reduced their ability to conjugate with sulfate (135).

H. Enantiomers

β_2-Agonists are administered as racemates; that is, equimolar mixtures of a pair of enantiomers. The physicochemical properties of the enantiomers are the same but they have different pharmacological potency. The more active enantiomer is termed the *eutomer* and the less active one is the *distomer*. Progress in bioanalytical methodology (28–30) has made it possible to study the pharmacokinetics of the separate enantiomers. The results achieved so far, particularly concerning the stereokinetics of terbutaline and albuterol, illustrate that the pharmacokinetics may differ within a pair.

Terbutaline

In vitro studies by Walle and Walle (136) showed that the sulfate conjugation of terbutaline by rat liver cytosol is stereoselective in that (+)-terbutaline, that is, the dextrorotatory distomer, was sulfated eight times more efficiently than (−)-terbutaline (the levorotatory eutomer). Experiments with human liver cytosol (137) demonstrated that the distomer was sulfated twice as fast as the eutomer. Studies by Pacifici et al. (51) confirmed and extended the findings by Walle and Walle (136) by measuring a higher sulfation rate of (+)-terbutaline in cytosolic fractions of human origin, not only from the liver but also from mucosal specimens of duodenum, ileum, ascending and sigmoid colon, and lung tissue.

The in vitro findings are reflected by the fate of the terbutaline enantiomers in humans. When oral terbutaline was administered repeatedly to human subjects, the AUC of (−)-terbutaline was about twice that of (+)-terbutaline (125,138). A study of each isomer given separately in humans showed that (−)-terbutaline had a lower clearance and a higher bioavailability than (+)-terbutaline. The higher bioavailability was not only a result of a smaller first-pass metabolism of the terbutaline eutomer but it was also absorbed to a greater extent than the distomer (139).

Albuterol

Concerning albuterol, the opposite situation exists. When albuterol was administered orally in two healthy subjects, an enrichment of unchanged (+)-isomer was found in the urine (140). After administration of a single oral dose of albuterol to healthy subjects, the urine was enantioselectively analyzed (28). The eutomer was more conjugated than the distomer. After intravenous administration, the metabolic difference between the enantiomers was much smaller, indicating that most of the difference had arisen during first pass. Recently, after oral administration of racemic albuterol, Boulton and Fawcett (140a) reported about three times higher concentrations in plasma or amounts in urine of the albuterol distomer compared with the eutomer. A considerably smaller difference was seen after intravenous administration. Walle et al. (141) found that the sulfation efficiency of the stereoselective enzyme (the M form of phenolsulfotransferase) and of human jejunal and platelet homogenates was about 10 times higher for (−)-albuterol than for (+)-albuterol. In liver cytosol, however, sulfation efficiency on average was only 75% higher for the (−)-enantiomer (142), suggesting the existence of endogenous inhibitors or an additional sulfation reaction in the crude liver cytosol (141).

Experiments using cells of the human hepatoma cell line Hep G2 for the sulfation of racemates of β-agonists revealed an about eightfold preference for (−)-albuterol vis-à-vis the (+)-form (143). Other studies with Hep G2 cells showed an about twofold preference for sulfation of the (+)-isomer of terbutaline (144). Based on the existing experience, the high sulfation of (−)-albuterol as compared with (+)-albuterol appears to be a unique property of this drug among the β-adrenoceptor agonists (141).

Enantiomeric vs. Racemic Kinetics

A complicating factor in the stereokinetics of terbutaline and albuterol is that the behavior of the racemic mixture cannot always be predicted from the individual kinetics of the enantiomers estimated in separate studies. Interaction between the enantiomers occurs. For instance, clearance of racemic terbutaline in humans is about the same as for the (+)-isomer, and absorption of the racemate equals the absorption of the (−)-isomer (139). The sulfation rate of racemic albuterol is usually similar to that of (−)-albuterol (141,143). However, in human liver cytosol, the racemate of albuterol is metabolized considerably slower than both the enantiomers (142). Nonetheless, the kinetic studies administering racemates in humans (28,125,138–140a) qualitatively confirm the trends observed with the individual enantiomers. Thus, several difficulties that have been met in attempts to correlate plasma concentrations of "mixed" β_2-agonist with pharmacological action now seem to have been explained. Also, the different sulfation patterns of terbutaline and albuterol enantiomers rationalize, at least partly, why "therapeutic" plasma concentrations of albuterol after oral administration are higher than those after terbutaline despite similar volumes of distribution (cf. below).

Fenoterol

In hepatic and intestinal microsomes as well as in hepatocytes and enterocytes from the rat, glucuronidation of fenoterol (two glucuronides formed at a constant proportion) proceeded faster with the S,S(+)-enantiomer; that is, the distomer (145). In humans, fenoterol is sulfated, but preliminary data from measurements in human urine suggest a higher amount of the eutomer of fenoterol; this would then imply that sulfate conjugation of fenoterol is stereoselective too and proceeds in the same direction as shown for terbutaline (146).

Bambuterol

Additional stereoselective processes have been identified for the terbutaline prodrug bambuterol, which also is a racemate. One metabolic pathway to the active moiety terbutaline is hydrolysis of bambuterol by plasma cholinesterase. In vitro experiments in human plasma have shown that the (–)-isomer of bambuterol during 3 hr produced more than twice as much terbutaline as the (+)-isomer (147). This may explain why during treatment with bambuterol the ratio of active to inactive terbutaline in plasma was as high as 2.8:1.0 (125), that is, a higher ratio than when terbutaline was given as such (125,138). However, like with the terbutaline enantiomers, different absorption of the enantiomers of bambuterol might be another factor contributing to the positive skewing of the enantiomeric ratio.

Tissue Distribution

The terbutaline enantiomers are taken up at a similar rate by human erythrocytes (111). In platelets, their uptake rates do not differ (148). This suggests that their distribution is governed by their physicochemical properties and not by steric structure. Likewise, their protein binding is similar, and, as a measure of their overall distribution, they have virtually the same V_{ss} (139). As a consequence of the differences in clearance though, the half-life of (–)-terbutaline tended to be slightly longer (139).

I. Interactions

Enantiomers in a racemic pair can interact so that the pharmacokinetics of the racemate might not be predictable from the individual kinetic parameters of the enantiomers (139,141–143). Otherwise few interactions of importance are reported with β_2-agonists. In a 19-month-old infant, albuterol infusion about doubled the clearance of infused theophylline (149). In contrast, only a modest increase (+14%) of theophylline clearance was seen in adults with oral albuterol and no effect with inhaled albuterol (150). In a steady-state study with oral dosing of SR theophylline and SR terbutaline sulfate alone or in combination, an 11% reduction of plasma theophylline during the night was measured with the combination (124). Terbutaline kinetics were not influenced by theophylline. Theophylline clearance was not changed by plain terbutaline sulfate 5 mg every 8 hr (151). The terbutaline prodrug bambuterol did not significantly change steady-state plasma theophylline levels (152). The kinetics of bambuterol or generated terbutaline were not influenced by theophylline.

Evidently interaction between β_2-agonists and theophylline is modest or not even seen in adults but is possibly greater in younger patients. Concerning concomitant treatment with corticosteroids and β_2-agonists, no interaction in either direction was found between bambuterol and oral prednisolone (153).

Adrenergic stimulation retards gastric emptying (42). As a result, albuterol reduced absorption rate of paracetamol (154) and of sulfamethoxazole (155).

The prodrug bambuterol had bioequivalent kinetics at different dietary conditions (156). Fasting or fed conditions did not differ regarding extent of absorption of albuterol from SR preparations (Volmax, Proventil Repetabs, Glaxo Wellcome) (157,158). The rate of absorption from Volmax was, however, slower with food. Fasting increases the bioavailability of terbutaline from plain tablets by about 50% by increasing the absorbed amount (50).

J. Pharmacokinetics in Children

Bioavailability of terbutaline in children after oral administration is about the same as in adults (159). Calculated on body weight, the kinetics of terbutaline after intravenous administration show only a small difference between the two age groups (160). Likewise, preterm neonates about 2–3 months after birth had weight-normalized volume of distribution and clearance of albuterol similar to what has been found in adults (161).

V. Pharmacokinetics of Individual β_2-Agonists

A. Resorcinolamines

Fenoterol

Fenoterol is a racemic pair of two enantiomers having (R,R)- or (S,S)-configuration at two centers of asymmetry (5). The absorption of oral fenoterol is roughly 60% (34), but extensive first-pass metabolism reduces the bioavailable fraction of an oral dose to 1.5% (162). Fenoterol is rapidly conjugated even after intravenous administration (34). The main metabolite in humans is the sulfate conjugate (90).

After intravenous administration of tritiated fenoterol in humans, radioactivity was found in the feces (about 15%) (34) which should reflect secretion or biliary excretion of fenoterol or metabolites into the gut.

In rats, fenoterol is rapidly conjugated with glucuronic acid, but autoradiography soon (30 min) after intravenous injection showed 2.6 times higher radioactivity per gram tissue in the lungs than in the blood (163), suggesting an affinity of the intact drug to lung tissue. Other autoradiographic studies shortly after intravenous administration in rats (164) showed no measurable radioactivity in the brain. This suggests that fenoterol, like other hydrophilic β_2-agonists, has a limited access to the central nervous system. The protein binding in human serum is in the order of 50%, and the concentration in erythrocytes is nearly the same as in plasma (165). The total volume of distribution in humans (V_{ss}) is 1.9–2.7 L/kg body weight (90, 162).

Total clearance of fenoterol in humans is very high; in the order of 1 L/min (90) or even higher (162). One reason for the high clearance is that the fenoterol molecule offers phenolic groups for conjugation at both ends (Fig. 1). Renal clearance of fenoterol is about 270 mL/min (162), indicating a considerable component of tubular secretion. Fenoterol is known to be a short-acting bronchodilator, which is supported by the finding of a terminal half-life of only about 3 hr (90,162).

Drug particles in a fenoterol PMDI (Berotec, Boehringer, Ingelheim, Germany) were labeled with ^{99m}Tc and the deposition in the body was studied in a group of healthy subjects (74). As much as 33% of the body deposition was found in the lungs if inhalation was slow and made from half the vital capacity. As about 15–20% of a metered dose is usually retained in the actuator of a PMDI on inhalation by healthy subjects (166–168), this value probably corresponds to about 27% of the metered dose. In another study measuring plasma concentrations of fenoterol by a radioimmunoassay method, the bioavailability of fenoterol from the aerosol could be judged to be at the most 9% (90). Differences in inhalation technique might explain the conflicting results.

Terbutaline

Presystemic and Systemic Fate

The average absorption of terbutaline after oral administration is about 50% in fasting subjects (50). About two-thirds of the absorbed drug is first-pass metabolized (169), so the bioavailability of oral terbutaline is 10–15%; the lower figure is seen during fed conditions, which reduce absorption (50). Terbutaline is metabolized predominantly by sulfate conjugation (11,55).

The volume of distribution of terbutaline (V_{ss}) is 1.6 L/kg (50). The plasma protein binding is low ($\sim$20%) (109), and the erythrocyte/plasma concentration ratio is about 2 (111–113). Autoradiographic studies in mice (170) revealed no terbutaline in the brain, but subsequent studies in humans showed that the steady-state concentration in cerebrospinal fluid is 1/5 of that in plasma (171).

Metabolic clearance accounts for one-third of the body clearance of intact terbutaline, with the latter being about 3 ml/min/kg body weight (50); the remaining two-thirds reflect renal excretion, as systemically available terbutaline and metabolites are excreted virtually only in the urine. Negligible amounts of terbutaline were found in human bile (172) which is an observation that is further supported by the finding of only 2–3% of the dose in the feces after parenteral administration to healthy subjects (11). Renal clearance of terbutaline in young healthy adults is about 140 ml/min (92). This is higher than the glomerular filtration rate (GFR) even without correction for protein binding; evidently active secretion of terbutaline in the kidneys must exist.

The access to sensitive analytical methods has made it possible to measure terbutaline in plasma and urine for long periods after cessation of dosing. In that way, a terminal half-life of 17.0 ± 4.5 hr (SD) was revealed in young healthy subjects (92). However, this half-life determines only about half the AUC; therefore, dosing of systemic terbutaline must be more frequent than terminal half-life to avoid too much fluctuation of the plasma concentration over time.

Oral Sustained-Release Tablets

SR terbutaline tablets extend the profile of drug plasma concentration versus time sufficiently to admit dosing twice daily. They have a bioavailability which is three-quarters of that of plain tablets (92). Nonsymmetrical dosing with terbutaline SR tablets, that is, 5 mg in the morning and 10 mg in the evening, was successful in protecting patients against early-morning dyspnea and maintained plasma levels of terbutaline above 9 nmol/L during 24 hr in all patients (173).

Transdermal Administration

A transdermal delivery system for terbutaline in the form of an adhesive patch has been developed. It is capable of delivering the drug through the skin for a long time at a constant rate (103). A product delivering 45 μg terbutaline sulfate per hour was tested in asthmatic patients. Plasma concentrations of terbutaline reached a plateau after 6 hr and remained steady until the patch was removed after 24 hr. The plateau value, 12 nmol/L, can be calculated to correspond to a bioavailability of about 75%; that is, the drug must have been absorbed with small or negligible first-pass metabolism.

Inhalation

Absorption from a commercial Freon-driven aerosol was measured with and without blocking of gut absorption by swallowed activated charcoal (78). In a subgroup of five healthy subjects, total bioavailability was 16.5% of the delivered dose. With charcoal protection in the total of 11 subjects, absorption by the lungs was found to be 9.1% (subgroup: 9.8%) of the delivered dose. Absorption in the lungs when terbutaline was given by a new powder inhaler (Turbuhaler) to six healthy subjects was 21% of the metered dose (32).

Instillation

Terbutaline sulfate has been encapsulated in liposomes and administered by instillation at the tracheal bifurcation in guinea pigs (174). The residence time of terbutaline in the lungs could be prolonged up to a 10 times as compared with the situation when the drug was given without encapsulation.

Children

Children 7–13 years of age received about 20% higher plasma concentrations than adults during repeated administration of terbutaline SR tablets, 5 mg b.i.d. (175). A solution of terbutaline had an absorption of 33% and a bioavailability of 9.5% in children 8–12 years old (159). Children of the same age had a terbutaline bioavailability of 11% with a SR granulate (176).

The children have only slightly higher body and renal clearances of terbutaline than adults if the parameters are normalized to body weight (160).

B. Albuterol and Pirbuterol

Albuterol*

Presystemic and Systemic Fate

After oral administration, albuterol is well or completely absorbed (10,37,38, 126) but about one-half is metabolized during first pass (38,56). The bioavailability from the gastrointestinal tract of readily soluble albuterol is therefore about 50% (56). Albuterol is predominantly conjugated with sulfate (46), forming a virtually inactive metabolite (38).

Volume of distribution during terminal phase (V_β) was reported to be about 2.5 L/kg body weight (56). However, data from Goldstein et al. (177) allow for calculation of V_{ss} by recognized equations giving a value of 1.6 L/kg; that is, the same as found for the more hydrophilic terbutaline. Binding to plasma proteins is 8% and the concentration ratio between erythrocytes and plasma is about unity (56). Studies in rats given single oral doses of tritiated drug showed more and longer remaining radioactivity in fat than in muscle (10). In rat brain, after a high intravenous dose (10 mg/kg), the time-averaged concentration of albuterol was only 4% of that in plasma, but in the pituitary and the pineal glands (i.e., structures outside the blood-brain barrier), concentrations were six to eight times those in plasma (24).

The body clearance of albuterol in humans is comparatively high: 470–480 ml/min (56,177). This together with a distribution volume of moderate size

---

*Names of dosage forms referred to in this section are trademarks of Glaxo Wellcome, UK.

explains the rather short half-life of the substance: 4–7 hr has been reported (12,56,98,105,177,178). The fact that a steady state was reached already after 24 hr with oral albuterol (56) indicates that there should be no longer, undetected half-life of quantitative importance.

Renal clearance of albuterol in healthy humans is about 290 ml/min (56); that is, 60% of total clearance and much higher than glomerular filtration rate implying a considerable component of tubular secretion.

A study of intravenous albuterol in patients with renal function impairment, creatinine clearance being 7–53 (mean 24) ml/min (179), indicated that body clearance as compared with healthy subjects was more than halved. Because volume of distribution was very reduced too, the half-life was in the usual range for albuterol. Nevertheless, the reduced clearance calls for dosage consideration in renal impairment.

Oral Sustained-Release Preparations

Several oral SR formulations of albuterol have been developed. The earliest one, Spandets, in comparison with conventional tablets had an extended profile of plasma concentration versus time with a lower peak concentration but with preserved bioavailability as judged from the AUCs (180). Another product, Proventil Repetabs, given repeatedly every 12 hr had the same AUC and a similar fluctuation of the albuterol plasma concentrations as conventional albuterol tablets given every 6 hr (123). Still another preparation, Volmax, has a dissolution rate of albuterol which appears to control absorption rate very well (181). When compared during repeated dosing twice daily with standard albuterol tablets given four times daily, Volmax had similar minimal albuterol plasma concentrations as the standard tablets but lower concentration peaks (104,134). AUC from Volmax was the same as from the plain tablets (104) or somewhat reduced (134). In another steady-state comparison (105), there was no difference between Volmax twice daily and plain tablets four times daily either in AUC or maximal and minimal concentrations. A single-dose comparison between Proventil Repetabs and Volmax showed the same AUC of the preparations but a tendency toward more prolonged absorption with Volmax (158); a trend that became evident during multiple dosing (182).

Another way of prolonging the absorption phase of albuterol is a SR capsule formulation currently under development that contains the drug as sulfate salt and floats on the top of the gastric fluid (183).

Transdermal Administration

Experiments with albuterol applied in pads on the skin of rhesus monkeys showed that the dose liberated from the pad during 24 hr was well absorbed and underwent no substantial first-pass metabolism (184).

Inhalation

Measurements of albuterol deposition after inhalation have been made with gamma camera imaging methods after labeling of the drug with ^{99m}Tc. With a good inhalation technique, around 20% of the metered-dose albuterol from a PMDI is deposited in the lungs (166–168). The deposition of albuterol from Diskhaler, a dry-powder inhaler, is about half of that from the PMDI (167, 168). Another dry-powder inhaler, Rotahaler, had almost the same deposition as the PMDI but gave less improvement of FEV_1 (64).

Children

In children 5–14 years of age, an estimate of the terminal half-life from data after single administration of albuterol suppositories containing 2 mg of the drug (88) gives a value of 3.9 hr, which is in the range found in adults. Absorption was rapid as judged by the occurrence of plasma concentration peaks already after 1 hr in the majority of the children. Mean maximum concentration was 25 nmol/L compared with the range found in adults given a single 4-mg tablet: 30–60 nmol/L (41,98).

Pirbuterol

Pirbuterol is a β_2-agonist that has become profiled against lung problems associated with cardiovascular disease rather than being used as a bronchodilator. Absorption of pirbuterol in humans after oral administration of the hydrochloride salt should be at least 60%, as about 50% of the dose was recovered in the urine as sulfate conjugate and about 10% as unchanged substance (120). The elimination half-life is short: 1–2 hr in rat and dog and 2–3 hr in humans (120,185).

The rat metabolizes pirbuterol exclusively by conjugation with glucuronic acid, but in the dog, at least five metabolites are formed. Predominant in the dog is the 3-O-sulfate ester; little glucuronide is found (120).

After inhalation of 800 μg pirbuterol acetate (four puffs), half the dose was collected in urine as unchanged drug and conjugate in 24 hr (185). It is not known how much of this originated from deposition in the lungs.

C. Halogen-Substituted Phenyl Ring

As shown in Figure 1, halogen substituents and not phenolic hydroxyl groups are present in the phenyl ring of clenbuterol, mabuterol, and tulobuterol. This substitution makes clenbuterol and mabuterol very lipophilic substances with a long duration of action.

Clenbuterol

Clenbuterol is a potent bronchodilator with oral twice-daily doses as low as 20 or 40 μg (hydrochloride salt). The absorption after oral administration is complete and first-pass metabolism is low; for instance, 75% of the maximum plasma concentration after a single dose is intact drug (35). Steady-state plasma concentrations during a regimen of 20 μg twice daily are only about 1 nmol/L (96).

As a lipophilic substance, clenbuterol has a large distribution volume in the body: A value of 350 L (V_β) has been reported in healthy subjects (187). This was found in spite of a plasma protein binding of 90% or more (96). After intravenous administration in rats, concentrations in the brain were higher than in skeletal muscle and even somewhat higher than in heart muscle (188). In the dog, concentrations of clenbuterol were three to four times higher in bronchi and lungs than in plasma (107). Very high and long-lasting concentrations were measured in calf eyes (189).

The metabolism of clenbuterol has been thoroughly elucidated (186). In dogs, a total of 12 metabolites were identified, although several in minute quantities. Intact clenbuterol made up one-fourth of the recovery, and the principal metabolites were formed by side-chain degradation plus conjugation of the aliphatic and the aromatic nitrogen. Qualitatively, humans and dogs show a similar metabolic pattern (186), but the metabolism of clenbuterol in humans is slower as shown by the excretion of a larger fraction of intact drug in cumulated urine collections from humans (35,96,186).

In humans, clenbuterol and metabolites are eliminated in the urine with a negligible fecal excretion (35). The high plasma protein binding reduces glomerular filtration and hepatic clearance. If complete absorption and a negligible first-pass metabolism are assumed, data from Couet et al. (190) can be used to calculate a total body clearance of clenbuterol in humans of only about 120 ml/min and a renal clearance of about 35 ml/min. The latter value corresponds to an unbound renal clearance of ≥350 ml/min, which considerably exceeds the GFR and thus implies active secretion in the tubules.

The low body clearance of clenbuterol combined with a large distribution volume explains the long terminal half-life of the substance: 26–35 hr (96,190).

Mabuterol

Mabuterol is completely absorbed and undergoes little first-pass metabolism. As a result, bioavailability after oral administration is about 90% (36). This together with its pharmacological properties makes mabuterol a very potent drug with twice-daily oral therapeutic doses of 40–60 μg (hydrochloride salt).

Mabuterol has a large volume of distribution. If a 10% first-pass metabolism is adjusted for, a V_β in humans of 6.6 L/kg can be calculated from the data of Guentert et al. (36). The concentration ratio between erythrocytes and plasma is about unity (36); no value of protein binding in humans has been reported. In rats after intravenous administration of ^{14}C-labeled mabuterol (191), equilibrium concentrations were about 10 times higher in lung tissue than in plasma. Shortly after the dose, the concentration in rat brain was higher than in plasma, but after 4 hr, the concentrations were the same. Concentrations and time courses of mabuterol in brain and skeletal muscle were very similar. Much drug was located to secretory organs; the lacrimal gland among others. In general, the distribution of mabuterol in rats was similar to that of clenbuterol (188).

In the rat (192), mabuterol is metabolised predominantly by oxidative deamination and subsequent oxidation of the remaining side chain. It appears that the aromatic ring is resistant to metabolism. An appreciable amount of intact mabuterol was excreted in the rat urine and, in addition, six metabolites were identified. One of these, found in a minor amount, had the t-butyl group hydroxylated and showed pharmacological activity, although 2–10 times lower than mabuterol itself.

The results of metabolic studies in humans are conflicting, probably because of methodological differences and difficulties. Measurements of mabuterol with an enzyme immunoassay resulted in as much as 64% of the dose being intact in cumulated urine (27), whereas studies with tritiated substance gave only one-fourth of the dose as intact mabuterol in the urine (36). In plasma, intact (tritiated) mabuterol was 46% of the peak concentration, but metabolites could not be identified except for a small (<5% of intact mabuterol) concentration of the active hydroxylated t-butyl metabolite. In urine, that metabolite and its conjugate were responsible for about 5 and 8%, respectively, of the radioactivity to be compared with 30% from intact mabuterol. Conjugated mabuterol made up about 16% of the urinary radioactivity (36).

Mabuterol has a moderate body clearance; an estimate from the data of Guentert et al. (36) is 3.2 ml/min/kg. Since the distribution volume is great, the half-life of mabuterol is long: 20–23 hr (27,36). Virtually all mabuterol and metabolites are excreted in urine; the excretion via feces is negligible (36). If then one-fourth of the dose is excreted intact (cf. above), renal clearance would be about 1 ml/min/kg.

Tulobuterol

Tulobuterol has only one halogen substituent in its aromatic ring and is therefore less lipophilic than clenbuterol and mabuterol. Data from several species show incomplete absorption (193). In humans, as judged from the excretion in urine (194), absorption is in the mean order of 40% with a substantial interindividual variation.

Autoradiographic studies in rats after oral administration of 14C-labeled tulobuterol (195) at tissue equilibrium showed low concentrations in the brain and eye and nothing in the pituitary. Concentrations in the lungs were lower than in plasma.

The metabolism of tulobuterol shows large interspecies variation. In humans, considerable metabolic variability exists; in a study with three healthy male subjects, one conjugated tulobuterol to a high degree and formed little hydroxylated metabolites and the two others formed less conjugates of the intact substance but primarily formed metabolites hydroxylated in the aromatic ring, which were conjugated to a high extent (194). The formation of the 4-hydroxy metabolite (HOKU-81) is noteworthy, as it is more potent than tulobuterol itself on isolated guinea pig trachea (196) and therefore may give a contribution to the clinical effect and duration (97). The urinary excretion of free intact tulobuterol in humans was on average 14% of the administered dose. About 6% of the dose was excreted as the 4-hydroxy metabolite mainly in conjugated form. The half-life of tulobuterol in humans has been estimated to 2–3 hr (97,197).

D. Substances with a Heterocyclic Ring

Broxaterol

Broxaterol is claimed to have an enhanced metabolic stability in comparison with phenolic β_2-agonists and a high oral bioavailability (198). Clinical experience might support that claim, as in cumulative studies in asthmatic patients, broxaterol given orally was greater than 10 times more potent than albuterol, whereas its potency at inhalation was rather less than that of albuterol (199).

Procaterol

Procaterol is a racemic mixture of two enantiomers having (R,S)- or (S,R)-configuration at two centers of asymmetry (7). Procaterol has a high affinity to β_2-receptors in mammalian tissues (200) and an extremely high functional β_2-selectivity in isolated organs (201,202). The substance is very potent: Oral doses of 50–75 μg (hydrochloride salt) three times daily are recommended therapy.

Studies in beagle dogs indicated an absorption of orally given procaterol of about 70% (203) and bioavailability was about 40%, as judged from the urinary excretion (24 hr) of intact drug after single oral and intravenous administrations. In humans, net absorption should be in the order of 70%, as judged from the 24-hr recoveries of a tritium-labeled dose in urine and feces (204).

Autoradiograms of beagle dogs showed no distribution of procaterol to the eyeballs or the brain (203). Data after intravenous administration (205) allow calculation of a V_{ss} of about 1.4 L/kg in the dog and thus are similar to the values found in humans for albuterol and terbutaline.

Studies in rats (206) identified six metabolites of procaterol. Procaterol was conjugated to a great extent with glucuronic acid and very little with sulfuric acid. Other metabolites were formed by successive degradation of the side chain and conjugation of a formyl-containing metabolite. In the dog, conjugation is the predominating metabolic pathway. About 90% of the conjugates are formed with procaterol itself. Again, more glucuronide than sulfate is formed (203).

Also in humans procaterol is predominantly conjugated with glucuronic acid. Metabolites resulting from side-chain degradation have been identified too (47). Thus, qualitatively, metabolism of procaterol is similar in the investigated species.

In healthy adult humans, about 20% of an oral dose was recovered intact in urine (99,207). Renal clearance is 100–170 ml/min (99,204,207). Concerning body clearance of procaterol in humans, reported values are inconsistent.

The half-life of procaterol is 0.7 hr in the rat and about 2 hr in the dog (203,205). Its half-life in humans is about 4 hr (204,207).

E. Inhaled Long-Acting Substances

Formoterol and salmeterol have a very long effect duration after inhalation. Both substances are lipophilic, but the distribution coefficient between octanol and water at pH 7.4 is 20–30 times higher for salmeterol than for formoterol (8). As a possible consequence of the lipophilicity, both substances resist washing after administration to tracheal preparations, with salmeterol being somewhat more resistant (208).

Salmeterol was tailored according to a theory of nonspecific anchoring of a long side chain to a hydrophobic site ("exoreceptor") near the β_2-receptor (209,210). Formoterol might exert its long duration of action by being retained in the plasmalemma lipid bilayer of airway smooth muscle from which site it can leach out and reach the receptor (211).

One factor that may affect the onset of action and prolong the effect duration of relatively big and lipophilic drug molecules, such as formoterol and salmeterol, is solubility in the liquid layer of the airways. The volume of liquid is small and might not be able to dissolve the substances but slowly as lung uptake progresses.

Formoterol

Formoterol is a racemic mixture of two enantiomers having (R,R)- or (S,S)-configuration at two chiral centers (6). Common inhaled and oral doses of formoterol fumarate are as low as 12 and 80 μg, respectively, twice daily. However, on oral administration, the duration of the effect offers no advantage over albuterol (212).

Presystemic and Systemic Fate

Studies in rats and dogs (213) indicate that formoterol is well absorbed in these species. In humans, absorption after oral administration is said to be 60% (214), a surprisingly low figure in light of the experience in the animals and the drug's lipophilic character. The rat seems to first-pass metabolize formoterol heavily, whereas in the dog, the fraction of intact drug in plasma is similar after oral and intravenous administration (213). About 20% of an oral dose was found intact in the urine of dogs (213) and almost 10% in human urine collected during 24 hr after administration (14).

The protein binding of formoterol is moderate. By ultrafiltration in the concentration range 10–500 nmol/L, the binding of the RR-enantiomer was found to be 46% and that of the SS-enantiomer 58% (K. Tegnér, personal communication). Autoradiography performed during the first 3–10 min after intravenous administration of formoterol in rats showed wide distribution of the drug within the body but little in the central nervous system or the eyes (215).

Like with procaterol, the major metabolite in rat, dog, and human is a glucuronide formed with the phenolic hydroxyl group (6,48,213). The ability to conjugate decreases in the order rat > dog > human (48). The ratio intact drug/glucuronide was about 0.7:1.0 in human urine collected for 10 hr after a single oral dose (6).

The half-life of formoterol is about 2 hr in rats and 4–6 hr in dogs (213). In humans, a half-life of 3.4 hr has been reported from plasma concentration measurements up to 8 hr after an oral dose (216), but prolonged measurement after inhalation gives a value of 8 hr (J. Rosenborg, personal communication).

Inhalation

The uptake of formoterol in the airways can be judged to be as good as with other bronchodilators, because during a 12-hr period, as much as 24% of an inhaled dose was recovered as intact drug plus glucuronide in the urine (217).

Salmeterol

The customary therapeutic dose of salmeterol is 50 μg of the xinafoate inhaled twice daily.

Presystemic and Systemic Fate

After oral administration, salmeterol is well absorbed in rats and dogs and seemingly also in humans (218).

In albino rats, salmeterol appears to be extensively metabolized during first pass, but in beagle dogs most of the absorbed drug reaches the systemic blood intact (219). Also in humans, first-pass metabolism is probably small (218).

Salmeterol has a high plasma protein binding of about 95% in all investigated species and distributes equally between erythrocytes and plasma. Autoradiographic studies showed long-lasting binding of radioactive material to the uveal tract and melanin of the eye (218).

Phenolic glucuronidation is an important metabolic pathway of salmeterol in the rat (219). In the dog, the predominant metabolite is a conjugate, not unequivocally identified but apparently a sulfate. In humans, the main metabolite is an aliphatic alcohol formed by oxidation at the carbon α to the phenyl ring of the phenylbutoxy side chain (218). This metabolite is said to be equipotent to salmeterol (220).

After intravenous administration, 60–70% of the dose was recovered in the feces from rats and dogs. Most of that fraction originated from the bile. In humans, 23% of an oral radioactive dose was found in urine and 57% in feces, with a significant fraction of the fecal recovery being the aliphatic alcohol (218).

A salmeterol clearance of almost 100 ml/min/kg in rats and about 30 ml/min/kg in dogs was found after intravenous administration (218). The plasma half-life of salmeterol was estimated to 5–6 hr in rats and about 2 hr in dogs (219). In humans, it is said to be in the same order as that of albuterol (i.e., 4–6 hr [221]); the half-life of the active alcohol metabolite has not been reported.

The drug is presented as salt with hydroxynaphtoic acid (xinafoate). This counterpart has a half-life of about 2 weeks and is largely bound to plasma proteins (more than 99%) with a very small distribution volume of about 7 L. As a result, steady-state plasma concentrations of hydroxynaphtoic acid are about 1000 times higher (400–500 nmol/L) than those of salmeterol during maintenance treatment. The acid is devoid of intrinsic pharmacological activity (110).

Inhalation

About 10% of the inhaled dose of salmeterol from the device Diskhaler is said to be deposited in the lungs (222).

F. Prodrugs

A prodrug is a substance usually inactive in itself that is metabolized to an active drug (parent compound) in the body (223). Prodrugs may give the active substance improved pharmacokinetic properties; for example, better absorption, less first-pass metabolism, a more favorable distribution to or within the target organ, or prolonged stay in the body. Concerning β_2-agonists, only bitolterol and bambuterol represent progress as compared with the parent compound. Bitolterol is the bis-p-toluate ester of colterol, a catechol ethanolamine, and bambuterol is the bis-N,N-dimethylcarbamate of terbutaline (Fig. 3). Bitolterol is comparatively easily hydrolyzed with a high first-pass metabolism. Therefore, bitolterol is more useful as an aerosol for inhalation than for oral administration. On the contrary, bambuterol is very stable against metabolism and therefore functions well orally but poorly as an inhaled drug.

Bitolterol

Presystemic and Systemic Fate

The active moiety in bitolterol, colterol (N-*tert*-butylarterenol) (see Fig. 1), has a very low bioavailability partly because of incomplete absorption and partly because of a high first-pass metabolism. Esterification of the phenolic hydroxyl groups of colterol increases its bioavailability (224,225).

In humans, the absorption of an oral dose of bitolterol is almost complete, although there is some hydrolysis to colterol already in the gastrointestinal tract. First-pass metabolism is high, giving a low bioavailability of the intact prodrug; in fact, only 1% of the plasma contents is bitolterol 1 hr after oral dosing (43).

At 4.5 hr after intravenous administration of radiolabeled bitolterol in dogs, the concentrations of radioactivity in the lungs were about 30 times higher than in blood and even higher than in the liver and the kidneys. Of the lung radioactivity, one-fourth to one-half was from intact bitolterol (43).

No intact bitolterol and virtually no colterol were found in human urine after oral administration or bitolterol. Hydrolysis to colterol occurs through esterases in plasma and tissues and colterol is subject to COMT 3-O-methylation. The methylcolterol thus formed and colterol itself are conjugated to a large extent (43).

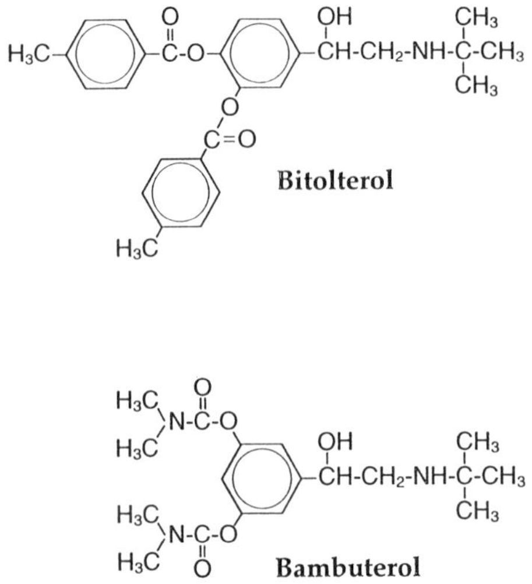

Figure 3 Structural formulae of bitolterol and bambuterol, prodrugs to the β_2-agonists colterol and terbutaline.

The specific half-life of bitolterol or colterol has not been reported.

Inhalation

Lung tissue hydrolyses bitolterol at a rate of 4.8 μmol/g/hr, which is more than twice the rate in plasma (43). The recommended dose of bitolterol for inhalation is about 1–2 μmol. Thus, enough colterol is produced to give an onset of action already within 5 min. Then continuous hydrolysis of remaining bitolterol in the lungs contributes to the relatively long duration of action: up to 8 hr (226).

Bambuterol

Previous experiences with prodrugs of terbutaline (227) led to the conclusion that only extremely stable ones would be able to resist first-pass metabolism. One such substance is bambuterol, the bis-N,N-dimethylcarbamate of terbutaline (see Fig. 3). Together with intermediary metabolites, bambuterol functions as a depot in body tissues releasing terbutaline slowly enough to allow for one-daily dosing (122).

About 20% of an oral bambuterol dose is absorbed in humans (228). The remainder is found in the feces, with 80% of that recovery being unchanged prodrug. After some hours, absorption becomes slower than elimination (128) and determines the terminal phase of bambuterol plasma concentrations. As much as two-thirds of the absorbed fraction survives first-pass metabolism (228). The metabolised third is transformed mainly to intermediary metabolites, which are still prodrugs to terbutaline (86). Terbutaline is predominantly generated systemically, and its bioavailability is about 10% of the administered dose; that is, the same as when terbutaline is given as such (50). The plasma concentration profile of generated terbutaline shows little fluctuation during the 24-hr dosing interval (122,128).

The volume of distribution, V_{ss}, of bambuterol in humans is 1.6 L/kg, which is the same as that of terbutaline (128). The plasma protein binding of bambuterol is 40–50% and the concentration is about the same in erythrocytes and plasma (K. Tegnér, personal communication). Equilibrium concentrations of bambuterol in human cerebrospinal fluid are one-tenth of those in plasma (171). Studies in mice show a high affinity of bambuterol and intermediary hydroxylated bis-carbamates to lung tissue (227).

Bambuterol is metabolized to terbutaline by hydrolysis catalysed by plasma cholinesterase (EC 3.1.1.8) or by oxidation probably brought about by cytochrome P-450–dependent enzymes (86). Seven metabolites between bambuterol and terbutaline, formed by hydroxylation, demethylation, and hydrolysis, have been identified (86,229). Hydrolysis of bambuterol in humans is capacity-limited as demonstrated in plasma samples at bambuterol concentrations above 30 nmol/L (230).

Table 1 Systemic Pharmacokinetics of a Number of β_2-Agonists in Humans

	D_{oct} (pH 7.4)	fu (%)	Abs (%)	F (%)	V_{ss} (L/kg)	CL (mL/min)	fCL_{ren}	$t_{1/2}$ (hr)
Terbutaline	<0.016	~80	50	15	1.6	200	2/3	15–20
Salbutamol	0.016	92	100	50	1.6	500	0.6	4–7
Fenoterol	0.74	50	60	1–2	1.9–2.7	≥1000	1/4	3
Procaterol	—	—	70	40	1.4	—	—	4
Formoterol	2.6	~50	60(?)	30(?)	—	—	1/3(?)	8
Clenbuterol	4.8	≥10	100	>75	High	120(?)	~1/3	~30
Salmeterol	63	5	100	"High"	High(?)	—	—	4–6(?)
Bitolterol	—	—	~100	Low	—	High	—	—
Bambuterol	—	50–60	20	12	1.6	1250	1/10	9–15

Symbols: D_{oct} = Distribution coefficient between octanol and water; fu = Fraction of drug not bound to plasma proteins; Abs = Fraction of oral dose absorbed; F = Fraction of oral dose reaching the systemic blood; V_{ss} = Distribution volume at steady state (tissue equilibrium); CL = Total body clearance; fCL_{ren} = Fraction of CL due to renal elimination; $t_{1/2}$ = Terminal plasma half-life.

Bambuterol is a potent (IC_{50} = 17 nmol/L) but reversible ($t_{1/2}$ = 75–80 min) inhibitor of plasma cholinesterase (231). Maximum plasma concentrations of bambuterol in clinical practice are usually below 20 nmol/L, and in no subject with therapeutic doses has the activity of plasma cholinesterase been completely abolished (86). Inhibition of the esterase is not known to interfere with normal life, but during treatment with bambuterol, the muscle relaxant suxamethonium gets longer duration of effect because of slower hydrolytic inactivation (232–235). Occasionally (1 of 2500), subjects have a genetically variant, atypical cholinesterase with considerably reduced affinity to the pro-drug (236). Still, in such individuals, terbutaline is formed to the same extent as in normal subjects (237).

Total body clearance of bambuterol in humans is 1.25 L/min, of which about 90% is nonrenal (127,128). About 20% of an intravenous dose was recovered in the feces as bambuterol and metabolites (228) which suggests transport over the gut wall into the lumen. The terminal half-life of intravenous bambuterol is only 2–3 hr (127) compared with 9–15 hr after oral administration where absorption is the rate-determining step. Steady-state plasma concentrations of bambuterol increase more than predicted by dose increments. However, bambuterol is not toxic even at high concentrations. Not until concentrations reach the *micro*molar range would inhibition of acetylcholinesterase (IC_{50} = 41,000 nmol/L) occur (231).

Although bambuterol kinetics are nonlinear, generation of terbutaline occurs proportionally to dose with therapeutic doses (238). The terminal half-life of generated terbutaline has been found to be about 20 hr (128), which is slightly longer than found with terbutaline given as such (92) which probably reflects the prolonged absorption of bambuterol.

VI. Conclusions

This chapter has evaluated and summarized the scattered and heterogeneous knowledge of the pharmacokinetics of β_2-adrenoceptor–stimulating drugs. Table 1 gives a very condensed survey. Facts about their fate in the body, including that of the enantiomers, should facilitate the choice of administration route and improve dosage in general. However, much pharmacokinetic information is still lacking, which should be an exciting provocation to continued research.

Acknowledgments

Drs. Kerstin Tegnér and Bertil Waldeck are gratefully acknowledged for generous advice and constructive criticism.

References

1. Persson K, Persson K. The metabolism of terbutaline in vitro by rat and human liver O-methyltransferases and monoamine oxidases. Xenobiotica 1972; 2:375–382.
2. Johansson L-H, Persson H, Rosengren E. β_2-Adrenoceptor selectivity in four series of β-adrenoceptor agonists. Eur J Pharmacol 1986; 130:97–103.
3. Johansson L-H, Linder Eliasson E, Persson H, Rosengren E. An analysis of the β_2-adrenoceptor selectivity in three series of β-adrenoceptor agonists. Pharmacol Toxicol 1990; 66:203–208.
4. Cahn RS, Ingold CK, Prelog V. The specification of asymmetric configuration in organic chemistry. Experientia 1956; 12:81–124.
5. Beale JP, Stephenson NC. X-ray analysis of Th 1165a and salbutamol. J Pharm Pharmacol 1972; 24:277–280.
6. Tasaka K. Formoterol (Atock®): a new orally active and selective β-receptor stimulant. Drugs of Today 1986; 22:505–519.
7. Yoshizaki S, Manabe Y, Tamada S, et al. Isomers of *erythro*-5-(1-hydroxy-2-isopropylaminobutyl)-8-hydroxycarbostyril, a new bronchodilator. J Med Chem 1977; 20:1103–1104.
8. Jeppsson A-B, Löfdahl C-G, Waldeck B, Widmark E. On the predictive value of experiments in vitro in the evaluation of the effect duration of bronchodilator drugs for local administration. Pulm Pharmacol 1989; 2:81–85.
9. Conway PG, Tejani-Butt S, Brunswick DJ. Interaction of beta adrenergic agonists and antagonists with brain beta adrenergic receptors in vivo. J Pharmacol Exp Ther 1987; 241:755–762.
10. Martin LE, Hobson JC, Page JA, Harrison C. Metabolic studies of salbutamol-^{3}H: a new bronchodilator, in rat, rabbit, dog and man. Eur J Pharmacol 1971; 14:183–199.

11. Nilsson HT, Persson K, Tegnér K. The metabolism of terbutaline in man. Xenobiotica 1972; 2:363–373.
12. Lin C, Magat J, Calesnick B, Symchowicz S. Absorption, excretion and urinary metabolic patterns of ^{3}H-albuterol aerosol in man. Eur J Pharmacol 1971; 14:183–199.
13. Briant RH, Blackwell EW, Williams FM, et al. The metabolism of sympathomimetic bronchodilator drugs by the isolated perfused dog lung. Xenobiotica 1973; 3:787–799.
14. Yokoi K, Murase K, Shiobara Y. The development of a radioimmunoassay for formoterol. Life Sci 1983; 33:1665–1672.
15. Jacobsson S-E, Svensson L-Å. Quantitative gas chromatography mass spectrometry (GC-MS) of terbutaline in urine using deuterated internal standard. 35th International Congress of Pharmaceutical Sciences, Dublin, 1975.
16. Martin LE, Rees J, Tanner RJN. Quantitative determination of salbutamol in plasma, as either its trimethylsilyl or t-butyldimethylsilyl ether, using a stable isotope multiple ion recording technique. Biomed Mass Spectrom 1976; 3:184–190.
17. Falkner FC, McIlhenny HM. Selected ion monitoring assay for the bronchodilator pirbuterol. Biomed Mass Spectrom 1976; 3:207–211.
18. Leferink JG, Wagemaker-Engels I, Maes RAA, et al. Quantitative analysis of terbutaline in serum and urine at therapeutic levels using gas chromatography–mass spectrometry. J Chromatogr 1977; 143:299–305.
19. Clare RA, Davies DS, Baillie TA. The analysis of terbutaline in biological fluids by gas chromatography electron impact mass spectrometry. Biomed Mass Spectrom 1979; 6:31–37.
20. Jacobsson SE, Jönsson S, Lindberg C, Svensson L-Å. Determination of terbutaline in plasma by gas chromatography chemical ionization mass spectrometry. Biomed Mass Spectrom 1980; 7:265–268.
21. Edholm L-E, Kennedy B-M, Bergquist S. Automated analysis of terbutaline (Bricanyl®) in human plasma with liquid chromatography and electrochemical detection using column-switching (multidimensional chromatography). Chromatographia 1982; 16:341–344.
22. Oosterhuis B, van Boxtel CJ. Determination of salbutamol in human plasma with bimodal high-performance liquid chromatography and a rotated disc amperometric detector. J Chromatogr Biomed Appl 1982; 232:327–334.
23. Hutchings MJ, Paull JD, Morgan DJ. Determination of salbutamol in plasma by high performance liquid chromatography with fluorescence detection. J Chromatogr Biomed Appl 1983; 227:423–426.
24. Caccia S, Fong MH. Kinetics and distribution of the β-adrenergic agonist salbutamol in rat brain. J Pharm Pharmacol 1984; 36:200–202.
25. Tan YK, Soldin SJ. Determination of salbutamol in human serum by reversed phase high performance liquid chromatography with amperometric detection. J Chromatogr Biomed Appl 1984; 311:311–317.
26. Yamamoto I, Iwata K. Enzyme immunoassay for clenbuterol, a β_2-adrenergic stimulant. J Immunoassay 1982; 3:155–171.
27. Yamamoto I, Matsuura E, Horiba M, et al. Enzyme immunoassay for mabuterol, a selective β_2-adrenergic stimulant in the trachea. J Immunoassay 1985; 6:261–276.

28. Tan YK, Soldin SJ. Analysis of salbutamol enantiomers in human urine by chiral high-performance liquid chromatography and preliminary studies related to the stereoselective disposition kinetics in man. J Chromatogr Biomed Appl 1987; 422: 187–195.

29. Edholm L-E, Lindberg C, Paulson J, Walhagen A. Determination of drug enantiomers in biological samples by coupled column liquid chromatography and liquid chromatography-mass spectrometry. J Chromatogr Biomed Appl 1988; 424:61–72.

30. Walhagen A, Edholm L-E, Kennedy B-M, Liu Chang-Xiao. Determination of terbutaline enantiomers in biological samples using liquid chromatography with coupled columns. Chirality 1989; 1:20–26.

31. Van den Berg W, Leferink JG, Maes RAA, et al. Correlation between terbutaline serum levels, c-AMP plasma levels and FEV_1 in normals and asthmatics after subcutaneous administration. Ann Allergy 1980; 44:235–239.

32. Borgström L, Newman S, Weisz A, Morén F. Pulmonary deposition of inhaled terbutaline: comparison of scanning gamma camera and urinary excretion methods. J Pharm Sci 1992; 81:1–3.

33. Davies DS. Pharmacokinetics of terbutaline after oral administration. Eur J Respir Dis 1984; 65(suppl 134):111–117.

34. Rominger KL, Pollmann W. Vergleichende Pharmakokinetik von Fenoterol-Hydrobromid bei Ratte, Hund und Mensch. Arzneimittelforschung 1972; 22:1190–1196.

35. Zimmer A, Bücheler A. Einmalapplikation, Mehrfachapplikation und Metabolitenmuster von Clenbuterol beim Menschen. Arzneimittelforschung 1976; 26: 1446–1450.

36. Guentert TW, Buskin JN, Galeazzi RL. Single dose pharmacokinetics of mabuterol in man. Arzneimittelforschung 1984; 34:1691–1696.

37. Kennedy MCS, Simpson WT. Human pharmacological and clinical studies on salbutamol: a specific β-adrenergic bronchodilator. Br J Dis Chest 1969; 63:165–174.

38. Evans ME, Walker SR, Brittain RT, Paterson JW. The metabolism of salbutamol in man. Xenobiotica 1973; 3:113–120.

39. Hörnblad Y, Ripe E, Magnusson PO, Tegnér K. The metabolism and clinical activity of terbutaline and its prodrug ibuterol. Eur J Clin Pharmacol 1976; 10:9–18.

40. Powell ML, Weisberg M, Gural R, et al. Comparative bioavailability and pharmacokinetics of three formulations of albuterol. J Pharm Sci 1985; 74:217–219.

41. Jonkman JHG, Freie HMP, van der Boon WJV, Grasmeijer G. Single dose absorption profiles and bioavailability of two different salbutamol tablets. Arzneimittelforschung 1986; 36:1133–1135.

42. Rees MR, Clark RA, Holdsworth CD, et al. The effect of beta-adrenoceptor agonists and antagonists on gastric emptying in man. Br J Clin Pharmacol 1980; 10: 551–554.

43. Shargel L, Dorrbecker SA. Physiological disposition and metabolism of [^{3}H]bitolterol in man and dog. Drug Metab Dispos 1976; 4:72–78.

44. George CF. Drug metabolism by the gastrointestinal mucosa. Clin Pharmacokinet 1981; 6:259–274.

45. Back DJ, Rogers SM. Review: first-pass metabolism by the gastrointestinal mucosa. Aliment Pharmacol Ther 1987; 1:339–357.

46. Lin C, Li Y, McGlotten J, et al. Isolation and identification of the major metabolite of albuterol in human urine. Drug Metab Dispos 1977; 5:234–238.

47. Shimizu T, Mori H, Tabusa E, Nakagawa K. The metabolites of procaterol HCl in urine and faeces of dog and man. Xenobiotica 1978; 8:705–710.
48. Kamimura H, Sasaki H, Higuchi S, Shiobara Y. Quantitative determination of the β-adrenoceptor stimulant formoterol in urine by gas chromatography mass spectrometry. J Chromatogr Biomed Appl 1982; 229:337–345.
49. Pacifici GM, Franchi M, Gervasi PG, et al. Profile of drug-metabolizing enzymes in human ileum and colon. Pharmacology 1989; 38:137–145.
50. Nyberg L. Pharmacokinetic parameters of terbutaline in healthy man. An overview. Eur J Respir Dis 1994; 65(suppl 134):149–160.
51. Pacifici G, Eligi M, Giuliani L. (+) and (−) terbutaline are sulphated at a higher rate in human intestine than in the liver. Eur J Clin Pharmacol 1993; 45:483–487.
52. Conway WD, Singhvi SM, Gibaldi M, Boyes RN. The effect of route of administration on the metabolic fate of terbutaline in the rat. Xenobiotica 1973; 3:813–821.
53. George CF, Blackwell EW, Davies DS. Metabolism of isoprenaline in the intestine. J Pharm Pharmacol 1974; 26:265–267.
54. Ilett KF, Dollery CT, Davies DS. Isoprenaline conjugation—a "true first-pass effect" in the dog intestine. J Pharm Pharmacol 1980; 32:362.
55. Davies DS, George CF, Blackwell E, et al. Metabolism of terbutaline in man and dog. Br J Clin Pharmacol 1974; 1:129–136.
56. Morgan DJ, Paull JD, Richmond BH, et al. Pharmacokinetics of intravenous and oral salbutamol and its sulphate conjugate. Br J Clin Pharmacol 1986; 22:587–593.
57. Jeppsson A-B, Roos C, Waldeck B, Widmark E. Pharmacodynamic and pharmacokinetic aspects on the transport of bronchodilator drugs through the tracheal epithelium of the guinea-pig. Pharmacol Toxicol 1989; 64:58–63.
58. Newman SP. Therapeutic aerosols. In: Clarke SW, Pavia D, eds. Aerosols and the Lung: Clinical and Experimental Aspects. London: Butterworths, 1984:197–224.
59. Kerrebijn KF. Beta agonists. In: Kaliner MA, ed. Asthma: Its Pathology and Treatment. New York: Marcel Dekker, 1991:523–559.
60. Davies DS. Pharmacokinetics of inhaled substances. Postgrad Med J 1975; 51 (suppl 7):69–75.
61. Davies DS. Pharmacokinetic studies with inhaled drugs. Eur J Respir Dis 1982; 63 (suppl 119):67–72.
62. Shenfield GM, Evans ME, Walker SR, Paterson JW. The fate of nebulized salbutamol (albuterol) administered by intermittent positive pressure respiration to asthmatic patients. Am Rev Respir Dis 1973; 108:501–505.
63. Shenfield GM, Evans ME, Paterson JW. The effect of different nebulizers with and without intermittent positive pressure breathing on the absorption and metabolism of salbutamol. Br J Clin Pharmacol 1974; 1:295–300.
64. Zainudin BMZ, Biddiscombe M, Tolfree SEJ, et al. Comparison of bronchodilator responses and deposition patterns of salbutamol inhaled from a pressurised metered dose inhaler, as a dry powder, and as a nebulised solution. Thorax 1990; 45: 469–473.
65. Schanker LS. Drug absorption from the lung. Biochem Pharmacol 1978; 27:381–385.
66. Enna SJ, Schanker LS. Absorption of drugs from the rat lung. Am J Physiol 1972; 223:1227–1231.

67. Schanker LS, Mitchell EW, Brown Jr RA. Species comparison of drug absorption from the lung after aerosol inhalation or intratracheal injection. Drug Metab Dispos 1986; 14:79–88.
68. Herrmann DR, Olsen KM, Hiller FC. Nicotine absorption after pulmonary instillation. J Pharm Sci 1992; 81:1055–1058.
69. Summers QA. Inhaled drugs and the lung. Clin Exp Allergy 1991; 21:259–268.
70. Hultquist C, Wollmer P, Eklundh G, Jonson B. Effect of inhaled terbutaline sulphate in relation to its deposition in the lungs. Pulm Pharmacol 1992; 5:127–132.
71. Shenfield GM, Evans ME, Paterson JW. Absorption of drugs by the lung. Br J Clin Pharmacol 1976; 3:583–589.
72. Laros CD, van Urk P, Rominger KL. Absorption, distribution and excretion of the tritium-labelled β_2 stimulator fenoterol hydrobromide following aerosol administration and instillation into the bronchial tree. Respiration 1977; 34:131–140.
73. Newman SP, Pavia D, Morén F, et al. Deposition of pressurised aerosols in the human respiratory tract. Thorax 1981; 36:52–55.
74. Köhler D, Fleischer W, Matthys H. New method for easy labeling of beta-2-agonists in the metered dose inhaler with Technetium[99m]. Respiration 1988; 53:65–73.
75. Newman SP, Clark AR, Talaee N, Clarke SW. Pressurised aerosol deposition in the human lung with and without an "open" spacer device. Thorax 1989; 44:706–710.
76. Newman SP, Morén F, Trofast E, et al. Deposition and clinical efficacy of terbutaline sulphate from Turbuhaler, a new multi-dose powder inhaler. Eur Respir J 1989; 2:247–252.
77. Summers QA, Clark AR, Hollingworth A, et al. The preparation of a radiolabelled aerosol of nedocromil sodium for administration by metered-dose inhaler that accurately preserves particle size distribution of the drug. Drug Invest 1990; 2: 90–98.
78. Borgström L, Nilsson M. A method for determination of the absolute pulmonary bioavailability of inhaled drugs: terbutaline. Pharm Res 1990; 7:1068–1070.
79. Ilowite JS, Bennett WD, Sheetz MS, et al. Permeability of the bronchial mucosa to ^{99m}Tc-DTPA in asthma. Am Rev Respir Dis 1989; 139:1139–1143.
80. Jeppsson A-B, Sundler F, Luts A, et al. Hydrogen peroxide-induced epithelial damage increases terbutaline transport in guinea-pig tracheal wall: implications for drug delivery. Pulm Pharmacol 1991; 4:73–79.
81. Schmekel B, Borgström L, Wollmer P. Difference in pulmonary absorption of inhaled terbutaline in healthy smokers and non-smokers. Thorax 1991; 46:225–228.
82. Schmekel B, Borgström L, Wollmer P. Exercise increases the rate of pulmonary absorption of inhaled terbutaline. Chest 1992; 101:742–745.
83. Dahl AR. Metabolic characteristics of the respiratory tract. In: McClellan RO, Henderson RF, eds. Concepts in Inhalation Toxicology. New York: Hemisphere, 1989:141–162.
84. McManus ME, Boobis AR, Pacifici GM, et al. Xenobiotic metabolism in the human lung. Life Sci 1979; 26:481–487.
85. Whitnack E, Knapp DR, Holmes JC, et al. Demethylation of nortriptyline by the dog lung. J Pharmacol Exp Ther 1972; 181:288–291.
86. Svensson L-Å, Tunek A. The design and bioactivation of presystemically stable prodrugs. Drug Metab Rev 1988; 19:165–194.

87. Ryrfeldt Å, Bodin N-O. The physiological disposition of ibuterol, terbutaline and isoproterenol after endotracheal instillation to rats. Xenobiotica 1975; 5:521–529.

88. Stemmann EA, Wolff GE. Salbutamol (Aerosol und Zäpfchen) bei Kindern mit Asthma bronchiale. Monatsschr Kinderheilkd 1980; 128:89–92.

89. Lipworth BJ, Clark RA, Dhillon DP, et al. Pharmacokinetics, efficacy and adverse effects of sublingual salbutamol in patients with asthma. Eur J Clin Pharmacol 1989; 37:567–571.

90. Hochhaus G, Schmidt EW, Rominger KL, Möllmann H. Pharmacokinetic/dynamic correlation of pulmonary and cardiac effects of fenoterol in asthmatic patients after different routes of administration. Pharm Res 1992; 9:291–297.

91. Fuglsang G, Pedersen S, Borgström L. Dose-response relationships of intravenously administered terbutaline in children with asthma. J Pediatr 1989; 114:315–320.

92. Nyberg L, Kennedy B-M. Pharmacokinetics of terbutaline given in slow-release tablets. Eur J Respir Dis 1984; 65(suppl 134):119–139.

93. Lipworth BJ, Clark RA, Dhillon DP, et al. Single dose and steady-state pharmacokinetics of 4 mg and 8 mg oral salbutamol controlled-release in patients with bronchial asthma. Eur J Clin Pharmacol 1989; 37:49–52.

94. Stålenheim G, Lindström B, Lönnerholm G. Oral terbutaline alone and in combination with theophylline: dose, plasma concentration, and effect in long-term treatment of bronchial asthma. Eur Respir J 1989; 2:861–867.

95. Lönnerholm G, Foucard T, Lindström B. Dose, plasma concentration, and effect of oral terbutaline in long-term treatment of childhood asthma. J Allergy Clin Immunol 1984; 73:508–515.

96. Yamamoto I, Iwata K, Nakashima M. Pharmacokinetics of plasma and urine clenbuterol in man, rat and rabbit. J Pharmacobiodyn 1985; 8:385–391.

97. Chasseaud LF, Wood SG. Pharmacokinetics of the bronchodilator tulobuterol in man after repeated oral doses. J Int Med Res 1986; 14:223–227.

98. Powell ML, Chung M, Weisberger M, et al. Multiple-dose albuterol kinetics. J Clin Pharmacol 1986; 26:643–646.

99. DeVries TM, Blake DS, Coon MJ, et al. Pharmacokinetics of procaterol for single- and multiple-dose administration of Pro-air® tablets in healthy subjects. Pharm Res 1990; 7(suppl):S-209.

100. Van den Berg W, Leferink JG, Tabingh Suermondt W, et al. Terbutaline serum concentrations related to different lung function parameters and beta-receptor function. Int J Clin Pharmacol Ther Toxicol 1983; 21:24–30.

101. Oosterhuis B, Braat MCP, Roos CM, et al. Pharmacokinetic-pharmacodynamic modeling of terbutaline bronchodilation in asthma. Clin Pharmacol Ther 1986; 40:469–475.

102. Billing B, Dahlqvist R, Garle M, et al. Separate and combined use of terbutaline and theophylline in asthmatics. Eur J Respir Dis 1982; 63:399–409.

103. Jain SK, Vyas SP, Dixit VK. A new approach towards the development of a transdermal terbutaline releasing system. J Control Release 1992; 22:117–124.

104. Maesen FPV, Smeets JJ. Comparison of a controlled-release tablet of salbutamol given twice daily with a standard tablet given four times daily in the management of chronic obstructive lung disease. Eur J Clin Pharmacol 1986; 31:431–436.

105. Sykes RS, Reese ME, Meyer MC, Chubb JM. Relative bioavailability of a controlled-release albuterol formulation for twice-daily use. Biopharm Drug Dispos 1988; 9:551–556.
106. Bengtsson B, Fagerström P-O. Extrapulmonary effects of terbutaline during prolonged administration. Clin Pharmacol Ther 1982; 31:726–732.
107. Saux MC, Girault J, Bouquet S, et al. Étude comparative des distributions tissulaires de deux β-mimétiques: le clenbutérol et le salbutamol chez le chien. J Pharmacol (Paris) 1986; 17:692–698.
108. Leferink JG, Wagemaker-Engels I, Maes RAA. Determination of terbutaline in postmortem human tissues by gas chromatography-mass spectrometry. J Anal Toxicol 1978; 2:86–88.
109. Ryrfeldt Å, Ramsay CH. Distribution of terbutaline. Eur J Respir Dis 1984; 65 (suppl 134):63–72.
110. Brogden RN, Faulds D. Salmeterol xinafoate. A review of its pharmacological properties and therapeutic potential in reversible obstructive airways disease. Drugs 1991; 42:895–912.
111. Borgå O, Lindberg C. Pharmacokinetic implications of slow equilibration of terbutaline between plasma and erythrocytes. Eur J Respir Dis 1984; 65(suppl 134):73–80.
112. Bergman B, Bokström H, Borgå O, et al. Transfer of terbutaline across the human placenta in late pregnancy. Eur J Respir Dis 1984; 65(suppl 134):81–86.
113. Delén A-M, Rosenborg J, Nyberg L. Distribution of bambuterol and terbutaline in whole blood during repeated administration of bambuterol. II. Baltic Meeting on Pharmacology and Clin Pharmacology. Tallinn, Estonia, Oct 3–4, 1990.
114. Martin DH, McDevitt DG. Salbutamol in the management of premature labour. Irish J Med Sci 1977; 146:424–429.
115. Dellenbach P, Guikovaty JP, Munch F, et al. Passage transplacentaire d'un anesthésique steroidien et d'un beta-mimétique: Intérêt des isotopes stables et de la spectrometrie de masse. Inserm 1977; 73:55–76.
116. Ingemarsson I, Westgren M, Lindberg C, et al. Single injection of terbutaline in term labor: placental transfer and effects on maternal and fetal carbohydrate metabolism. Am J Obstet Gynecol 1981; 139:697–701.
117. Svenningsen NW, Holmqvist P, Ingemarsson I, Westgren M. Postnatal effects of antenatal beta-receptor agonist treatment in preterm infants. In: Stern L, Bard H, Friis-Hansen B, eds. Intensive Care in the Newborn, IV. New York: Masson, 1983:19–26.
118. Von Mandach U, Huch A, Huch R. Pharmacokinetic studies on fenoterol in maternal and cord blood. Am J Perinatol 1989; 6:209–213.
119. Lindberg C, Boréus LO, de Château P, et al. Transfer of terbutaline into breast milk. Eur J Respir Dis 1984; 65(suppl 134):87–91.
120. McIlhenny HM, Ghaly MSD. Biotransformation of pirbuterol by the rat, dog, and human. Fed Proc 1979; 38:442.
121. Davies DS. Metabolism of isoprenaline and other bronchodilator drugs in man and dog. Bull Physiopathol Respir 1972; 8:679–682.
122. D'Alonzo G, Smolensky M, Feldman S, Gnosspelius G, Karlsson K. Bambuterol in the treatment of asthma. A placebo-controlled comparison of once-daily morning vs evening administration. Chest 1995; 107:406–412.

123. Powell ML, Weisberger M, Dowdy Y, et al. Comparative steady state bioavailability of conventional and controlled-release formulations of albuterol. Biopharm Drug Dispos 1987; 8:461–468.
124. Jonkman JHG, Borgström L, van der Boon WJV, de Noord OE. Theophylline-terbutaline, a steady state study on possible pharmacokinetic interactions with special reference to chronopharmacokinetic aspects. Br J Clin Pharmacol 1988; 26:285–293.
125. Rosenborg J, Nyberg L. Stereoselective pharmacokinetics of terbutaline and its prodrug bambuterol. Second Jerusalem Conference on Pharmaceutical Sciences and Clinical Pharmacology, Jerusalem, May 24–29, 1992.
126. Walker SR, Evans ME, Richards AJ, Paterson JW. The clinical pharmacology of oral and inhaled salbutamol. Clin Pharmacol Ther 1972; 13:861–867.
127. Nyberg L. Pharmacokinetic properties of bambuterol in solution and tablet—basis for once-daily dosage in asthma. Presentation at III World Conference on Clinical Pharmacology and Therapeutics. Abstract in Acta Pharmacol Toxicol 1986; 59(suppl 5):229.
128. Nyberg L, Rosenborg J, Weibull E, Jönsson S, Kennedy B-M, Nilsson M. Pharmacokinetics of bambuterol in healthy subjects. Submitted.
129. Taburet AM, Tollier C, Richard C. The effect of respiratory disorders on clinical pharmacokinetic variables. Clin Pharmacokinet 1990; 19:462–490.
130. Hutchings MJ, Paull JD, Wilson-Evered E, Morgan DJ. Pharmacokinetics and metabolism of salbutamol in premature labour. Br J Clin Pharmacol 1987; 24: 69–75.
131. Berg G, Lindberg C, Rydén G. Terbutaline in the treatment of preterm labour. Eur J Respir Dis 1984; 65(suppl 134):219–230.
132. Lyrenäs S, Grahnén A, Lindberg B, et al. Pharmacokinetics of terbutaline during pregnancy. Eur J Clin Pharmacol 1986; 29:619–623.
133. Tan WC, Lee HS. Pharmacokinetics of oral salbutamol controlled-release in Asian patients with asthma. Eur J Clin Pharmacol 1991; 41:495–496.
134. Milroy R, Carter R, Carlyle D, Boyd G. Clinical and pharmacological study of a novel controlled release preparation of salbutamol. Br J Clin Pharmacol 1990; 29:578–580.
135. Levy G, Matsuzawa T. Pharmacokinetics of salicylamide elimination in man. J Pharmacol Exp Ther 1966; 156:285–293.
136. Walle UK, Walle T. Stereoselective sulfation of terbutaline by the rat liver cytosol: evaluation of experimental approaches. Chirality 1989; 1:121–126.
137. Walle T, Walle UK. Stereoselective sulphate conjugation of racemic terbutaline by human liver cytosol. Br J Clin Pharmacol 1990; 30:127–133.
138. Borgström L, Liu Chang-Xiao, Walhagen A. Pharmacokinetics of the enantiomers of terbutaline after repeated oral dosing with racemic terbutaline. Chirality 1989; 1:174–177.
139. Borgström L, Nyberg L, Jönsson S, et al. Pharmacokinetic evaluation in man of terbutaline given as separate enantiomers and as the racemate. Br J Clin Pharmacol 1989; 27:49–56.
140. Baba S, Goromaru T, Kawaguchi I, Kishi K. Urinary excretion of salbutamol enantiomers in man by stable isotope tracer technique. Iyakuhin Kenkyu 1981; 12:84–90.

140a. Boulton DW, Fawcett JP. Enantioselective disposition of Salbutamol in man following oral and intravenous administration. Br J Clin Pharmacol 1996; 41: 35–40.

141. Walle UK, Pesola GR, Walle T. Stereoselective sulphate conjugation of salbutamol in humans: comparison of hepatic, intestinal and platelet activity. Br J Clin Pharmacol 1993; 35:413–418.

142. Pesola GR, Walle T. Enantiomeric interaction in the sulfate conjugation of the β₂-agonist drug albuterol by the human liver. Res Commun Chem Pathol Pharmacol 1992; 75:125–128.

143. Walle T, Walle UK, Thornburg KR, Schey KL. Stereoselective sulfation of albuterol in humans. Biosynthesis of the sulfate conjugate by HEP G2 cells. Drug Metab Dispos 1993; 21:76–80.

144. Shwed JA, Walle UK, Walle T. The Hep G2 cell line as a human model for sulfate conjugation of drugs. Xenobiotica 1992; 22:973–982.

145. Koster AS, Frankhuijzen-Sierevogel AC, Mentrup A. Stereoselective formation of fenoterol-para-glucuronide and fenoterol-meta-glucuronide in rat hepatocytes and enterocytes. Biochem Pharmacol 1986; 35:1981–1985.

146. Rominger KL, Mentrup A, Stiasni M. Radioimmunological determination of fenoterol. Part II: Antiserum and tracer for the determination of fenoterol. Arzneimittelforschung 1990; 40:887–895.

147. Tunek A, Kennedy B-M, Svensson A. Stereoselective interactions of bambuterol with human plasma cholinesterase. Recent Progress in Extrahepatic Drug Metabolism, Ronneby, Sweden, May 15–17, 1991.

148. Walle UK, Pesola GR, Shwed JA, Walle T. Temperature-dependent accumulation of terbutaline by the human platelet. Clin Pharmacol Ther 1992; 51:129.

149. Amirav I, Amitai Y, Avital A, Godfrey S. Enhancement of theophylline clearance by intravenous albuterol. Chest 1988; 94:444–445.

150. Amitai Y, Glustein J, Godfrey S. Enhancement of theophylline clearance by oral albuterol. Chest 1992; 102:786–789.

151. Lombardi TP, Bertino JS, Goldberg A, et al. The effects of a beta-2 selective adrenergic agonist and a beta-nonselective antagonist on theophylline clearance. J Clin Pharmacol 1987; 27:523–529.

152. Nyberg L, Weibull E, Rosenborg J. Lack of pharmacokinetic interaction between Bambec® tablets and theophylline. Eur Respir J 1991; 4(suppl 14):434s.

153. Rosenborg J, Nyberg L. Bambuterol and prednisolone do not interact. ERS Annual Congress, Florence, Italy, Sept 25–29, 1993.

154. Clark RA, Holdsworth CD, Rees MR, Howlett PJ. The effect on paracetamol absorption of stimulation and blockade of β-adrenoceptors. Br J Clin Pharmacol 1980; 10:555–559.

155. Adebayo GI, Ogundipe TO. Effects of salbutamol on the absorption and disposition of sulphamethoxazole in adult volunteers. Eur J Drug Metab Pharmacokinet 1989; 14:57–60.

156. Rosenborg J, Nyberg L, Delén A-M. Dietary habits do not influence the dosage of Bambec® tablets. Eur Respir J 1991; 4(suppl 14):434s.

157. Bolinger AM, Young KY, Gambertoglio JG, et al. Influence of food on the absorption of albuterol Repetabs. J Allergy Clin Immunol 1989; 83:123–126.

158. Hussey EK, Donn KH, Powell JR, et al. Albuterol extended-release products: effect of food on the pharmacokinetics of single oral doses of Volmax and Proventil Repetabs in healthy male volunteers. J Clin Pharmacol 1991; 31:561–564.

159. Hultquist C, Lindberg C, Nyberg L, et al. Kinetics of terbutaline in asthmatic children. Eur J Respir Dis 1984; 65(suppl 134):195–203.

160. Hultquist C, Lindberg C, Nyberg L, et al. Pharmacokinetics of intravenous terbutaline in asthmatic children. Dev Pharmacol Ther 1989; 13:11–20.

161. Kirpalani H, Koren G, Schmidt B, et al. Respiratory response and pharmacokinetics of intravenous albutamol in infants with bronchopulmonary dysplasia. Crit Care Med 1990; 18:1374–1377.

162. Rominger KL, Hermer M. Neuere Ergebnisse zur Pharmakokinetik von Fenoterol. In: Jung H, Feudel H, Karl C, eds. Neuste Ergebnisse über Betamimetika. Darmstadt: Steinkopff Verlag, 1986:6–12.

163. Kojima S, Kubodera A, Otani M, et al. Studies on the absorption, distribution, metabolism and excretion of 1-(3,5-dihydroxyphenyl)-1-hydroxy-2-[(4-hydroxyphenyl)isopropylamino]-ethane hydrobromide (Th 1165a, fenoterol hydrobromide) in rats. Pharmacometrics 1980; 20:55–66.

164. Kramer I, Klingspohr HJ. Ganztierautoradiographische Untersuchungen über die Verteilung und die diaplazentare Passage von Fenoterol-hydrobromid (Th 1165a) an Ratten. Arzneimittelforschung 1974; 24:1210–1213.

165. Heckner RM. Systematische Untersuchungen zur Proteinbindung biologisch wirksamer Substanzen. Pharmatherapeutica 1979; 2:177–186.

166. Newman SP, Weisz AWB, Talaee N, Clarke SW. Improvement of drug delivery with a breath actuated pressurised aerosol for patients with poor inhaler technique. Thorax 1991; 46:712–716.

167. Biddiscombe M, Melchor R, Mak V, et al. The lung deposition of salbutamol, directly labelled with technetium-99m, delivered by pressurised metered dose and dry powder inhalers. Int J Pharm 1993; 91:111–121.

168. Melchor R, Biddiscombe MF, Mak VHF, et al. Lung deposition patterns of directly labelled salbutamol in normal subjects and in patients with reversible airflow obstruction. Thorax 1993; 48:506–511.

169. Tegnér K. Nilsson HT, Persson CGA, et al. Elimination pathways of terbutaline. Eur J Respir Dis 1984; 65(suppl 134):93–100.

170. Bodin NO, Hansson E, Ramsay CH, Ryrfeldt Å. The tissue distribution of ^{3}H-terbutaline (Bricanyl®) in mice. Acta Physiol Scand 1972; 84:40–47.

171. Rosberg B, Schröder C, Nyberg L, et al. Bambuterol and terbutaline in human cerebrospinal fluid and plasma. Eur J Clin Pharmacol 1993; 45:147–150.

172. Nilsson HT, Persson CGA, Tegnér K, et al. Biliary excretion of ^{3}H-terbutaline in man. Biochem Pharmacol 1973; 22:3128–3129.

173. Postma DS, Koëter GH, Keyzer JJ, Meurs H. Influence of slow-release terbutaline on the circadian variation of catecholamines, histamine, and lung function in nonallergic patients with partly reversible airflow obstruction. J Allergy Clin Immunol 1986; 77:471–477.

174. Fielding RM, Abra RM. Factors affecting the release rate of terbutaline from liposome formulations after intratracheal instillation in the guinea pig. Pharm Res 1992; 9:220–223.

175. Wettrell G, Anehus S, Hattevig G, Kjellman B. Terbutaline slow-release tablets in children with bronchial asthma. Allergy 1986; 41:418–422.
176. Fuglsang G, Hertz B, Holm EB, Borgström L. Absolute bioavailability of terbutaline from a CR-granulate in asthmatic children. Biopharm Drug Dispos 1990; 11:85–90.
177. Goldstein DA, Tan YK, Soldin SJ. Pharmacokinetics and absolute bioavailability of salbutamol in healthy adult volunteers. Eur J Clin Pharmacol 1987; 32:631–634.
178. Fairfax AJ, McNabb WR, Davies HJ, Spiro SG. Slow-release oral salbutamol and aminophylline in nocturnal asthma: relation of overnight changes in lung function and plasma drug levels. Thorax 1980; 35:526–530.
179. Rey E, Luquel L, Richard MO, et al. Pharmacokinetics of intravenous salbutamol in renal insufficiency and its biological effects. Eur J Clin Pharmacol 1989; 37: 387–389.
180. Maconochie JG, Fowler P. Plasma concentrations of salbutamol after an oral slow-release preparation. Curr Med Res Opin 1983; 8:634–639.
181. Civiale C, Ritschel WA, Shiu GK, et al. In vivo–in vitro correlation of salbutamol release from a controlled release osmotic pump delivery system. Methods Find Exp Clin Pharmacol 1991; 13:491–498.
182. Hussey EK, Donn KH, Powell JR. Albuterol extended-release products: a comparison of steady-state pharmacokinetics. Pharmacotherapy 1991; 11:131–135.
183. Babu VBM, Khar RK. In vitro and in vivo studies of sustained-release floating dosage forms containing salbutamol sulfate. Pharmazie 1990; 45:268–270.
184. Gokhale R, Schmidt C, Alcorn L, et al. Transdermal drug delivery systems of albuterol: In vitro and in vivo studies. J Pharm Sci 1992; 81:996–999.
185. Pitts NE, Borger AP, Ghaly MS, et al. Pirbuterol—a new selective beta-agonist. Royal Society of Medicine: International Congress and Symposium Series 1983; 56:1–31.
186. Schmid J, Prox A, Zimmer A, et al. Biotransformation of clenbuterol. Fresenius J Anal Chem 1990; 337:121.
187. Girault J. Le couplage chromatographique gaz-liquide spectrométrie de masse: application à la détermination de femtomoles de Clenbutérol (NAB 365 Cl) dans les milieux biologiques. PhD dissertation, Faculty of Pharmacy, University of Poitiers, France, 1986.
188. Kopitar Z, Zimmer A. Pharmakokinetik und Metabolitenmuster von Clenbuterol bei der Ratte. Arzneimittelforschung 1976; 26:1435–1441.
189. Meyer HH, Rinke LM. The pharmacokinetics and residues of clenbuterol in veal calves. J Anim Sci 1991; 69:4538–4544.
190. Couet W, Girault J, Reigner BG, et al. Steady-state bioavailability and pharmacokinetics of ambroxol and clenbuterol administered alone and combined in a new oral formulation. Int J Clin Pharmacol Ther Toxicol 1989; 27:467–472.
191. Yuge T, Hase T, Takayanagi Y, et al. Pharmacokinetic studies of mabuterol, a new selective β_2-stimulant. I: Studies on the absorption, distribution and excretion in rats. Arzneimittelforschung 1984; 34:1659–1667.
192. Horiba M, Murai T, Nomura K, et al. Pharmacokinetic studies of mabuterol, a new selective β_2-stimulant. II: Urinary metabolites of mabuterol in rats and their pharmacological effects. Arzneimittelforschung 1984; 34:1668–1679.

193. Matsumura K, Kubo O, Sakashita T, et al. Studies on the metabolism of tulo-buterol·HCl. Identification of basic urinary metabolites in the dog, rat, rabbit, and guinea pig. Drug Metab Dispos 1982; 10:537–541.

194. Matsumura K, Kubo O, Sakashita T, et al. Quantitative determination of tu-lobuterol and its metabolites in human urine by mass fragmentography. J Chro-matogr Biomed Appl 1981; 222:53–60.

195. Uesaka I, Aratani T, Nishide K, et al. Studies on the metabolic fate of o-cloro-α-(*tert*-butylaminomethyl) benzylalcohol hydrochloride (C-78). I. Absorption, dis-tribution and excretion of C-78 in rats. Iyakuhin Kenkyo 1976; 7:548–557.

196. Gomi Y, Shirahase H, Funato H. Effects of 1-(2-chloro-4-hydroxyphenyl)-*t*-buty-laminoethanol (Hoku-81), a new bronchodilator, on isolated trachea and atria of guinea pig. Jpn J Pharmacol 1979; 29:515–524.

197. Matsumura K, Kubo O, Tsukada T, et al. Determination of tulobuterol in human serum by electron-capture gas-liquid chromatography. J Chromatogr Biomed Appl 1982; 230:148–153.

198. Grassi C. Broxaterol: a new β_2-adrenoceptor agonist for the treatment of revers-ible airways disease. Opening remarks. Respiration 1989; 55(suppl 2):1–3.

199. Löfdahl C-G, Sigvaldasson A, Skoogh B-E, Svedmyr N. Broxaterol, a new β_2-ad-renoceptor agonist compared to salbutamol in asthmatics, oral and inhalation treatment. Respiration 1989; 55(suppl 2):15–19.

200. Minneman KP, Hedberg A, Molinoff PB. Comparison of beta adrenergic recep-tor subtypes in mammalian tissues. J Pharmacol Exp Ther 1979; 211:502–508.

201. Yabuuchi Y. The β-adrenoceptor stimulant properties of OPC-2009 on guinea-pig isolated tracheal, right atrial and left atrial preparations. Br J Pharmacol 1977; 61:513–521.

202. Waldeck B, Jeppsson A-B, Widmark E. Partial agonism and functional selectivity: a study on β-adrenoceptor mediated effects in tracheal, cardiac and skeletal mus-cle. Acta Pharmacol Toxicol 1986; 58:209–218.

203. Yasuda Y, Fujisawa N, Morita S, Kohri H. Metabolic fate of a new β_2-adrenergic stimulant procaterol (OPC-2009). Absorption, distribution, metabolism and ex-cretion in the beagle dog. Arzneimittelforschung 1979; 29:261–265.

204. Eldon MA, Battle MM, Coon MJ, et al. Clinical pharmacokinetics and relative bioavailability of oral procaterol. Pharm Res 1993; 10:603–605.

205. Ishigami M, Saburomaru K, Niino K, et al. Pharmacokinetics of procaterol in the rat, rabbit and beagle dog. Arzneimittelforschung 1979; 29:266–270.

206. Shimizu T, Mori H, Tabusa E, et al. The metabolism of a bronchodilator pro-caterol HCl in the rat in vitro and in vivo. Xenobiotica 1978; 8:349–358.

207. Eldon MA, Blake DS, Coon MJ, et al. Clinical pharmacokinetics of procaterol: dose proportionality after administration of single oral doses. Biopharm Drug Dispos 1992; 13:663–669.

208. Ullman A, Bergendal A, Lindén A, et al. Onset of action and duration of effect of formoterol and salmeterol compared to salbutamol in isolated guinea pig tra-chea with or without epithelium. Allergy 1992; 47:384–387.

209. Brittain RT, Dean CM, Jack D. Sympathomimetic bronchodilator drugs. Phar-macol Ther 1976; 2:423–462.

210. Bradshaw J, Brittain RT, Coleman RA, et al. The design of salmeterol. A long-acting selective β_2-adrenoceptor agonist. Br J Pharmacol 1987; 92:590P.

211. Anderson G, Lindén A, Rabe K. Why are long-acting beta-adrenoceptor agonists long-acting? Eur Respir J 1994; 7:569–578.

212. Löfdahl C-G, Svedmyr N. Formoterol fumarate, a new β_2-adrenoceptor agonist. Acute studies of selectivity and duration of effect after inhaled and oral administration. Allergy 1989; 44:264–271.

213. Sasaki H, Kamimura H, Shiobara Y, et al. Disposition and metabolism of formoterol fumarate, a new bronchodilator, in rats and dogs. Xenobiotica 1982; 12: 803–812.

214. Maesen FPV, Smeets JJ, Gubbelmans HLL, Zweers PGMA. Bronchodilator effect of inhaled formoterol vs salbutamol over 12 hours. Chest 1990; 97:590–594.

215. Sasaki H, Kamimura H, Enjoji Y, Shiobara Y. Absorption and distribution of formoterol fumarate in rats. Pharmacometrics 1983; 25:981–991.

216. Braat M, Portier E, Van den Berg B, et al. Formoterol detection and pharmacokinetics in human subjects after an oral dose of 168 microgram. Am Rev Respir Dis 1992; 145(4):A60.

217. Firkusny L, Deeg M, Gradin-Frimmer G, et al. Untersuchung zur Pharmakodynamik und Resorption des β_2-Sympathikomimetikums Formoterol nach Inhalation an gesunden Probanden. Klin Wochenschr 1990; 68(suppl XIX):42.

218. Manchee G, Barrow A, Kulkarni S, et al. Disposition of salmeterol xinafoate in laboratory animals and humans. Drug Metab Dispos 1993; 21:1022.

219. Colthup PV, Young GC, Felgate CC. Determination of salmeterol in rat and dog plasma by high-performance liquid chromatography with fluorescence detection. J Pharm Sci 1993; 82:323–325.

220. Drug monograph: Serevent (Salmeterol). Swedish Medical Agency Information No. 31, 1992 (in Swedish).

221. Ullman A, Svedmyr N. Salmeterol, a new long acting inhaled β_2-adrenoceptor agonist: comparison with salbutamol in adult asthmatic patients. Thorax 1988; 43:674–678.

222. Glaxo product information. "This is Serevent" (in Swedish).

223. Sinkula AA, Yalkowsky SH. Rationale for design of biologically reversible drug derivatives: prodrug. J Pharm Sci 1975; 64:181–210.

224. Tullar BF, Minatoya H, Lorenz RR. Esters of N-*tert*-butylarterenol. Long-acting new bronchodilators with reduced cardiac effects. J Med Chem 1976; 19:834–838.

225. Minatoya H. Studies on bitolterol, di-p-toluate ester of n-*tert*-butylarterenol: a new long-acting bronchodilator with reduced cardiovascular effects. J Pharmacol Exp Ther 1978; 206:515–527.

226. Friedel HA, Brogden RN. Bitolterol. A preliminary review of its pharmacological properties and therapeutic efficacy in reversible obstructive airways disease. Drugs 1988; 35:22–41.

227. Svensson L-Å. A prodrug approach to a long-acting beta$_2$ agonist. Drug News & Perspectives 1991; 4:544–549.

228. Tunek A, Borgström L, Nyberg L. Metabolism in man of ^{3}H-bambuterol: a carbamate ester prodrug of terbutaline. Acta Pharmacol Toxicol 1986; 59(suppl 5): 214.

229. Lindberg C, Roos C, Tunek A, Svensson L-Å. Metabolism of bambuterol in rat liver microsomes: identification of hydroxylated and demethylated products by liquid chromatography mass spectrometry. Drug Metab Dispos 1989; 17:311–322.

230. Tunek A, Levin E, Svensson L-Å. Hydrolysis of ^{3}H-bambuterol, a carbamate prodrug of terbutaline, in blood from humans and laboratory animals in vitro. Biochem Pharmacol 1988; 37:3867–3876.

231. Tunek A, Svensson L-Å. Bambuterol, a carbamate ester prodrug of terbutaline, as inhibitor of cholinesterases in human blood. Drug Metab Dispos 1988; 16:759–764.

232. Fisher DM, Caldwell JE, Sharma M, Wirén J-E. The influence of bambuterol (carbamylated terbutaline) on the duration of action of succinylcholine-induced paralysis in humans. Anesthesiology 1988; 69:757–759.

233. Bang U, Viby-Mogensen J, Wirén J-E, Theil Skovgaard L. The effect of bambuterol (carbamylated terbutaline) on plasma cholinesterase activity and suxamethonium-induced neuromuscular blockade in genotypically normal patients. Acta Anaesthesiol Scand 1990; 34:596–599.

234. Bang U, Viby-Mogensen J, Wirén J-E. The effect of bambuterol on plasma cholinesterase activity and suxamethonium-induced neuromuscular blockade in subjects heterozygous for abnormal plasma cholinesterase. Acta Anaesthesiol Scand 1990; 34:600–604.

235. Staun P, Lennmarken C, Eriksson LI, Wirén J-E. The influence of 10 mg and 20 mg of bambuterol on the duration of succinylcholine-induced neuromuscular blockade. Acta Anaesthesiol Scand 1990; 34:498–500.

236. Tunek A, Hjertberg E, Viby-Mogensen J. Interactions of bambuterol with human serum cholinesterase of the genotypes E_uE_u (normal), E_aE_a (atypical) and E_uE_a. Biochem Pharmacol 1991; 41:345–348.

237. Bang U, Nyberg L, Rosenborg J, Viby-Mogensen J. Pharmacokinetics of bambuterol in subjects homozygous for the atypical gene for plasma cholinesterase. Submitted.

238. Holstein-Rathlou N-H, Laursen LC, Madsen F, et al. Bambuterol: dose response study of a new terbutaline prodrug in asthma. Eur J Clin Pharmacol 1986; 30:7–11.

6

Mechanisms of Duration of Action of Inhaled Long-Acting Beta₂-Adrenoceptor Agonists

KLAUS F. RABE

Zentrum für Pneumologie und
  Thoraxchirurgie
Krankenhaus Grosshanssdorf
Landesversicherungsanstalt Hamburg
Grosshansdorf, Germany

ANDERS LINDÉN

Institute of Heart and Lung Disease
Gothenburg University
Gothenburg, Sweden

I. Introduction

Long-acting beta₂-adrenoceptor agonists are now frequently used for the treatment of reversible obstructive airways disease. The mechanisms behind the long duration of bronchodilatory action for the currently available β_2-adrenoceptor agonists with extended duration of action, formoterol and salmeterol, are only partially understood. This chapter compares the pharmacological characteristics of long-acting with those of short-acting β_2-adrenoceptor agonists in human and animal airways. The available experimental evidence suggests that, for β_2-adrenoceptor agonists, long duration of action may depend on several factors: both formoterol and salmeterol display a higher lipophilicity and have a higher affinity and selectivity than most short-acting agonists at the β_2-adrenoceptor. Of these factors, the lipophilicity may be one of the most important ones by determining the amount of drug entering into the cell membrane in the vicinity of the β_2-adrenoceptor. However, the receptor affinity, maximum relaxant effect (efficacy or intrinsic activity), potency, and receptor selectivity may also be of importance in determining how much β_2-adrenocep- tor agonist needs to remain at the receptor for sustained action.

The β_2-adrenoceptor agonists formoterol (Foradil) and salmeterol (Ser- event) represent a significant improvement in the treatment of reversible air- way obstruction in terms of long-lasting bronchodilation (1,2). The rapidly increasing clinical use of these new β_2-agonists is, however, contrasted by the limited understanding of the mechanisms behind the long-lasting bronchodi- lation. Because these mechanisms may have applications not only for the de- sign of new bronchodilators but also for other types of drugs, it might be bene- ficial to consider the increasing basic pharmacological data on long-acting β_2-adrenoceptor agonists in detail.

II. Physicochemical Properties of Formoterol and Salmeterol

Formoterol is a diasteriomer comprising a 1:1 mixture of the (RR)- and (SS)- enantiomers of 2-hydroxy-5-[(1RS)-hydroxy-2-(p-methoxyphenyl)-1-methyl- ethyl]amino]-ethyl]formanilide formulated as the fumarate dihydrate salt. Salmeterol, on the other hand, is a steriomer comprising a 1:1 mixture of the (R)- and (S)-enantiomers of (4-hydroxy-alpha[[[6-[4-phenylbutyl)oxy]hexyl]amino] methyl]-1,3-benzenedimethanol formulated as the xinofoate (hydroxynaph- thoate) salt. Both these drugs are derivatives of phenylethanolamine (3,4) (Fig. 1).

The pronounced lipophilicity of salmeterol is believed to be due to its aliphatic side chain (3,5–7). In spite of its apparently long side chain, salmet- erol is thought to be only twice the length (25 Å) of formoterol at a neutral pH (3). For formoterol, without any aliphatic side chain, the lipophilicity is less pronounced (3,7). Compared with shorter-acting salbutamol, however, both long-acting β_2-adrenoceptor agonists display significantly more lipophilicity, as indicated by the octanol/water distribution (7).

III. Animal Airways

A. Formoterol and Salmeterol at the β_2-Adrenoceptor In Vitro

Potency

Many in vitro studies on the pharmacology of formoterol and salmeterol deal with only one of these drugs using short-acting salbutamol as a reference. There is, however, one study comparing the potency of formoterol and salmet- erol with that of short-acting salbutamol at various levels of basal airway smooth-muscle tone within the same guinea pig model (8,9) (Fig. 2). This study indicates that formoterol is significantly more potent than salmeterol and

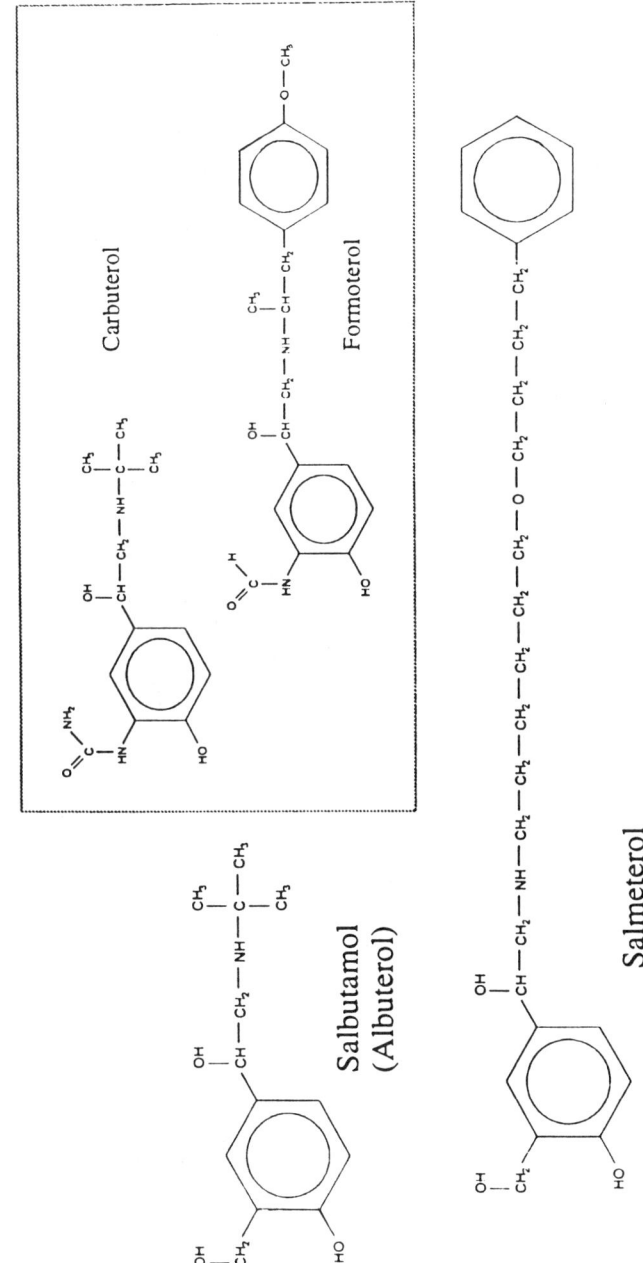

Figure 1 The chemical structures of the saligenin β-adrenoceptor agonists salbutamol and salmeterol and the anilide derivatives carbuterol and formoterol.

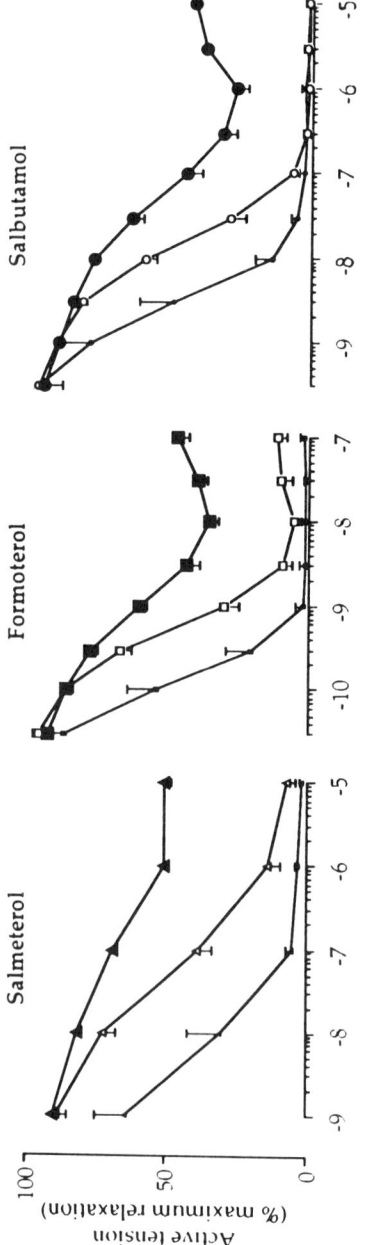

Figure 2 Concentration response curves for β-adrenoceptor agonists salmeterol (triangles), formoterol (squares), and salbutamol (circles) at various levels of carbachol-induced precontraction (small filled symbols, 60 nM; intermediate open symbols, 0.3 μM; large filled symbols, 3 μM) in the guinea pig trachea. The data are presented as mean (s.e.m.) percentage of the difference in active tension between the precontraction level and the level in the presence of 2.2 mM theophylline. Airways were pretreated with 10 μM indomethacin. (From Ref. 8.)

salbutamol at all levels of smooth muscle tone using muscarinic precontraction. For formoterol and its analogue BD40A and for salbutamol, the difference in potency is also demonstrated in other studies on the guinea pig trachea using moderate or severe precontraction induced by carbachol, histamine, methacholine, or prostaglandin $F_{2\alpha}$ ($PGF_{2\alpha}$) (10–12). The higher potency of formoterol compared with salmeterol is also evident in another study using one moderate level of muscarinic precontraction in the guinea pig trachea (13). Some data on the guinea pig trachea suggest that salmeterol is slightly more potent than salbutamol as well using precontraction caused by prostaglandin $F_{2\alpha}$ (14,15). This rank order of potency for formoterol, salmeterol, and salbutamol is unchanged when tested against neurally mediated cholinergic contraction in the guinea pig trachea (12). Using various means of inducing precontraction, formoterol thus appears more potent than salbutamol and salmeterol in animal airways.

It is generally accepted that as the basal smooth muscle tone is increased from a low to a high level, the concentration response curve to a smooth muscle relaxant, such as theophylline, shifts to the right (16,17). This functional antagonism has now also been examined for long-acting β₂-agonists. Using increasing carbachol-induced smooth muscle contraction, data on the guinea pig trachea show that the concentration response curve to formoterol, salmeterol, and short-acting salbutamol shifts rightward without any pronounced drug-related difference (8,9) (see Fig. 2). The results on animal airways are thus consistent with a similar functional antagonism against muscarinic smooth muscle contraction for long- and short-acting β₂-agonists.

Selectivity

The standard procedure to estimate adrenoceptor selectivity for β-agonists is to compare the potency for relaxation of airway smooth muscle with the potency for an increase in rate in atrial muscle, assuming that these tissues are dominated by β₂- and β₁-adrenoceptors, respectively (4,18–21). Using this technique on guinea pig trachea and atria, formoterol appears to be slightly more selective for β₂-adrenoceptors than salmeterol, whereas the corresponding selectivity for short-acting salbutamol is far less (20). Formoterol is also more selective than short-acting salbutamol, as estimated by the ratio for the inhibition of binding of the selective β₂-antagonist ICI 118,551 in lung membranes and of the selective β₁-antagonist CGP 12,177 in atria of the guinea pig (11).

Salmeterol, on the other hand, is claimed to be more selective than formoterol in one study using the guinea pig trachea and rat atrium (22). There are also data showing a concentration-dependent increase in the contractile force of rat atria for formoterol but not to salmeterol (23), but this was observed using formoterol concentrations beyond those required for relaxation of the guinea pig trachea. In rat atria, salmeterol also displays less shift of the concentration response curve to the nonselective β-agonist isoprenaline when compared with salbutamol. Furthermore, salmeterol displays more potency than salbutamol in the human bronchus and in the guinea pig trachea as well (4). This also suggests that salmeterol is more selective than salbutamol at β₂-adrenoceptors. In other words, although the rank order for formoterol and salmeterol can be questioned, both these long-acting drugs appear to be more selective for β₂-adrenoceptors in animal airways than short-acting salbutamol.

Affinity

Formoterol has a higher binding affinity for the β₂-adrenoceptor than short-acting salbutamol in guinea pig lung membranes, as indicated by the capability to inhibit binding of the selective β₂-antagonist ICI 118,551 (11). In rat lung membranes, however, the difference in affinity for formoterol and salmeterol is small, as indicated by the capability to inhibit binding of the β-antagonist iodopindolol (24). In this latter model, short-acting salbutamol displays a considerably lower inhibitory potency against iodopindolol binding than both long-acting β-agonists. There are also data on inhibition of pindolol binding in guinea pig lungs, suggesting that salmeterol has a higher affinity for the β-adrenoceptor than short-acting salbutamol (25,26). Tentatively, both formoterol and salmeterol do display a higher degree of β-adrenoceptor affinity in animal airways than does short-acting salbutamol.

Maximum Relaxant Effect (Efficacy, Intrinsic Activity)

In the guinea pig trachea, long-acting formoterol and short-acting salbutamol produce a greater maximum relaxant effect than long-acting salmeterol using maximally effective muscarinic precontraction (8,9) (Fig. 2), and these results have been confirmed independently (27). There are also data showing that very high concentrations of salmeterol produce relaxation which cannot be overcome by β-blockade in correspondingly high concentrations (9) (Fig. 3). The possibility of a non–β-adrenoceptor–mediated relaxant effect must therefore be considered. This possibility is also highlighted by data on the ferret trachea (28) (Fig. 4). Using postganglionic neural activation to induce precontraction, formoterol and salmeterol produce more relaxation than short-acting salbutamol in the ferret trachea. However, in contrast to formoterol and short-acting salbutamol, the relaxation induced by salmeterol is not inhibited by β-adrenoceptor blockade. Using matched postjunctional muscarinic precontraction, however, the relaxant effect of salmeterol is far less pronounced and it is also inhibited by β-blockade (Fig. 4). For formoterol and salbutamol, β-blockade does inhibit the relaxant effect on postjunctional precontraction. Most likely, these data indicate that postganglionic cholinergic nerves are more

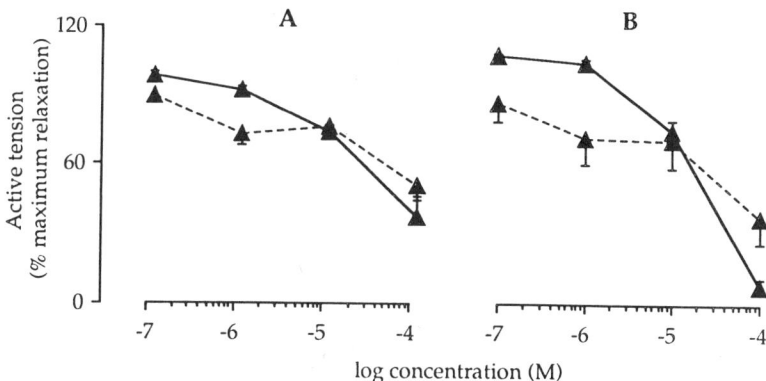

Figure 3 Concentration response curve for β-adrenoceptor agonist salmeterol with (solid line) and without (filled line) β-blockade with either 0.1 mM (A) or 1 mM (B) sotalol in the isolated guinea pig trachea. The airways were pretreated with 10 μM indomethacin and precontracted with 3 μM carbachol. Data are presented as the mean (s.e.m.) percentage of the difference in active tension between the precontraction level and the level in the presence of 2.2 mM theophylline. (From Ref. 9.)

sensitive to the non–β-adrenoceptor–mediated relaxant effect than airway smooth muscle.

It thus appears as if formoterol and salbutamol produce more β-adrenoceptor–mediated relaxant effect than salmeterol in animal airways. Salmeterol, on the other hand, may also produce non–β-adrenoceptor–mediated relaxation (9,28). It remains to be established whether the non–β-adrenoceptor–mediated relaxation can be produced by other lipophilic β-adrenoceptor agonists than salmeterol.

Second-Messenger Production

There are limited data on the ability of the long-acting β-agonists to increase the second-messenger levels. However, in line with salmeterol being a partial agonist, the adenylate cyclase activation is smaller with salmeterol than with formoterol at the β₂-adrenoceptor using guinea pig lung membranes (11). In this model, isoprenaline produces more cyclic AMP than either of the long-acting β-agonists. Because isoprenaline is relatively short-acting compared with salmeterol against contraction induced PGF$_{2\alpha}$ and postganglionic cholinergic activation in the guinea pig trachea (4,14,29), these data suggest that the level of second-messenger production is not critical for long duration of action. This is provided that a threshold increase in second messenger is obtained.

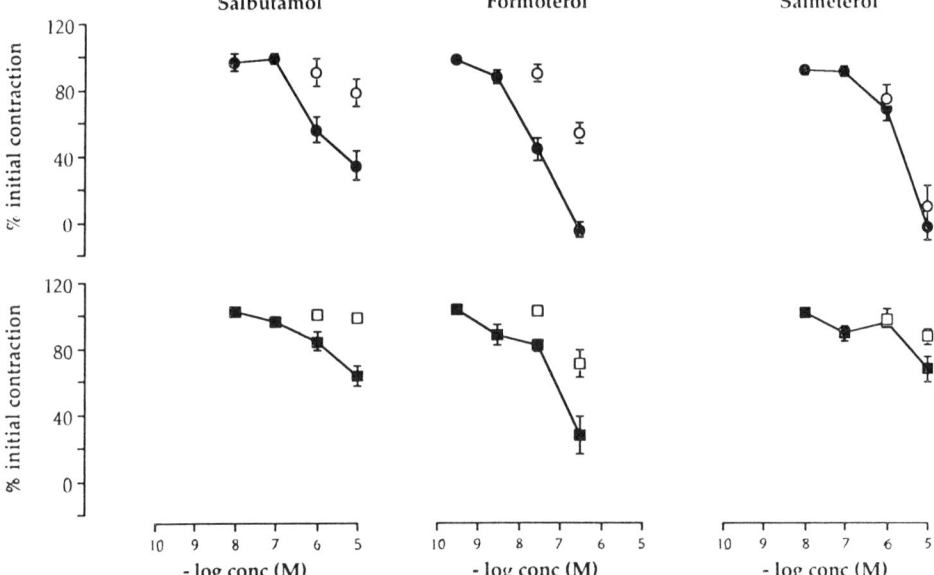

Figure 4 Inhibition of contraction induced by electrical field stimulation (2 Hz, 700 mA; upper panel) or by acetylcholine (0.5 μM; lower panel) in the isolated ferret trachea. Filled symbols represent increasing concentrations of the β-adrenoceptor agonists salbutamol, formoterol, and salmeterol and open symbols represent corresponding values after sotalol (10 μM). The data are presented as mean (s.e.m.) percent of initial baseline contraction. (From Ref. 28.)

The importance of the duration of cyclic adenosine monophosphate (cAMP) production remains to be evaluated.

B. Formoterol and Salmeterol at the β₂-Adrenoceptor In Vivo

Formoterol is significantly more potent than salmeterol, which in turn is more potent than salbutamol as an inhibitor of histamine-induced bronchoconstriction in anesthetised or conscious guinea pigs (12,30). For salmeterol and salbutamol, however, the difference in potency might be small as measured against a serotonin-induced increase in tracheal pressure or histamine-induced bronchoconstriction using intraduodenal administration in the anesthetised cat and aerosol administration in conscious guinea pigs, respectively (15). Evidently, with respect to the potency in animal airways in vivo, the rank order for formoterol, salmeterol, and salbutamol is similar to that observed in vitro.

Summarizing the basic pharmacological characteristics at the β_2-adrenoceptor in animals, it appears as if long-acting formoterol and salmeterol display higher potency, affinity, and selectivity in vitro as well as in vivo than does short-acting salbutamol. Formoterol and salmeterol are also more lipophilic than salbutamol. In contrast to formoterol, salmeterol appears to be a partial agonist in comparison with short-acting salbutamol.

C. Duration of Action for Salmeterol and Formoterol In Vitro

Salmeterol

In vitro, salmeterol induces a relaxation which persists significantly longer than that of salbutamol using the guinea pig trachea precontracted by prostaglandins (4,5). This is indicated by an approximately fourfold longer time to 50% offset of action using the concentration required for 50% of the maximum drug response.

Lipophilic salmeterol but not hydrophilic salbutamol produce β-adrenoceptor activation which persists significantly after washout followed by muscarinic stimulation in the guinea pig trachea (7). In a corresponding way, the relaxant effect of lipophilic salmeterol also reasserts itself after β-blockade followed by repeated washout using the guinea pig trachea and muscarinic precontraction (31,32) (Fig. 5). Similar results have been obtained using salmeterol against postganglionic cholinergic activation in the guinea pig isolated

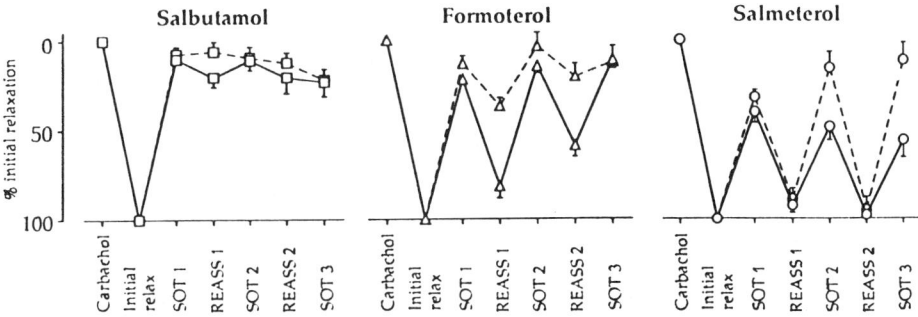

Figure 5   Reassertion of relaxant effects after β-adrenoceptor blockade followed by washout for formoterol, salbutamol, and salmeterol in the guinea pig isolated trachea. Baseline contraction was established by 0.2 μM carbachol, and the data are presented as mean (s.e.m.) percentage of the initial relaxation caused by the β-adrenoceptor agonist before β-adrenoceptor blockade with 10 μM sotalol. (From Ref. 8.)

trachea (33,34). As demonstrated in Figure 5, the reassertion phenomenon of salmeterol appears both at the maximally effective concentration and at a concentration 10 times as high and a recent study demonstrates salmeterol's reasserted relaxant effect even at submaximally effective concentrations (31). Using postganglionic neural activation by electrical field stimulation, the relaxant effect of salmeterol also reasserts itself after superfusion and β-blockade (4,24). All these findings are consistent with the idea that salmeterol remains in the vicinity of the β_2-adrenoceptor and that its long duration does not require constant attachment to the catecholamine site of the receptor (1,18).

In correspondence with its slower offset of action, salmeterol displays a slower onset of action than short-acting salbutamol in the guinea pig trachea precontracted by carbachol (7,13,31). This rank order in time to onset of action may, as the offset of action, relate to the lipophilicity as measured by the octanol/water distribution ratio. Recent data on the guinea pig trachea suggest that an increase in salmeterol's concentration does not significantly reduce the time to onset of action (31). This is similar to the weak influence of the drug concentration on the reassertion of salmeterol's relaxant effect after β-blockade followed by washout (32) (see Fig. 5).

In addition to the functional studies on salmeterol, there are data on the time course of salmeterol's dissociation from the β_2-adrenoceptor in rat lung membranes. These data, based on the replacement of salmeterol by the β-antagonist pindolol, indicate that salmeterol persists at the receptor for more than 1 hr, whereas salbutamol dissociates to a major part within 15 min (22,25, 29). According to data on the guinea pig trachea, salmeterol's duration of action is similar with and without removal of the airway mucosa at the pars membranacea (13).

Formoterol

Clinically, long-acting formoterol (1) clearly illustrates the limitations of and difficulties in experimental pharmacology by displaying a relatively short duration of action in several in vitro studies. Formoterol is thus inferior to salmeterol in causing reasserted relaxation in the guinea pig trachea using precontraction by postganglionic cholinergic activation (24). Its time to 50% recovery of baseline precontraction is, however, threefold that of clinically short-acting salbutamol when used in high concentrations (24).

Although formoterol is surprisingly short acting in some in vitro models, there are data showing that formoterol's relaxant effect reasserts itself significantly after β-blockade followed by repeated washout (31,32). These data were obtained on the guinea pig trachea (Fig. 5). At equieffective concentrations, the degree of reasserted effect is less pronounced for formoterol than for salmeterol but more pronounced for formoterol than for salbutamol. This finding is in agreement with formoterol producing β-adrenoceptor activation after washout followed by muscarinic stimulation but to a lesser degree than for salmeterol (7).

In contrast to formoterol's significantly longer time to offset of action, formoterol displays a time to onset of action which is similar to that of short-acting salbutamol at near-maximum equieffective concentrations in the guinea pig trachea (7,13,31). However, this rank order in onset of action appears, as the offset of action, to relate with the lipophilicity as measured by the octanol/water distribution. Recent data on the guinea pig trachea also suggest that the time to onset of action is reduced as formoterol's concentration is increased (31). For formoterol, this relationship is thus similar to the influence of the drug concentration on the reassertion of relaxant effect after β-blockade followed by washout.

Measuring replacement at the β_2-adrenoceptor by the β_2-antagonist pindolol in rat lung membranes, there is also one study suggesting that formoterol dissociates from the β_2-adrenoceptor almost as rapidly as salbutamol (22,25, 33). For formoterol, as for salmeterol, the duration of action is similar with and without removal of the airway mucosa at the pars membranacea using the guinea pig trachea (13).

In summary, measuring the reassertion of relaxant effect after β-block-ade and washout at micromolar β_2-agonist concentrations reveals a property shared by clinically long-acting salmeterol and formoterol but not by clinically short-acting salbutamol (31,32). The fact that the measurement of the time to 50% offset of initial relaxation is a less reproducible method to demonstrate formoterol's long duration might be explained in terms of choosing an adequate drug concentration. This latter possibility is suggested by the fact that, for formoterol but not for salmeterol, a near-maximally effective concentration appears to be required for a significant reassertion of relaxant effect after β-blockade and washout (31,32).

D. Duration of Action for Salmeterol and Formoterol In Vivo

The in vivo data regarding duration of action for long-acting β_2-agonists is limited, especially for formoterol. In one study on conscious guinea pigs, salmeterol produces twice as long inhibition of histamine-induced bronchoconstriction as does formoterol (12). Both salmeterol and formoterol do, however, produce longer lasting inhibition of histamine-induced bronchoconstriction than does salbutamol according to the referred study.

Unexpectedly, orally administered salmeterol and salbutamol both display a 12-hr duration of relaxation of histamine-induced bronchoconstriction using conscious guinea pigs (15). When inhaled, however, salbutamol's duration of action is shorter, approximately 1 hour, and is concentration dependent.

Inhaled salmeterol, on the other hand, displays a similar duration of action for various doses and its duration of action is at least threefold that of salbutamol (15). The discrepancy in duration of action between inhalation and oral administration for salbutamol is opposite to that of formoterol in human subjects (1). In anesthetized cats, the time to 50% recovery of initial bronchodilation is also significantly longer for salmeterol than for clinically shorter-acting clenbuterol, isoprenaline, and salbutamol, measuring the time course for changes in tracheal pressure with doses producing 50% of the maximum drug response (15). Surprisingly, there is also one study on anesthetized guinea pigs demonstrating a similar time course for formoterol and clinically short-acting salbutamol regarding inhibition of a histamine-induced increase in lung resistance (30).

In summary, there are in vivo studies on animal airways suggesting that formoterol and salmeterol are long acting, but there are contradictory data as well. At present, there is a lack of conclusive data on animal airways in vivo highlighting the mechanisms behind the long duration of action for these β_2-agonists.

IV. Human Airways

Several long-acting β-adrenoceptor agonists, including procaterol (35,36), bambuterol (37,38), formoterol, and salmeterol, have been developed for clinical use in bronchial asthma (1,4,39,40). Until now, however, limited data have been available on the in vitro pharmacology of these compounds in human lung (41–43) and airway smooth muscle (4,44–47). Furthermore, there are limited comparative data using formoterol and salmeterol in the same in vitro model of human bronchi.

Potency

Data on the human isolated bronchus indicate that formoterol is either similarly or more potent than salmeterol as a relaxant of the spontaneous smooth muscle tone and of tone induced by carbachol, respectively, which is compatible with the data on guinea pig trachea (44–48). In the human bronchus, both long-acting β-agonists are more potent than salbutamol and terbutaline using moderate or severe precontraction (44–48).

Maximum Relaxant Effect (Efficacy, Intrinsic Activity)

Using a high level of muscarinic precontraction in the human isolated bronchus, formoterol and terbutaline produce almost complete relaxation, whereas salmeterol relaxes this tone by approximately 40% (48). In a similar experimental model, formoterol's relaxant effect is more than 80% of that of isoprenaline and epinephrine (adrenaline) (45). Salmeterol, on the other hand, displays approximately 70% of the maximum relaxant effect of isoprenaline in the human bronchus precontracted by $PGF_{2\alpha}$ (4). Yet another study on the human isolated bronchus also demonstrated significant differences between isoprenaline and salmeterol, with salmeterol producing only 30% of isoprenaline's relaxation against spontaneous tone compared with 50% for salbutamol (49).

In human airways, it thus appears as if long-acting formoterol and salmeterol are more potent than shorter-acting salbutamol. As in animal airways, salmeterol seems to be a partial agonist compared with formoterol and short-acting β₂-adrenoceptor agonists.

A. Estimation of Duration of Action In Vivo and In Vitro

In clinical practice, both formoterol and salmeterol for inhalation afford long-lasting bronchodilation and protection against exogenous stimuli (50) (Fig. 6). In the human isolated bronchus, salmeterol displays at least a 40-fold longer time to offset of action than salbutamol using spontaneous smooth muscle tone and measuring time to 50% offset of action for the concentration required for 50% of the maximum drug response (44,47). Using the drug concentration required for 50% of the maximum drug response in the same airway model,

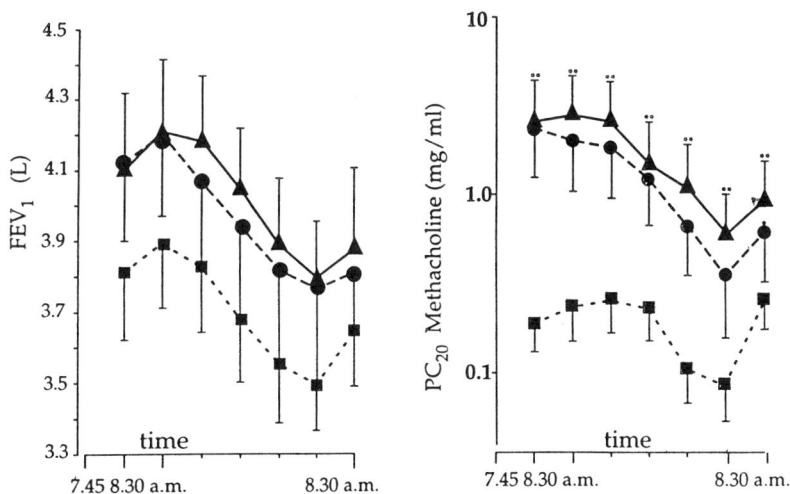

Figure 6   Comparison of the effects of 50 μg salmeterol (▲) and 12 μg formoterol (●), given by a metered-dose inhaler, on airway tone and responsiveness over 24 hr in patients with mild bronchial asthma. (From Ref. 50.)

formoterol displays a 40-fold shorter time than salmeterol to 50% recovery of the spontaneous tone (44,47). This gives formoterol a position similar to salbutamol in terms of duration in vitro in contrast to the clinical data. For formoterol, there is also a discrepancy in duration of action between inhalation and oral administration in human subjects, with only the inhaled route producing a long duration of effect (1).

B. Factors Influencing Duration of Action

Drug Concentration

The duration of action of formoterol, fenoterol, isoprenaline, and salbutamol has recently been assessed in relation to the concentration applied (3,46,47). For these β_2-agonists, it appears as if increasing concentrations increase their duration of action (46,47) (Fig. 7). As will be discussed below, salmeterol represents an exception in this type of experiments, because even moderate concentrations achieve a long duration of action in a similar way as the reasserted relaxant effect in the isolated guinea pig trachea (31,32).

As for animal airways, there is now also data on reassertion of relaxation after β-blockade and washout in human isolated airways (Fig. 8) with both salmeterol and formoterol (51). This reassertion of effect can also be demonstrated with high concentrations of fenoterol but not with salbutamol. As in animal airways, the β-adrenoceptor agonists which produce significant reassertion of effect after β-blockade and washout in human airways display a high degree of lipophilicity (7).

Duration of Administration

Using superfused human bronchi in vitro, the onset and duration of action as well as the maximum effect of formoterol—and shorter acting β-agonists—appears to depend on the duration of drug administration (3,46). This cannot be demonstrated with salmeterol; at least not within the 4.5 hr of observation. For salmeterol, increasing times of drug administration will influence the onset of action but not the maximum effect nor the duration of action during the observation time in vitro.

Figure 7 Relaxant effect versus time after peak drug response for increasing concentrations of the β-adrenoceptor agonists (a) salbutamol (open circles 10 nM, closed circles 100 nM, open triangles 1000 nM); (b) formoterol (open circles 1 nM, closed circles 10 nM, open triangles 100 nM); and (c) salmeterol (open circles 1 nM, closed circles 10 nM) in the human isolated bronchus under superfusion conditions. Data are presented as mean (s.e.m.) percentage of the maximum isoprenaline-induced relaxation of the initial spontaneous tone. (From Ref. 47.)

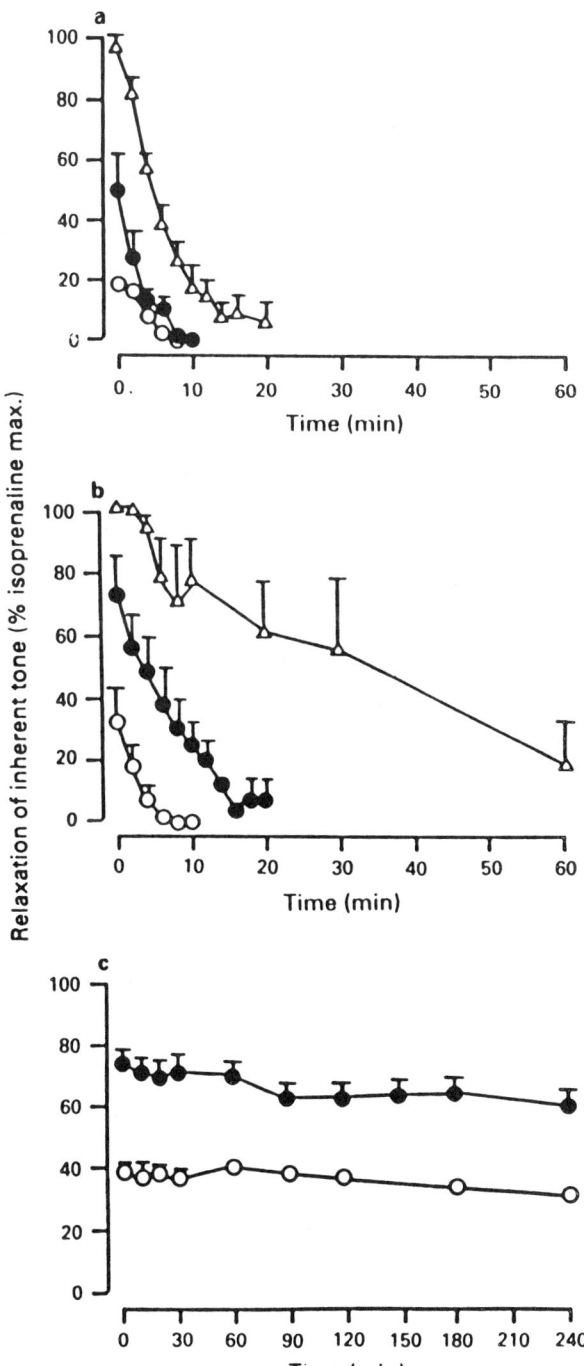

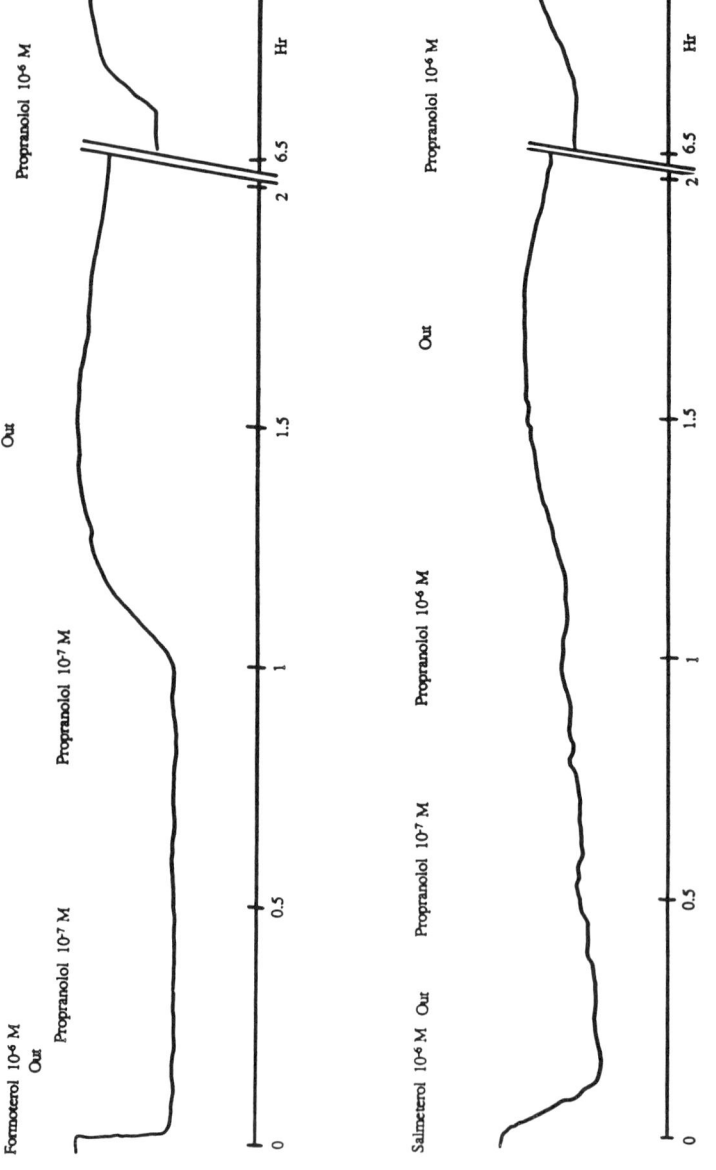

Figure 8 Original recording of the reassertion of relaxant effect after β-blockade with 0.1 μM propranolol followed by a washout in the superfused human isolated bronchus for the β-adrenoceptor agonists formoterol (1 μM, top trace) and salmeterol (1 μM, bottom trace). (From Ref. 51.)

C. Onset of Action

In human isolated bronchi, as in the guinea pig isolated trachea, the time to full onset of action is longer for salmeterol than for other β-agonists, and this onset of action remains similar as the drug concentration is increased (3,46). For isoprenaline, fenoterol, and formoterol, although these β-agonists display a more rapid onset of action, an increase in the drug concentration seems to significantly reduce the time to onset of action (3).

V. Hypothesis on Long Duration of Action

From the available in vitro data on the duration of relaxant effects and their reassertion after β-blockade and washout, it has been suggested that the long-acting but not the intermediate- or short-acting β-agonists remain accessible in the vicinity of, but not at, the catecholamine-binding site of the β_2-adrenoceptor (29, 31,32). The hypothesis of an "exosite" was first formulated for salmeterol and is based on the assumption that an agonist and an antagonist cannot be present at the same time at the β-adrenoceptor. This concept additionally raises the question how formoterol and salmeterol remain accessible at an exosite in the vicinity of the β_2-adrenoceptor and whether the basis for this ability differs for formoterol and salmeterol.

A. Is There an Exosite?

With reference to its reasserted relaxant effect after β-blockade and washout in isolated airways, it is has originally been suggested that salmeterol anchors at a specific exosite, an "exoreceptor," which is thought to be distinct from the β_2-adrenoceptor (5,25,29,47,52). This anchorage is supposed to be due to the long aliphatic side chain of salmeterol. There is still, however, no conclusive pharmacological or structural evidence that this exosite is constituted by a specific receptor. Furthermore, also because of formoterol's much shorter side chain, only slightly longer than that of salbutamol, the idea of a specific exoreceptor explaining the long duration of action for formoterol has been questioned. The formoterol molecule may not be long enough to anchor outside the β_2-adrenoceptor (31). At least for formoterol, an alternative mechanism of action might thus be required to explain the long duration of action. A more recent concept for the mechanisms of long duration of action for salmeterol suggests that the exosite is situated within the β_2-adrenoceptor, which binds the pharmacologically inactive long aliphatic side chain with high affinity, allowing the active saligenin head structure to angle on and off within the receptor in a manner that would allow a β-adrenoceptor antagonist, such as sotalol, access to the active receptor site (53).

In a recent study (54), the exosite hypothesis was tested using three analogues of salmeterol, which preserved the molecular structure of the aliphatic
side chain but had zero or low efficacy at the β₂-adrenoceptor. The investigators hypothesized that structural mimics of the side chain of salmeterol would
be likely to affect the capacity of salmeterol to exert relaxation reassertion if
smooth muscle was preincubated with these analogues. The side chain analogues CGP 54103 and D2543 (Fig. 9), at concentrations up to 10-fold that of
salmeterol, did not affect the relaxation reassertion, although these compounds
are not proven to directly interact with the β-adrenoceptor. A third compound,
CGP 59162, with an identical molecular formula to that of salmeterol, differing
only in the relative position of the substituents on the saligenin head group
(Fig. 9), showed weak efficacy at the β-adrenoceptor and also demonstrated
limited relaxation reassertion properties. Biophysical studies also revealed that
this compound had comparable lipophilicity (logP) and lipid membrane affinity (Kp$_{mem}$), and computer-assisted molecular modeling (CAMM) suggested
almost identical conformation to salmeterol, with the obvious exception of the

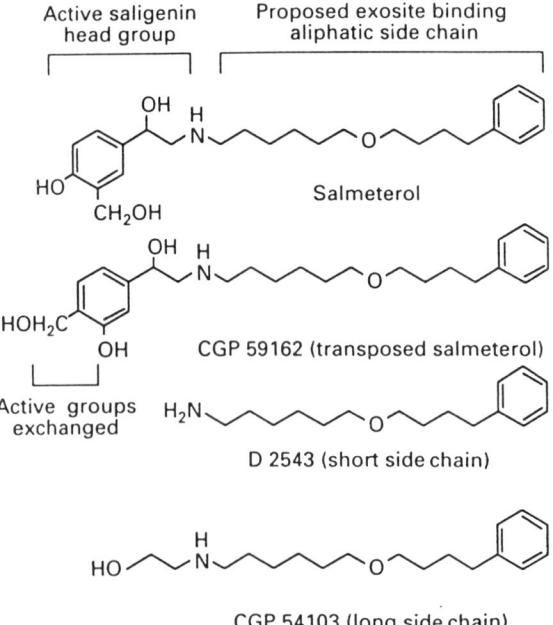

Figure 9   Molecular structure of salmeterol and its synthesized analogues indicating
the structural differences of the compounds used in the study of Bergendal et al. (54).

functional groups on the saligenin head. CGP 59162, however, also had no effect on the reassertion relaxation exerted by salmeterol even when preincubated in 10-fold molar excess. The investigators concluded that their findings do not support the existence of a distinct exosite recognizing the aliphatic side chain of salmeterol mediating reassertion, although the study did not provide direct evidence of the actual mechanism underlying salmeterol-induced reassertion.

As the long-acting β-agonists may remain not at, but in, the vicinity of the β₂-adrenoceptor, it appears not convincing that their very high and durable adrenoceptor affinity is the sole explanation for their long duration. Furthermore, the high potency and selectivity of these drugs can hardly alone explain the long duration of action, since these parameters are at least partially shared by short-acting β-agonists. The magnitude of lipophilicity for formoterol and salmeterol is, however, not shared by short-acting β-agonists (3,6,7).

VI. Interactions with the Cell Membrane of Airway Smooth Muscle

A. Salmeterol

As suggested in the microkinetic diffusion theory, the high lipophilicity of formoterol and salmeterol might be crucial for the long duration of action of these bronchodilators (3,7,18,55) (Fig. 10). In the case of salmeterol, this theory focuses on the possibility that, owing to its lipophilicity, salmeterol diffuses into the cell membrane's phospholipid bilayers and that the cell membrane then acts as a depot without any specific exoreceptors being distinct from the β₂-adrenoceptor. In fact, this concept is compatible with recent data showing that salmeterol, and to a lesser extent also formoterol, partition into lipid bilayers significantly more than short-acting salbutamol (6).

Situated in the cell membrane, salmeterol may diffuse laterally and reach the β₂-adrenoceptor. Molecules of salmeterol will thus indirectly encounter the β₂-adrenoceptor and activate its transduction system after entering the cell membrane lipid bilayer. If salmeterol later dissociates from the β₂-adrenoceptor, it could remain within the cell membrane in the vicinity of the adrenoceptor owing to its high lipophilicity. This type of lateral diffusion could cause an increasing receptor activation by time just because of an increasing probability that salmeterol would reach the receptor as it moves within the cell membrane. As salmeterol reaches the β₂-adrenoceptor, it may possibly even accumulate at this site owing to its very high β-adrenoceptor affinity, although there is no evidence so far for this proposition. In this way, a continuously increasing adrenoceptor stimulation could occur even at low concentrations of salmeterol, which is in line with the recognized slow onset of action for salmeterol in vitro.

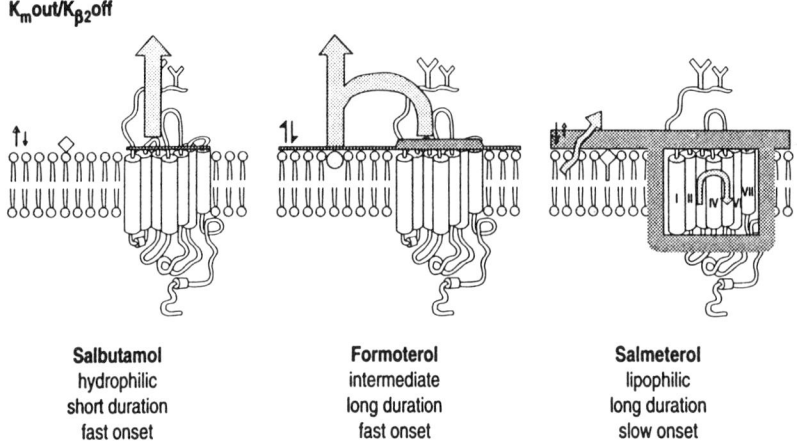

$K_m$out/$K_{β2}$off

Salbutamol
hydrophilic
short duration
fast onset

Formoterol
intermediate
long duration
fast onset

Salmeterol
lipophilic
long duration
slow onset

Figure 10 Microkinetic diffusion model. During association with the receptor, the interaction of salbutamol with membrane lipid ($K_m$in) is energetically unfavorable (dark shaded barrier) owing to its high hydrophilicity, and salbutamol associates directly with the receptor ($K_{β2}$on) from the aqueous biophase. Therefore, salbutamol exhibits rapid onset, but the drug diffuses from tissues rapidly causing a short duration of effect. The association of formoterol with both receptor and lipid is thermodynamically favorable allowing fast onset. Formoterol is retained in the lipid to be released over an extended period and continually activating the β-adrenoceptor. Salmeterol associates predominantly with lipid, and its interaction with the β-adrenoceptor is proposed to be energetically unfavorable causing slow onset of action. (From Ref. 3.)

The fact that salmeterol is a partial $β_2$-adrenoceptor agonist could thus be compensated for by the molecule's ability to persist in the vicinity of the $β_2$-adrenoceptor (9,27).

Lateral diffusion may also explain why a true concentration response relationship for airway smooth muscle relaxation is difficult to obtain with salmeterol in human airways (3). Low concentrations of salmeterol may cause a similar relaxant effect as much larger concentrations if the relaxant response is followed long enough (46,47). The effect of an increased concentration of salmeterol may thus not be causing a true, direct concentration-response effect, since a stable equilibrium between the biophase and the receptor may be difficult to achieve at low drug concentrations owing to the vast amount of cell membrane lipid bilayers. An increased salmeterol concentration may only slightly increase the statistical probability of an energetically unfavorable salmeterol-receptor interaction event to occur. This idea may also explain why there is a weak relationship between drug concentration and onset of action for salmeterol (31). However, further experimental studies are required to confirm this.

B. Formoterol

In the case of formoterol, its less pronounced lipophilicity might be compensated for by other factors (7,27). The extremely high potency of this drug combined with a pronounced β_2-adrenoceptor affinity and selectivity may substitute for the less pronounced lipophilicity. In addition to these factors, a topically high concentration could markedly contribute to formoterol's long duration of action. In fact, this idea is in line with formoterol displaying less reasserted relaxant effect after β-blockade and washout than does salmeterol and that this reassertion is dependent on a relatively high drug concentration in relation to the maximally effective concentration (31,32). Furthermore, the clinical observation that formoterol by inhalation produces a long duration of action, whereas formoterol by the oral route does not, also suggests that a topically high concentration of this drug is required for its long duration of effect (1). As indicated in vitro, this may not be the case for salmeterol (31,32). Unfortunately, very little is known about the actual drug concentration surrounding airways smooth muscle in vivo, and these aspects need to be addressed in future in vivo studies.

C. Short-Acting β-Adrenoceptor Agonists

For isoprenaline, fenoterol, and salbutamol, as for formoterol, not only the duration of action but also the time to onset of relaxation appears to depend on the concentration of the agonist at the smooth muscle site as measured in human as well as in guinea pig airways in vitro (31,47). This is also compatible with the theory on microkinetic diffusion (3,18,55). This is because, when present in very high concentrations, a fraction of a β-agonist with a moderate lipophilicity may enter into the cell membrane of the smooth muscle cell and then lateral diffusion to the β-adrenoceptor may occur. This reasoning may explain why clenbuterol, which has a lower potency than salmeterol and a lipophilicity in between salmeterol and most short-acting β_2-agonists, displays a duration of action in between salmeterol and salbutamol (56).

VII. Role of Non–β-Adrenoceptor–Mediated Relaxation?

Several studies on the guinea pig trachea show that salmeterol may produce non–β-adrenoceptor–mediated smooth muscle relaxation and this should also be considered when evaluating the mechanisms behind its long duration of action (9,27,28). Based on recent data, however, it has been suggested that non–β-adrenoceptor–mediated smooth muscle relaxation is not important for salmeterol's long duration. The basis for this suggestion is the finding that the (S)-enantiomer of salmeterol causes only short-lasting effects in the presence of the β-adrenoceptor blocker propranolol (57). Furthermore, it is unclear whether the topical drug concentration in human airways may reach the level which produces significant non–β-adrenoceptor–mediated effects. The importance of non–β-adrenoceptor–mediated relaxation therefore remains uncertain, and this issue is in need of further investigation in human subjects.

VIII. Conclusions

The mechanisms underlying the duration of effect for the long-acting β_2-adrenoceptor agonists formoterol and salmeterol are still a matter of debate. Two major hypotheses, the exosite theory with lateral diffusion and the microkinetic diffusion model have been put forward to explain the pharmacological findings obtained with this new class of drugs. At present, it seems reasonable to assume that several factors may determine the duration of action, since none of the proposed models are unequivocally proven. The high lipophilicity of formoterol and salmeterol may prove to be a required but not a sufficient factor for prolonged duration of action. Additional factors such as affinity, potency, and the selectivity at the β_2-adrenoceptor as well as the maximum relaxant effect produced by the drug are also likely to be of importance, since they may determine the amount of drug necessary to remain in the vicinity of the β_2-adrenoceptor for significant and long-lasting smooth muscle relaxation. So far, the proposed models have neither convincingly unified all pharmacological data obtained nor all researchers involved. There is still a proposed distinction between those β_2-adrenoceptor agonists with a "common" extended duration of action which may depend on drug concentrations and those that are "inherently" long-acting. Hopefully, future studies of formoterol and salmeterol will help to clarify some of the remaining controversial issues, preferably by comparing both long-acting drugs within the same experimental systems. The understanding of the mechanisms and pharmacological basis for the long duration of inhaled long-acting β_2-adrenoceptor agonists may improve not only the therapy of reversible airway disease but will also most certainly provide further insights in the activation of cell membrane receptors and may also reveal principles applicable to a wider range of drugs.

References

1. Löfdahl CG, Svedmyr N. Formoterol fumarate, a new β_2-adrenoceptor agonist. Acute studies of selectivity and duration of effect after inhaled and oral administration. Allergy 1989; 44:264–271.

2. Ullman A, Svedmyr N. Salmeterol, a new long-acting inhaled β₂-agonist: comparison with salbutamol in adult asthmatic patients. Thorax 1988; 43:674–678.
3. Anderson GP, Lindén A, Rabe KF. Why are long acting beta-adrenoceptor agonists long acting? Eur Respir J 1994; 7:569–578.
4. Ball DI, Brittain RT, Coleman RA, et al. Salmeterol, a novel, long-acting β₂-adrenoceptor agonist: characterization of pharmacological activity in vitro and in vivo. Br J Pharmacol 1991; 104:665–671.
5. Bradshaw J, Brittain RT, Coleman RA, et al. The design of salmeterol, a long-acting selective β₂-adrenoceptor agonist. Br J Pharmacol 1987; 92:590P.
6. Jaeckel K, John E, Anderson G. Comparative biophysical analysis of interactions between formoterol, salbutamol or salmeterol and lipid bilayers. Eur Respir J 1993; 6:383s.
7. Jeppson AB, Löfdahl C-G, Waldeck B, Widmark E. On the predictive value of in vitro experiments in the evaluation of the effect duration of bronchodilator drugs for local administration. Pulm Pharmacol 1989; 2:81–85.
8. Lindén A, Bergendal A, Ullman A, Skoogh B-E, Löfdahl C-G. Long- and short-acting β₂-agonists in the isolated guinea-pig trachea—efficacy, potency and functional antagonism. Eur Respir J 1991; 4:199s.
9. Lindén A, Bergendal A, Ullman A, Skoogh B-E, Löfdahl C-G. Salmeterol, formoterol and salbutamol in the isolated guinea pig trachea: differences in maximum relaxant effect and potency but not in functional antagonism. Thorax 1993; 48:547–553.
10. Ida H. Comparison of the action of BD 40 A and some other β-adrenoceptor stimulants on the isolated trachea and atria of the guinea pig. Arzneim Forsch 1976; 26:839.
11. Lemoine H, Overlack C, Worth H, Reinhardt D. Increased muscarinic prestimulation of guinea-pig tracheal strips decreases potency and intrinsic activity (ISA) of synthetic β₂-sympathomimetics. Comparison of relaxation with receptor binding and adenylate cyclase stimulation. Naunyn Schmiedebergs Arch Pharm 1991; 343:R98.
12. Nials AT, Butchers PR, Coleman RA, Johnson M, Vardey CJ. Salmeterol and formoterol: are both long-acting β₂-adrenoceptor agonists? Br J Pharmacol 1990; 99:120P.
13. Ullman A, Bergendal A, Lindén A, Waldeck B, Skoogh B-E, Löfdahl C-G. Onset of action and duration of effect of formoterol and salmeterol compared to salbutamol in isolated guinea pig trachea with or without epithelium. Allergy 1992; 47:384–387.
14. Ball DI, Coleman RA, Denyer LH, Nials AT, Sheldrick KE. In vitro characterization of the β₂-adrenoceptor agonist salmeterol. Br J Pharmacol 1987; 88:591P.
15. Ball DI, Coleman RA, Denyer LH, Nials AT, Sheldrick KE. Bronchodilator activity of salmeterol, a long-acting β₂-adrenoceptor agonist. Br J Pharmacol 1987; 90:746P.
16. Karlsson JA, Persson CGA. Influence of tracheal contraction on relaxant effects in vitro of theophylline and isoproterenol. Br J Pharmacol 1981; 74:73–79.

17. Torphy TJ, Rinard GA Rietow MG, Mayer SE. Functional antagonism in canine tracheal smooth muscle: inhibition by methacholine of the mechanical and biochemical responses to isoproterenol. J Pharmacol Exp Ther 1983; 227:694–699.
18. Anderson GP. Molecular pharmacology of formoterol. In: Holgate ST, ed. Formoterol: Fast and Long-lasting Bronchodilatation. Brussels: Royal Society of Medicine Services, 1992.
19. Anderson G, Niedenhauser U, Bray M. Beta-adrenoceptor subtype selectivity and potency of highly purified enantiomers of formoterol in guinea-pig isolated trachea smooth muscle. Eur Respir J 1993; 6(suppl 17):590s.
20. Decker N, Quennedey MS, Rouot B, Schwartz J, Velly J. Effects of N-aralkyl substitution of beta agonists on alpha- and beta-adrenoceptor subtypes: pharmacological studies and binding assays. J Pharm Pharmacol 1982; 34:107–112.
21. Zaagsma J, van der Heijden PC, van der Schaar MW, Bank CM. Comparison of functional β-adrenoceptor heterogeneity in central and peripheral airway smooth muscle of guinea pig and man. J Recept Res 1983; 3:89–106.
22. Johnson M. The preclinical pharmacology of salmeterol: bronchodilator effects. Eur Respir Rev 1991; 1:253–256.
23. Nials AT, Coleman RA, Vardey CJ. The β-adrenoceptor selectivity profiles of salmeterol and formoterol. Am Rev Respir Dis 1993; 147:A176.
24. Coleman RA, Johnson M, Nials AT, Sumner MJ. Salmeterol, but not formoterol, persists at β₂-adrenoceptors in vitro. Br J Pharmacol 1990; 99:121P.
25. Brittain RT, Jack D, Sumner MJ. Further studies on the long duration of action of salmeterol, a new, selective beta₂-stimulant bronchodilator. J Pharm Pharmacol 1988; 40:93P.
26. Brittain R. Approaches to a long-acting, selective β₂-adrenoceptor stimulant. Lung 1990; 168(Suppl):111–114.
27. Jeppson AB, Waldeck B, Källström B-L. Studies on the interaction between formoterol and salmeterol in guinea-pig trachea in vitro. Pharmacol Toxicol 1992; 71:1–6.
28. Bergendal A, Lindén A, Lötvall J, Skoogh B-E, Löfdahl C-G. Inhibitory effects of formoterol, salmeterol and salbutamol on nerve-induced contractions in the ferret trachea. Br J Pharmacol 1995; 114:1478–1482.
29. Nials AT, Sumner MJ, Johnson M, Coleman RA. Investigations into factors determining the duration of action of the β₂-adrenoceptor agonist, salmeterol. Br J Pharmacol 1993; 108:507–515.
30. Tokuyama K, Lötvall J, Löfdahl C-G, Barnes PJ, Chung KF. Inhaled formoterol inhibits histamine-induced airflow obstruction and airway microvascular leakage. Eur J Pharmacol 1991; 193:35–39.
31. Anderson P, Lötvall J, Lindén A. Relaxation kinetics of formoterol and salmeterol in the guinea-pig trachea in vitro. Lung 1996; 174:159–170.
32. Lindén A, Bergendal A, Ullman A, Skoogh B-E, Löfdahl C-G. High concentration of formoterol & salmeterol in the isolated guinea pig trachea—reassertion of smooth-muscle relaxation after beta blockade followed by wash-out. Am Rev Respir Dis 1991; 143:A749.
33. Nials AT, Coleman RA. The interaction between salmeterol and β-adrenoceptor blocking drugs on guinea-pig isolated trachea. Br J Pharmacol 1988; 95:540P.

34. Nials AT, Coleman RA. The interaction between salmeterol and β-adrenoceptor blocking drugs on guinea-pig trachea in vitro. Am Rev Respir Dis 1992; 145: A391.

35. Taguchi O, Hida W, Nogami H, Inoue H, Takishima T. Possible site of bronchodilation due to inhaled procaterol aerosol in asthmatic patients. Eur J Clin Pharmacol 1988; 34:433–437.

36. Watanabe-Kohno S, Shimizu T, Mizuta J, et al. Effect of procaterol on the isolated airway smooth muscle and the release of anaphylactic chemical mediators from the isolated lung fragments. Arzneim Forschung 1990; 40:669–674.

37. Persson G, Gnosspelius Y, Anehus S. Comparison between a new once-daily, bronchodilating drug, bambuterol, and terbutaline sustained release, twice daily. Eur Respir J 1988; 1:223–226.

38. Wempe JB, Tammeling EP, Postma DS, et al. Effects of budesonide and bambuterol on circadian variation of airway responsiveness and nocturnal symptoms of asthma. J Allergy Clin Immunol 1992; 90:349–357.

39. Brogden RN, Faulds D. Salmeterol xinafoate: a review of its pharmacological properties and therapeutic potential in reversible obstructive airways disease. Drugs 1991; 42:1–18.

40. Rabe KF, Chung KF. The challenge of long acting beta-adrenoceptor agonists. Respir Med 1991; 85:5–9.

41. Butchers P, Cousins SA, Vardey CJ. Salmeterol: a potent and long-acting inhibitor of the release of inflammatory and spasmogenic mediators from human lung. Br J Pharmacol 1987; 92:745.

42. Butchers PR, Vardey CJ, Johnson M. Salmeterol: a potent and long-acting inhibitor of inflammatory mediator release from human lung. Br J Pharmacol 1991; 104:672–676.

43. Mita H, Takao S. Anti-allergic activity of formoterol, a new β₂-adrenoceptor stimulant, and salbutamol in human leukocytes and human lung tissue. Allergy 1983; 38:547–552.

44. Coleman RA, Nials T, Vardey C, Rabe KF, Magnussen H. Effect of salmeterol, albuterol and formoterol on human bronchial smooth muscle. Am Rev Respir Dis 1992; 145:A391.

45. Advenier C, Zhang Y, Naline E, Grandordy BM. Effects of formoterol in human isolated bronchus. Am Rev Respir Dis 1991; 143:A651.

46. Rabe KF, Bodtke K, Liebig S, Magnussen H. Modulation of inherent tone of human airways in vitro. Am Rev Respir Dis 1992; 145:A378.

47. Nials AT, Coleman RA, Johnson M, Magnussen H, Rabe KF, Vardey CJ. Effects of β-adrenoceptor agonists in human bronchial smooth muscle. Br J Pharmacol 1993; 110:1112–1116.

48. Källström B-L, Sjöberg J, Waldeck B. The interaction between salmeterol and β₂-adrenoceptor agonists with higher efficacy on guinea-pig trachea and human bronchus in vitro. Br J Pharmacol 1994; 113:687–692.

49. Nials AT, Coleman RA, Johnson M, Vardey CJ. Determination of intrinsic activities of a range of β₂-adrenoceptor agonist bronchodilators. Am J Respir Crit Care Med 1994; 149:A481.

50. Rabe KF, Jörres R, Nowak D, Behr N, Magnussen H. Effect of formoterol vs salmeterol on the circadian variation of airway tone and responsiveness in bronchial asthma. Am Rev Respir Dis 1993; 147:1436–1441.
51. Lindén A, Rabe KF, Löfdahl CG. Pharmacological basis for duration of effect: formoterol and salmeterol versus short-acting β_2-adrenoceptor agonists. Lung 1996; 174:1–22.
52. Nials AT, Vardey CJ, Coleman RA. Membrane microkinetic diffusion—does it explain the duration of action of salmeterol and formoterol? Am Rev Respir Dis 1993; 147:A178.
53. Johnson M. Salmeterol: a novel drug for the treatment of asthma. In: Anderson GP, Morley J, eds. New Drugs for Asthma. Basel: Birkhäuser Verlag, 1992:79–95.
54. Bergendal A, Lindén A, Skoogh BE, Gerspacher M, Anderson GP, Löfdahl CG. Salmeterol-mediated reassertion of relaxation persists in guinea-pig trachea pretreated with aliphatic side chain structural analogues. Br J Pharmacol 1996; 117: 1009–1015.
55. Löfdahl C. Basic pharmacology of new long-acting sympathomimetics. Lung 1990; 168:18–21.
56. Johnson M. The pharmacology of salmeterol. Lung 1990; 168:115–119.
57. Coleman RA, Nials AT, Johnson M, Vardey CJ. (S)-Salmeterol: duration of β- and non–β-adrenoceptor mediated responses in guinea-pig trachea. Am J Respir Crit Care Med 1994; 149:A484.

Discussion

GARY P. ANDERSON

The University of Melbourne, Parkville, Victoria, Australia

Although considerable progress has been made in gathering new information on the mechanism(s) underlying the extended duration of action of formoterol and salmeterol, no consensus of opinion can currently be built on available scientific information. The exosite model, at least in its original form where the aliphatic side chain of salmeterol binds to a structure distinct from the β_2-adrenoceptor, is clearly untenable. However, data presented by Liggett at this symposium provides support for a modified concept where salmeterol's interaction with the agonist recognition domains of the β_2-adrenoceptor is, at the least, dependent on the integrity of transmembrane-spanning domain 4 (TMD 4). Whether point mutation studies will confirm that a specific aliphatic side chain recognition site does indeed exist on TM 4, the new binding information presented by Liggett clearly confirms earlier indications that salmeterol may form an essentially irreversible, albeit low-efficacy, complex with the β_2-adrenoceptor.

The diffusion microkinetic model deals with the likelihood that the now well-characterized biophysical propensity of formoterol, and particularly salmeterol, to partition into lipid membranes is an important determinate of the onset of action, the duration of action and the reassertion characteristics of formoterol and salmeterol. Liggett's data now provides clear evidence in support of the fully articulated microkinetic model proposed by Anderson, Lindén, and Rabe (1). In this model, it was predicted specifically that salmeterol would gain access to the ligand-recognition domain by intercalating between TMD 4 and TMD 5 and then form a stable but low-efficacy complex.

At issue now is whether TMD 4 can be conceived of as an exosite-equivalent within the β_2-adrenoceptor (perhaps the term *introsite* more appropriately describes current knowledge). The recent studies of Bergendal et al. (2) argue strongly against the existence of an exosite/introsite on TMD 4 or elsewhere. By synthesizing analogues of salmeterol with greatly reduced efficacy at β_2-adrenoceptor, Bergendal et al. sought to create pharmacological probes capable of binding to what, by inference from the irreversible nature of salmeterol binding, must be a very high-affinity recognition site for the aliphatic side chain.

One molecule in particular, CGP 59162, which exactly preserves the chemical formula, biophysical properties, and side chain structure of salmeterol and selectively occupies the β_2-adrenoceptor, was found to have no effect on salmeterol-mediated relaxation or reassertion of airway smooth muscle (Fig. D-1). Further studies, particularly systematic point mutations of TMD 4 are clearly essential to resolve whether interposing the analogous domains from the β_1-adrenoceptor and β_3-adrenoceptor truly replaces an exosite/introsite of whether this macroscale manipulation of the β_2-adrenoceptor simply alters the "window of access" between TMD 4 and TMD 5 proposed in the microkinetic model to be a spatially constrained access point for salmeterol moving from lipid membrane to β_2-adrenoceptor active site.

Although data presented at this symposium does not directly address these points, it has stimulated two refinements to the original diffusion microkinetic model proposed here for the first time (Figs. D-2a and 2b).

The first of these is the mechanism underlying "reassertion" relaxation. Reassertion relaxation is the capacity of long-acting β_2-adrenoceptor agonists repeatedly to cause functional antagonism of induced tone in airway smooth muscle when this tissue is transiently exposed to, then washed free of, hydrophilic β-adrenoceptor antagonists such as sotalol. Since the ligand-binding studies of Liggett clearly suggest that salmeterol irreversibly complexes the β_2-adrenoceptor, one obvious explanation, originally proposed in the context of the microkinetic model, is that dual occupancy of adrenoceptor by both salmeterol and antagonist might occur shifting the β_2-adrenoceptor complex from a low-efficacy state to a zero-efficacy state. I propose that more complex solutions to the problem should be considered. It is unlikely that salmeterol occupies the entire pool of β_2-adrenoceptors available on airway smooth

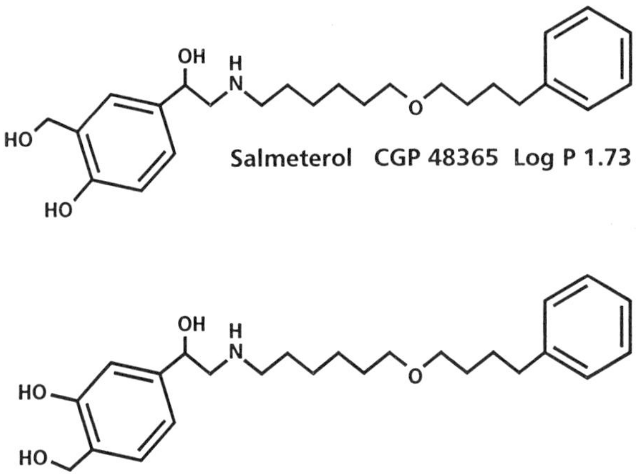

Figure D-1   Comparative structures of salmeterol and CGP 59162. These molecules have identical biophysical properties and spatial conformation of the aliphatic side chain. CGP 59162 is a weak and very low-efficacy β_2-adrenoceptor–selective agonist which manifests reassertion. The failure of CGP 59162 to attenuate salmeterol-induced effects has been interpreted as evidence against the existence of a distinct exosite. (Redrawn from Ref. 2.)

muscle. Indeed, data discussed in this symposium suggests that functional occupancy as low as 1–3% may be achieved after inhalation of therapeutic doses of salmeterol. Two distinct, but not mutually exclusive, possibilities are suggested by this information. The first is the possibility that reassertion may occur not by dual occupancy of the β_2-adrenoceptor but when β-adrenoceptor antagonists occupy free β_2-adrenoceptors not already complexed by salmeterol. This might occur, as suggested by the recent documentation of inverse agonism at the β-adrenoceptor, by a net reduction in the overall reduction in signal transduction efficiency from the β_2-adrenoceptor agonist complex, perhaps by reducing the net probability of G-proteins collision coupling with the receptor agonist complex or by perturbing membrane ionic conductances. A second possibility is that antagonists occupying noncomplexed adrenoceptors may reduce the net electromechanical coupling of inhaled airway smooth muscle cells, again resulting in a net reduction in signal transduction efficiency within the bundle of airway smooth muscle cells.

The fact that airway smooth muscle is arranged in clear bundles of fibers with adrenoceptors apparently evenly distributed within the bundle suggests a refinement to the microkinetic model explanation of the slow onset of action

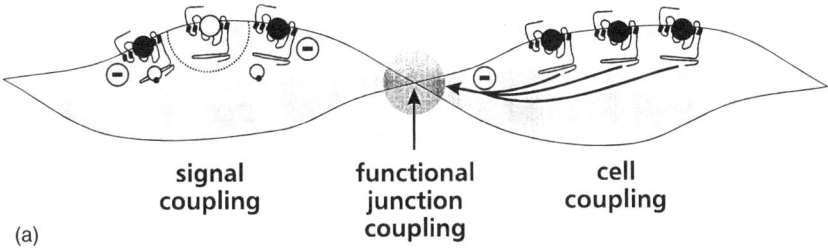

(a)

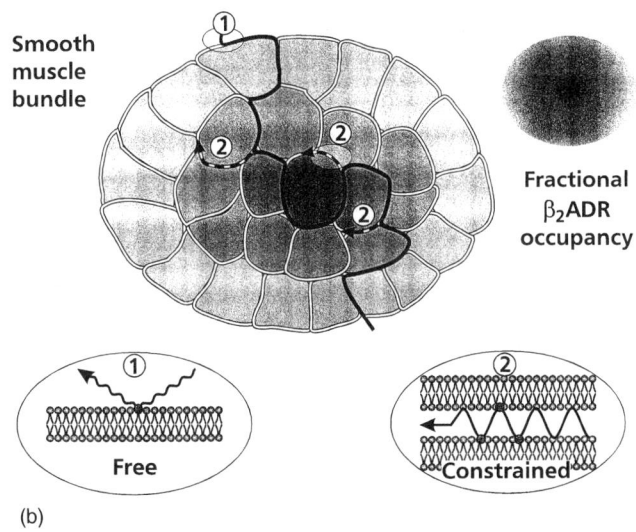

(b)

Figure D-2 (a) (Upper panel). Complex models of reassertion. The diagram shows two theoretical, not mutually exclusive, mechanisms which may cause reassertion. On the left side, β-adrenoceptor occupied by antagonist is shown reducing the net probability of randomly diffusing G-proteins encountering an agonist-occupied adrenoceptor. On the right side, antagonist-occupied adrenoceptors are shown reducing the functional coupling which exists in airways smooth muscle. Both mechanisms would lead to a net reduction in the efficiency of agonist-induced relaxation and would cause reassertion effects. (b) (Lower panel). The rate of diffusion of an agonist into the smooth muscle bundle is likely to determine the time to achieve a critical fractional occupancy of enough β₂-adrenoceptors from the total adrenoceptor pool to cause tissue relaxation. The diffusion path will be affected by the biophysical properties of the agonist where hydrophilic molecules move quickly through the aqueous biophase but aliphatic drugs move more slowly as a proportion of their diffusion time/path is impeded by partitioning into the plasmalemma cell membrane lipid pool.

of salmeterol. Although it is now clear that salmeterol may intercalate between TMD 4 and TMD 5 from the lipid membrane pool, the unfavorable thermo-dynamics of lateral diffusion *into* a protein alone may not be the sole determinant of salmeterol's slow onset of action, since in some single cell systems, salmeterol can activate β_2-adrenoceptors with significantly less lag time. Again, I feel that the concept of achieving an adequate fractional occupancy of β_2-adrenoceptor distributed within the smooth muscle cell bundle only after some time as salmeterol diffuses slowly into tissue must now be seriously considered.

Although insights have been gained into the mode of action of formoterol and salmeterol, it seems clear that much further work to extend our knowledge of drug biophysics to the receptor and subreceptor levels is now needed to understand completely how these bronchodilators achieve their undoubtedly advantageous clinical effects.

References

1. Anderson GP, Lindén A, Rabe K. Why are long acting beta-adrenoceptor agonists long acting. Eur Respir J 1994; 7:569–578.
2. Bergendal A, Linden A, Skoogh BE, Gerspacher M, Anderson BP, Lofdahl C-G. Extent of salmeterol-mediated reassertion of relaxation in guinea-pig trachea pretreated with aliphatic side chain structural analogues. Br J Pharmacol 1996; 117: 1009–1015.

7

Bronchodilatation

ERIC DEROM and ROMAIN PAUWELS

University Hospital
Ghent, Belgium

I. Introduction

Short-acting inhaled beta$_2$-agonists are the most useful medications for "rescue treatment" of asthma symptoms. They induce prompt symptomatic relief of wheezing, coughing, and breathlessness caused by exercise, cold air, inhalation of irritants or other bronchoconstrictor stimuli for 3–5 hr. They exhibit a rapid onset of action in comparison with other bronchodilators such as methylxanthines or anticholinergic agents. Moreover, their short-term use does not produce troublesome adverse effects, at least at doses that do not exceed recommended doses. Long-acting inhaled β_2-agonists are recommended as adjunct maintenance therapy together with anti-inflammatory therapy for the treatment of chronic asthma.

Selective β_2-agonists, such as salbutamol (albuterol), terbutaline, fenoterol, rimiterol, pirbuterol, procaterol, bitolterol, and broxaterol, provide a more prolonged bronchodilator effect (4–6 hr) than the nonselective β-agonists epinephrine (adrenaline) and isoproterenol, whose actions do not exceed 2 hr. Nevertheless, they are currently called short-acting β_2-agonists in order to distinguish them from the recently marketed drugs salmeterol and formoterol.

These are now considered to be long-acting β_2-agonists, since they are characterized by a duration of action of at least 12 hr.

II. Mechanisms Underlying the Bronchodilating Action

Airway narrowing can arise by a number of mechanisms, including direct activation of respiratory smooth muscle by locally generated mediators and by stimulation of neurogenic pathways in the airways, extravasation of plasma proteins into airway tissue leading to edema formation, loss of elastic recoil, and narrowing of the airway lumen. As studies performed in vitro and in asthmatic patients have pointed out that relaxation of human bronchial muscle is essentially mediated by β_2-receptors (1,2), the most successful approach to control bronchospasm has been through the administration of β_2-stimulant bronchodilators. These act as functional antagonists by several mechanisms, including the increase of intracellular cyclic adenosine monophosphate (AMP) in bronchial smooth muscle. Selective β_2-agonists are thus able to inhibit or reverse the contractile response irrespective of the constricting stimulus (3).

In animal preparations, β_2-adrenergic stimulation enhances mucociliary clearance (4), reduces microvascular hyperpermeability (5), suppresses the secretion of inflammatory mediators via the stimulation of β_2-receptors on mast cells and other inflammatory cells (6), and inhibits neurotransmission in parasympathetic ganglia (7), thereby opposing the airway effects of vagal nerve activation (bronchoconstriction and mucus hypersecretion). From a clinical point of view, the reduction in airway smooth muscle tone remains the most important therapeutic action of β_2-agonists in patients with asthma. The basic mechanisms through which the various β_2-agonists exert their effects are outlined in other chapters of this book.

III. Oral and Parenteral Administration of β_2-Agonists

Since it is the aim of bronchodilator therapy to produce optimal airway response with minimal systemic adverse effects, this will essentially be achieved with inhaled delivery of the drugs. If possible, parenteral or oral administration will be avoided or reserved for specific clinical situations, because side effects will always be less for any given degree of bronchodilatation obtained with the inhaled route than with systemic administration (8). In general, skeletal muscle tremor is the dose-limiting factor when β_2-agonists are given systemically (9).

A. Oral Administration

A comparative study in which the bronchodilating and systemic effects of orally administered salbutamol and fenoterol have been assessed has demonstrated that salbutamol 2, 6, and 18 mg and fenoterol 2.5, 5, and 15 mg resulted in similar increases in FEV_1, averaging 15, 35, and 50% of baseline, respectively (10). These substantial improvements in FEV_1 will never be attained in clinical practice, since the two highest doses of the two drugs induced a very disturbing tremor.

Important differences between the bronchodilator response of orally administered and inhaled β_2-agonists appear to exist. Indeed, in a controlled crossover study comparing inhaled and oral doses of salbutamol, inhalation of 200, 400, and 600 μg of salbutamol resulted in a bronchodilating effect similar to that obtained with an oral dose of 3, 9, and 17 mg. For a given increase in FEV_1, significantly less tremor was produced by inhalation than by the corresponding oral dose (11). In another study, inhalation of 200 μg of salbutamol produced a more rapid and substantially greater bronchodilator response than an oral dose of 2 mg, whereas decreases in serum potassium, tachycardia, and tremor were only observed after oral administration (12). Similar observations have been made with terbutaline (11). As a consequence, inhalation of a β_2-agonist from a metered-dose inhaler is superior to tablets in producing bronchodilatation without side effects.

In general, the rate of onset of action of the bronchodilator dose-response is much flatter with the oral route than with inhaled delivery (11,12), and the onset of action is around 15–30 min, with a peak effect between 1 and 2 hr (13).

Oral preparations still have some role in the treatment of asthmatic patients who are too young to use inhalation therapy conveniently. Sustained-release oral preparations reduce nocturnal bronchoconstriction in patients with asthma (14), but they are not as effective for this purpose as the long-acting inhaled β_2-agonists (15). Clinical efficacy in a once-daily dosing has also been reported with bambuterol, an ester of terbutaline, whose relatively slow activation in the liver eventually results in an enhanced terbutaline half-life of over 20 hr (16).

B. Parenteral Administration

Increasing dosages of intravenously administered terbutaline resulted in a bronchodilating effect in patients with asthma (8). However, even at levels that exceed the recommended serum levels, intravenous doses did not produce maximum bronchodilatation that can be attained via inhalation, whereas they did produce substantial increases in heart rate and muscle tremor. Nevertheless, the intravenous and subcutaneous administration of β_2-agonists has been advocated in the treatment of severe asthma and frequently prescribed in current practice. Although patients exhibiting severe bronchial obstruction may occasionally benefit from parenteral therapy (17,18), inhalation of β_2-agonists were as effective as parenteral administration for treating acute, severe asthma attacks in most patients (19). Moreover, several studies have demonstrated that even in patients with severe acute asthma attack, the efficacy to side effect ratio is better with inhaled treatment (20–22).

In asthmatic patients treated with subcutaneous injections of terbutaline, the bronchodilator effect follows closely the serum levels (23). Although 0.5 mg provides slightly greater bronchodilatation than 0.25 mg (24), 0.25 mg is generally considered to be the recommended dose (25). An additional dose of 0.25 mg after 20 min may be used if necessary (26). The duration of action of the 0.25-mg dose is 3–4 hr (27). Compared with terbutaline, an equal dosage of epinephrine produces a less intense bronchodilatation of shorter duration (28).

As peak levels decline precipitously after a single intravenous injection of 0.25 mg terbutaline administered over 5 min (29), terbutaline may be given as a continuous infusion (recommended dose 2.5–5.0 μg/min) to obtain a sustained bronchodilatation. For salbutamol, the suggested dose of 10 μg/min produced no significant increase in heart rate.

IV. Inhalation of β_2-Agonists

In asthmatic patients, the administration of a drug by inhalation has many advantages: The drug is directly delivered to the affected area, a rapid onset of action, and high efficacy can be obtained from a low dose, and the incidence of unwanted side effects can be reduced. The bronchodilator response to inhaled β_2-agonists can be described in terms of onset of action, duration, and magnitude of the bronchodilating effect. Such information provides a good basis for an intelligent choice of a specific β_2-agonist, dosage, and dosing interval in clinical practice. As onset of action, duration, and magnitude of the bronchodilator response are highly dependent on the intrinsic properties of the prescribed drug as well as on the dose that is eventually deposited in the lung, studies designed to compare these variables are only conclusive under the provision that measurements were obtained at "equivalent doses." Equivalent doses are defined as doses at which the bronchodilating effects of different β_2-agonists are of similar magnitude.

A. Dose Equivalence

It has been claimed that the failure to recognize that fenoterol had been marketed at a dose corresponding with two to four times the current dose of salbutamol or terbutaline (30) might be one of the reasons that fenoterol has been associated with increased morbidity in patients with asthma and possibly an increase in mortality in New Zealand (31). A good knowledge of the dose equivalence is thus critical in order to compare the bronchodilating properties of different β_2-agonists and determine the recommended doses. Dose equivalence can be calculated by comparing increasing doses of a new drug with increasing doses of an established drug on bronchodilating capacity and side effects. In such studies, it is critical to choose the lowest dose with great care in order to avoid the plateau of the dose-response curve after one or two doses (32). A recent study in which the bronchodilator response to cumulative doses of inhaled fenoterol (200 μg/puff), terbutaline (250 μg/puff), and salbutamol (100 μg/puff) was compared remained inconclusive, as the FEV_1 response already approached the top of the dose-response curve with the lowest doses of all three drugs (30).

Although a good understanding of the differences in potency in vitro is of great value to predict the dose equivalence of two different β_2-agonists, studies in asthmatic patients are always required to assess their exact dose equivalence for bronchodilatation. Using a dose-response curve for the bronchodilating effect, it has been demonstrated that inhalation from a pressurized metered-dose inhaler (pMDI) of 1330 μg orciprenaline (metaproterenol), 400 μg isoprenaline, and 2200 μg isoetharine resulted in a bronchodilator response of similar magnitude (33). The equivalent doses for the currently used selective β_2-agonists administered via pMDI are summarized in Table 1. Gray and co-workers compared inhaled fenoterol (100 μg/puff) and terbutaline (250 μg/puff) to a cumulative dose of 15 puffs in 12 asthmatic patients on regular inhaled β_2-agonists and showed bronchodilatory equivalence on a puff for puff basis (34). Other studies have pointed out that 100 μg of salbutamol and 250 μg of terbutaline are equivalent when given via the inhaled route (35–37).

Dose-response comparisons of formoterol and salbutamol in patients with asthma suggested that inhaled formoterol is 5 to 15 times as potent as inhaled salbutamol (32). Comparison of dose-response curves in nine asthmatic

Table 1 Equivalent Bronchodilating Doses for Inhalation of Some Selective β_2-Agonists on a Weight for Weight Basis Using Pressurized Metered-Dose Inhalers

β-agonist	μg
Salbutamol	100
Terbutaline	250
Fenoterol	100
Formoterol	12
Salmeterol	$\leq$25

patients showed that a cumulative dose of formoterol, 123 μg, produced a peak bronchodilator response equivalent to that of salbutamol, 1300 μg (38). Similar studies in children have suggested a 5- to 10-fold difference in potency (32). Studies in which dose-response curves of salmeterol and short-acting β_2-agonists are compared are scarce. Single dose comparisons of salbutamol at 50 and salbutamol at 200 μg have generally shown similar effects on FEV$_1$, heart rate, and tremor (39,40), leading to the view that 50 μg of salmeterol is roughly equivalent to 200 μg of salbutamol. Comparison of the bronchodilator response and the effects on heart rate, plasma potassium, and tremor of cumulative doses of salbutamol with that of noncumulative doses of salmeterol have, however, suggested an up to 10-fold difference in potency on a weight for weight basis (41).

Caution is necessary toward studies conducted to assess the equivalence of different β_2-agonists; in particular if data are expressed on a puff for puff or a milligram for milligram basis. Indeed, the bronchodilating effect is determined by the dose deposited in the airways, not by the nominal or actual dose released from the inhaler (42). We thus recently demonstrated that 500 μg of terbutaline inhaled from a pMDI is equivalent to 250 μg inhaled from Turbuhaler (43). Therefore, dose equivalence of different β_2-agonists should be based on studies in which the same inhalation device is used, or in which the doses are corrected for potential differences in deposition. This issue is further addressed in Chapter 10.

B. Rate of Onset

The onset of bronchodilatory action of most β_2-agonists occurs within 1–3 min, and no apparent differences among the currently available short-acting β_2-agonists have been reported. Indeed, it has been demonstrated that the time required for the onset of action of salbutamol and fenoterol is 0.8 and 1.1 min, respectively (44). Formoterol required 1.7 min to exert some effect, whereas the starting time for the other long-acting β_2-agonist, salmeterol, was clearly longer, averaging 17.6 min (45).

Older studies have shown that the catecholamines isoetharine and isoproterenol exerted their maximal level of effect within 5 min after aerosol administration (46,47). This contrasts with the noncatecholamines, such as salbutamol, fenoterol, and terbutaline, which produced about 75–80% of their maximum effect within 5 min but required 15–60 min before maximal bronchodilatation was achieved (48,49). This difference was attributed to a more rapid crossing of the catecholamines through the epithelial barriers (50). Inhaled formoterol exhibited a similar onset of action as the selective short-acting β_2-agonists, 80–90% of maximum bronchodilatation occurring within 5–10 min (83). In addition, we have found that, as with salbutamol, formoterol induced an increase in sGaw 1 min after inhalation, with a maximum increase in FEV_1 at 57 min for salbutamol, 200 μg, and 137, 141, and 161 min for formoterol, 12, 24 and 48 μg, respectively (83). Other investigators have subsequently confirmed the rapid onset of action of formoterol (52).

Conversely, studies with inhaled salmeterol have shown a tendency toward a somewhat slower onset of effect, but the peak bronchodilatation is reached 2–4 hr after inhalation, and some 90% of the maximum effect is seen at 1 hr (39,53). In another study, the ability of salmeterol and salbutamol to reverse methacholine-induced bronchoconstriction has been assessed. This represents just another way to compare the onset of action of different β-agonists. At 50 μg, salmeterol appeared to have a slower onset of action than salbutamol had at 200 μg, as recovery in FEV_1 to 90% of baseline occurred in 19.4 min with salmeterol and to 95% of baseline in 9.6 min with salbutamol (54).

C. Magnitude of Response

It has been previously shown that the magnitude of the response to inhaled β-agonists, as judged by the percentage increase in FEV_1 over baseline is linearly related to the logarithm of the inhaled dose, so that a 10-fold increase in the dose is needed to double the bronchodilating effect (33,55). This explains in part the "plateau" observed when nonlogarithmic scales are used to describe the dose-effect relationship in bronchodilator studies. Lipworth and co-workers have confirmed the linearity of the log dose-response in 14 asthmatics who inhaled cumulative doubling doses of inhaled salbutamol (100–4000 μg). Analysis of individual responses in their study revealed a wide interindividual variability in the magnitude of response; only one patient achieved maximal response with the conventional recommended dose of inhaled salbutamol (200 μg), and the majority of the patients required either 2000 μg or even 4000 μg in order to achieve maximal bronchodilatation (12). No correlation between baseline FEV_1 (expressed as a percentage predicted) and the dose required to produce maximal response could be detected, suggesting that the severity of asthma did not predict the dose needed to optimize the airway response. As expected, they observed a highly significant inverse correlation between baseline percentage predicted FEV_1 and the magnitude of response, expressed as a percentage of initial baseline value (12).

Using an identical protocol in healthy subjects, unlike asthmatic responses, a plateau in bronchodilatation already occurred at a much lower dose of salbutamol, 100 μg (56). This does not necessarily indicate that asthmatics are less sensitive to inhaled β_2-agonists, as direct comparison between healthy and asthmatic airways is complicated by differences in airway geometry.

D. Duration of Action

The mean duration of action of a given inhaled β₂-agonist is critically dependent on the dose deposited in the airways, the potency of drug on a milligram
for milligram (or puff for puff) basis, and the rate at which the effects of the
specific drug diminish with time. This third factor probably reflects the rate at
which the drug is eliminated from the vicinity of the β₂-receptors that mediate
airway relaxation.

It has been previously shown that the duration of action of equivalent
doses of inhaled orciprenaline (metaproterenol) was greater than of inhaled
isoetharine and isoprenaline: a 20% increase in FEV₁ lasted for 3 hr with
orciprenaline, but only for 90 and 60 min for isoetharine and isoprenaline,
respectively (26). By the inhaled route, the noncatecholamines terbutaline,
salbutamol, and fenoterol all had sustained activity for 4–6 hr, with orciprenaline (metaproterenol) being less long acting (57).

The results of the available studies are, however, often conflicting
and usually do not allow one to discern whether differences in apparent
duration of action of the inhaled β₂-agonist are related to differences in
magnitude of their initial effect, differences in the rate at which the effects of
the drugs decline, or both. Moreover, it cannot be ruled out that intersubject
and intrasubject variability in baseline pulmonary function status and in
potential for bronchodilator response may significantly obscure both the
magnitude of the initial effects and the rates at which effects diminish with
time.

Although the duration of bronchodilator activity of β₂-agonists is to some
degree related to the inhaled dose (58), and higher doses of the "short-acting"
inhaled bronchodilators at bedtime may be more effective than standard doses
in the prophylaxis of nocturnal bronchoconstriction, their duration of action
is often too short to last for the whole night even when given in high doses.
Prolonged bronchodilatation over 12 hr has, however, been demonstrated in
adults and in children after inhalation of salmeterol and formoterol.

In the first study with salmeterol (39), doses of 50, 100, and 200 μg were
shown to cause bronchodilatation for at least 12 hr, compared with 4–6 hr for
salbutamol at 200 μg. A similar prolongation of bronchodilatation has been
seen in studies in which the effect of salmeterol on airway reactivity was assessed (51,53). Inhaled formoterol, 12 and 24 μg, led to a sustained and prolonged improvement in pulmonary function over 12 hr in 12 patients with
asthma and in 13 children with asthma (59), a finding that has been confirmed
by others (60,83). It should be noted that the duration of effect may vary from
individual to individual, and some asthmatic patients seem to lose the effect
after 9–10 hr (61).

V. Comparison Between Bronchodilating Capacity of β₂-Agonists and Other Bronchodilating Drugs

A. Anticholinergic Drugs

There is evidence that the maximum bronchodilating response in patients with asthma is higher with β_2-agonists than with anticholinergics. In a placebo-controlled study, administration of cumulative doses of up to 16 inhalations of fenoterol (200 μg/puff) or ipratropium bromide (20 μg/puff) resulted in a final increase of 80% of baseline FEV_1 with the β_2-agonist, whereas the improvement did not exceed 35% of baseline with the highest doses of inhaled ipratropium (62). This difference in potency has been attributed to the different mechanisms through which anticholinergics and β_2-agonists act on the airways. It has been suggested that anticholinergics block acetylcholine, and consequently only the reflex-mediated bronchoconstriction (63), whereas β_2-agonists inhibit both the release and the smooth muscle contraction due to various mediators contributing to airway narrowing.

Studies in which the efficacy of both drugs were compared indicate that the onset of action of an anticholinergic is somewhat slower than that of a β_2-agonist; peak bronchodilation typically occurred 30–90 min after inhalation of ipratropium, as compared with 15–60 min with a short-acting β_2-agonist (64).

B. Methylxanthines

When monitoring twice-daily peak flow rates, regularly inhaled β_2-agonists have been shown to be as effective as sustained-release theophylline but not as good as the combination of both (65). The variable pharmacokinetics, the narrow therapeutic range, and the potentially dangerous concentration-related side effects makes theophylline less attractive as a bronchodilator drug than inhaled β_2-agonists.

As monotherapy, aminophylline was inferior to β-agonists in the emergency room treatment of asthma, as demonstrated by Rossing and colleagues in a randomized trial, in which the effects of nebulized isoproterenol and aminophylline given intravenously on FEV_1 and duration of therapy were compared (66).

VI. Combination of Short-Acting β₂-Agonists with Other Drugs

A. Short- and Long-Acting β₂-Agonists

Salmeterol is a partial agonist in vitro (67), and it might therefore be expected to act as a partial antagonist. This raises the theoretical possibility that salmeterol may occupy β-receptors and hence reduce the access and efficacy of short-acting β_2-agonists such as terbutaline (a full β_2-agonist) or salbutamol (which has less affinity for the β_2-receptor than salmeterol). A study in which cumulative doses of salbutamol were administered after pretreatment with salmeterol has pointed out that the effect of salbutamol was largely additive (41). The interaction between salbutamol and salmeterol is apparently not large enough to cause a clinically important reduction in the beneficial effects of salbutamol in patients taking salmeterol. Whether this potentially detrimental interaction may still occur in patients experiencing an acute asthma attack remains, however, to be investigated.

B. Anticholinergic Drugs and β_2-Agonists

Additional doses of a β_2-agonist, for example, salbutamol, after inhalation of ipratropium in asthmatic patients resulted in a further improvement that actually reflected the greater potency of the β_2 agonists (58,68). Conversely, when a maximal effect was achieved with a cumulative dose of 600 µg of salbutamol, ipratropium increased FEV_1 only slightly (69).

Similarly, several investigators have found that the addition of an anticholinergic drug (ipratropium bromide) further enhanced the bronchodilating effect of a nebulized β_2-agonist in acute asthma (70–72). In most of these studies, the choice of doses in the treatment was, however, somewhat questionable (71,72), and it cannot be ruled out that if the dose of β_2-agonist in the treatment alternative with only β_2-agonist had been higher, this could have produced the same bronchodilating effect as the combination alternative.

As inhaled ipratropium is virtually without systemic side effects, it has been suggested that the efficacy to side effect ratio is probably more favorable with this combination treatment than with inhaled β_2-agonists alone, especially in tremor-sensitive patients (73).

C. Theophylline and β_2-Agonists

When given by the systemic route, β_2-agonists and theophylline seem to have the same bronchodilating effect. It has been shown that the efficacy of inhaled terbutaline was increased by oral theophylline to the same degree as by oral terbutaline (74). This suggests that systemic bronchodilatation enhanced the effect of an inhaled bronchodilator, possibly by promoting a better distribution of the inhaled drug throughout the bronchial tree. The study did not show any pharmacological potentiation between theophylline and terbutaline, indicating that the combination had only an additive effect. Clinical studies have also pointed out that the effect of theophylline in combination with terbutaline aerosol was largely additive, particularly in the early morning (65).

The key question is, however, whether theophylline adds any further benefit on top of a maximized effect of β_2-agonist therapy. Few studies have approached this issue with a proper design. It appeared that the average group response to added theophylline was limited, whereas individual patients may still benefit from this combination (75,76).

It remains unclear whether the routine use of aminophylline should be recommended in patients with acute asthma, particularly since this drug can cause serious adverse effects when the dosage is not carefully adjusted on the basis of serum concentration measurements. In a meta-analysis, only a trend was detected favoring the addition of aminophylline to therapy with intravenously administered aminophylline (77). Two recently conducted double-blind, randomized, placebo-controlled studies have failed to answer this question. Indeed, in one trial, no additional improvement in peak expiratory flow was observed (78), whereas Huang and co-workers reported a faster rate of improvement in FEV_1 in patients treated with aminophylline than in patients receiving placebo (79). Further trials are thus needed to determine the exact place of theophylline in the management of acute exacerbations of asthma.

D. Corticosteroids and β_2-Agonists

The beneficial effects of corticosteroids in acute asthma are generally attributed to their anti-inflammatory actions. Although these do not occur within the first hours of administration, intravenous corticosteroids may nevertheless result in a clinical improvement within these very first hours, and rapid reversal of resistance to isoprenaline within 1 hr of treatment with corticosteroids has been reported (80). The latter observation is ascribed to an upregulation of bronchial β_2-receptors. This will increase the β_2-receptor density, which is eventually mirrored by an increased response to inhaled β_2-agonists (63). This hypothesis is supported by observations showing that prednisolone increased the β_2-receptor density on lymphocytes within 16 hr in asthmatic patients treated with inhaled β_2-agonists to levels found in healthy controls (81). Apparently, β_2-receptor upregulation does not occur with inhaled corticosteroids, since a 4-week treatment with high doses of beclomethasone dipropionate had no effect on the bronchodilator dose-response curve for inhaled salbutamol (82).

Acknowledgment

We gratefully thank C. Vandeven for typing the manuscript.

References

1. Nials ATRA, Coleman RA, Johnson M, Magnussen H, Rabe KF, Vardey CJ. Effects of β-adrenoreceptor agonists in human bronchial smooth muscle. Br J Pharmacol 1993; 110:1112–1116.

2. Zaagsma J, van der Heijden PJCM, van der Schaar MWG, Bank CMC. Differentiation of functional adrenoreceptors in human and guinea pig airways. Eur J Respir Dis 1984; 135(suppl):16–33.
3. Torphy TJ, Rinard GA, Rietola MG, Mayer SE. Functional antagonism in canine tracheal smooth muscle: inhibition by methacholine of the mechanical and biochemical responses to isoproterenol. J Pharmacol Exp Ther 1983; 227:694–699.
4. Phipps RJ, Williams IP, Richardson PS, Pell J, Pack RJ, Wright N. Sympathomimetic drugs stimulate the output of secretory glycoprotein from human bronchi in vitro. Clin Sci 1982; 63:23–28.
5. Erjefalt I, Persson CG. Pharmacologic control of plasma exudation into tracheobronchial airways. Am Rev Respir Dis 1991; 143:1008–1014.
6. Peters SP, Schulman ES, Schleimer RP, MacGlashan DW, Newball HH, Lichtenstein LM. Dispersed human lung mast cells. Pharmacologic aspects and comparison with human lung tissue fragments. Am Rev Respir Dis 1982; 126:1034–1039.
7. Skoogh BE. Transmission through airway ganglia. Eur J Respir Dis 1983; 131 (suppl):159–170.
8. Thiringer G, Svedmyr N. Comparison of infused and inhaled terbutaline in patients with asthma. Scand J Respir Dis 1976; 57:17–24.
9. Larsson S, Svedmyr N. Tremor caused by sympathomimetics is mediated by β_2-adrenoreceptors. Scand J Respir Dis 1977; 58:5–10.
10. Larsson S, Svedmyr N. Cumulative dose-response curves for comparison of oral bronchodilating drugs. A study of salbutamol and fenoterol. Ann Allergy 1977; 39:362–366.
11. Larsson S, Svedmyr N. Bronchodilating effect and side effects of β_2-adrenoreceptor stimulants by different modes of administration (tablets, metered aerosol, and combinations thereof). A study with salbutamol in asthmatics. Am Rev Respir Dis 1977; 116:861–869.
12. Lipworth BJ, Clark RA, Dhillon DP, Brown RA, McDevitt DG. β-Adrenoreceptor responses to high doses of inhaled salbutamol in patients with bronchial asthma. Br J Clin Pharmacol 1988; 26:527–533.
13. Boulet LP. Long- versus short-acting β_2-agonists. Drugs 1994; 47:207–222. (Erratum published in Drugs 1994; 48:326.)
14. Dahl R, Pedersen B, Hägglöf B. Nocturnal asthma: effect of treatment with oral sustained-release terbutaline, inhaled budesonide, and the two in combination. J Allergy Clin Immunol 1989; 83:811–815.
15. Brambilla C, Chastang C, Georges D, Bertin L. Salmeterol compared with slow-release terbutaline in nocturnal asthma. A multicenter, randomized, double-blind, double-dummy, sequential clinical trial. Allergy 1994; 49:421–426.
16. Vilsvik JS, Langaker O, Persson G, Ringdahl N, Schaanning J, Kvelstad G, Svensson K, Holthe S, Soliman S. Bambuterol: a new long acting bronchodilating prodrug. Ann Allergy 1991; 66:315–319.
17. Williams SJ, Winner SJ, Clark TJ. Comparison of inhaled and intravenous terbutaline in acute severe asthma. Thorax 1981; 36:629–632.
18. Appel D, Karpel JP, Sherman M. Epinephrine improves expiratory flow rates in patients with asthma who do not respond to inhaled metaproterenol sulfate. J Allergy Clin Immunol 1989; 84:90–98.

19. Van Renterghem D, Lamont H, Elinck W, Pauwels R, Van der Straeten M. Intravenous versus nebulized terbutaline in patients with acute severe asthma; a double-blind randomized study. Ann Allergy 1987; 59:313–316.
20. Noseda A, Yernault JC. Sympathomimetics in acute severe asthma: inhaled or parenteral, nebulizer or spacer? Eur Respir J 1989; 2:377–382.
21. Crompton GK. Nebulized or intravenous β_2-adrenoreceptor agonist therapy in acute asthma (editorial). Eur Respir J 1990; 3:125–126.
22. FitzGerald JM, Hargreave FE. The assessment and management of acute life-threatening asthma. Chest 1989; 95:888–894.
23. van den Bergh W, Leferink JG, Maes RAA, Fokkens JK, Kreukniet J, Bruynzeel PLB. The effects of oral and subcutaneous administration of terbutaline in asthmatic patients. Eur J Respir Dis 1984; 65(suppl):181–193.
24. Dulfano MJ, Glass P. The bronchodilator effects of terbutaline: route of administration and patterns of response. Ann Allergy 1976; 37:357–366.
25. Pierce RJ, Payne CR, Williams SJ, Denison DM, Clark TJH. Comparison of intravenous and inhaled terbutaline in the treatment of asthma. Chest 1981; 79:506–511.
26. Freedman BJ, Hill GB. Comparative study of duration of action and cardiovascular effects of bronchodilator aerosols. Thorax 1971; 26:46–50.
27. Freedman BJ. Trial of new bronchodilator, terbutaline, in asthma. Br Med J 1971; 1:633–636.
28. Schwarz HJ, Trautlein JJ, Goldstein AR. Acute effects of terbutaline and epinephrine on asthma. Double-blind crossover placebo study. J Allergy Clin Immunol 1976; 58:516–522.
29. Bengtsson B, Fagerstom PO. Extrapulmonary effects of terbutaline during prolonged administration. Clin Pharmacol Ther 1982; 31:726–732.
30. Wong CS, Pavord ID, Williams J, Britton JR, Tattersfield AE. Bronchodilator, cardiovascular, and hypokalaemic effects of fenoterol, salbutamol and terbutaline in asthma. Lancet 1990; 336:1396–1399.
31. Grainger J, Woodman K, Pearce N, Crane J, Burgess C, Keane A, Beasley R. Prescribed fenoterol and death from asthma in New Zealand. 1981–7: a further case-control study. Thorax 1991; 46:105–111.
32. Tattersfield AE. Clinical pharmacology of long-acting β-receptor agonists. Life Sci 1993; 52:2161–2169.
33. Freedman BJ, Meisner P, Hill GB. A comparison of the actions of different bronchodilators in asthma. Thorax 1968; 23:590–597.
34. Gray BJ, Frame MH, Costello JF. A comparative double-blind study of the bronchodilator effects and side-effects of inhaled fenoterol and terbutaline administered in equipotent doses. Br J Dis Chest 1982; 76:341–350.
35. Freedman BJ. Trial of a terbutaline aerosol in the treatment of asthma and a comparison of its effects with those of a salbutamol aerosol. Br J Dis Chest 1972; 66:222–229.
36. Simonsson BG, Stiksa J, Ström B. Double-blind trial with increasing doses of salbutamol and terbutaline aerosols in patients with reversible airways obstruction. Acta Med Scand 1972; 192:371–376.
37. Bennis J, Svedmyr N. A controlled comparison of salbutamol and terbutaline inhaled by IPPV in asthmatic patients: a dose-response study. Scand J Respir Dis 1977; 101(suppl):113–117.

38. Löfdahl CG, Svedmyr N. Formoterol fumarate, a new β_2-adrenoreceptor agonist. Allergy 1989; 44:264–271.
39. Ullman A, Svedmyr N. Salmeterol, a new long acting inhaled β_2-adrenoreceptor agonist: comparison with salbutamol in adult asthmatic patients. Thorax 1988; 43:674–678.
40. Ullman A, Hedner J, Svedmyr N. Inhaled salmeterol and salbutamol in asthmatic patients. An evaluation of asthma symptoms and the possible development of tachyphylaxis. Am Rev Respir Dis 1990; 142:571–575.
41. Smyth ET, Pavord ID, Wong CS, Wisniewski AFZ, Williams J, Tattersfield AE. Interaction and dose equivalence of salbutamol and salmeterol in patients with asthma. Br Med J 1993; 306:543–545.
42. Derom E, Pauwels R. Bioequivalence of inhaled drugs. Eur Respir J 1995; 8:1634–1636.
43. Borgström L, Derom E, Ståhl E, Wåhlin-Boll E, Pauwels R. The inhalation device influences lung deposition and bronchodilating effect of terbutaline. Am J Respir Crit Care Med 1996; 153:1636–1640.
44. Jeppsson AB, Löfdahl CG, Waldeck B, Widmark E. On the predictive value of experiments in vitro in the evaluation of the effect and duration of bronchodilator drugs for local administration. Pulm Pharmacol 1989; 2:81–85.
45. Ullman A, Bergendal A, Linden A, Waldeck B, Skoogh BE, Löfdahl CG. Onset of action and duration of effect of formoterol and salmeterol compared to salbutamol in isolated guinea pig trachea with or without epithelium. Allergy 1992; 47:384–387.
46. Ahrens RC, Smith GD. Albuterol: an adrenergic agent for use in the treatment of asthma; pharmacology, pharmacokinetics and clinical use. Pharmacotherapy 1984; 4:105–121.
47. Svedmyr N. Fenoterol: a β_2-adrenergic agonist for use in asthma. Pharmacology, pharmacokinetics, clinical efficacy, and adverse effects. Pharmacotherapy 1985; 5:109–126.
48. Lemanske RF, Joad J. β_2-Receptor agonists in asthma: a comparison. J Asthma 1990; 27:101–109.
49. Lipworth BJ, Clark RA, Dhillon DP, Moreland TA, Struthers AD, Clarck GA, McDevitt DG. Pharmacokinetics, efficacy and adverse effects of sublingual salbutamol in patients with asthma. Eur J Clin Pharmacol 1989; 37:567–571.
50. Jack D. An introduction to salbutamol and other modern β-adrenoreceptor stimulants. Postgrad Med J 1971; 47(suppl):8–11.
51. Derom EY, Pauwels RA, Van Der Straeten ME. The effect of inhaled salmeterol on methacholine responsiveness in subjects with asthma up to 12 hours. J Allergy Clin Immunol 1992; 89:811–815.
52. Wegener T, Hedenström H, Melander B. Rapid onset of action of inhaled formoterol in asthmatic patients. Chest 1992; 102:535–538.
53. Campos Gongora H, Wisniewski AFZ, Tattersfield AE. A single-dose comparison of inhaled albuterol and two formulations of salmeterol on airway reactivity in asthmatic subjects. Am Rev Respir Dis 1991; 144:626–629.
54. Beach JR, Young CL, Stenton SCV, Avery AJ, Walters EH, Hendrick DJ. A comparison of the speeds of action of salmeterol and salbutamol in reversing methacholine-induced bronchoconstriction. Pulm Pharmacol 1992; 5:133–135.

55. Nelson HS. β-Adrenergic bronchodilators. N Engl J Med 1995; 333:499–506.

56. Lipworth BJ, McDevitt DG, Struthers AD. Systemic β-adrenoreceptor responses to salbutamol given by metered-dose inhaler alone and with pear-shaped spacer attachment: comparison of electrocardiographic, hypokalaemic and haemodynamic effects. Br J Clin Pharmacol 1989; 27:837–842.

57. Weber RW. Role of long-acting β₂-agonists in asthma. Ann Allergy 1992; 69:381–384.

58. Ruffin RE, FitzGerald JD, Rebuck AS. A comparison of the bronchodilator activity of Sch 1000 and salbutamol. J Allergy Clin Immunol 1977; 59:136–141.

59. Graff-Lonnevig V. Twelve hours' bronchodilating effect of inhaled formeterol in children with asthma: a double blind, cross-over study versus salbutamol. Clin Exp Allergy 1990; 20:429–432.

60. Maesen FPV, Smeets JJ, Gubbelmans HL, Zweers PG. Bronchodilator effect of inhaled formoterol vs salbutamol over 12 hours. Chest 1990; 97:590–594.

61. Sykes AP, Ayres JG. A study of the duration of the bronchodilator effect of 12 micrograms and 24 micrograms of inhaled formoterol and 200 micrograms inhaled salbutamol in asthma. Respir Med 1990; 84:135–138.

62. Marlin GE, Bush DE, Berend N. Comparison of ipratropiumbromide and fenoterol in asthma and chronic bronchitis. Br J Clin Pharmacol 1978; 6:547–549.

63. Svedmyr N. Action of corticosteroids on β-adrenergic receptors. Clinical aspects. Am Rev Respir Dis 1990; 141:S31–S38.

64. Ruffin RE, Obminski G, Newhouse MG. Aerosol salbutamol administration by IPPB: lowest effective dose. Thorax 1978; 33:689–693.

65. Smith JA, Weber RW, Nelson HS. Theophylline and aerosolized terbutaline in the treatment of bronchial asthma. Double-blind comparison of optimal doses. Chest 1980; 78:816–818.

66. Rossing TH, Fanta CH, Goldstein DH, Snapper JR, McFadden ER Jr. Emergency therapy of asthma: comparison of the acute effects of parenteral and inhaled sympathomimetics and infused aminophylline. Am Rev Respir Dis 1980; 122:365–371.

67. Ball DI, Brittain RT, Coleman RA, Denyer LH, Jack D, Johnson M, Lunts LH, Nials AT, Sheldrick KE, Skidmore IF. Salbutamol, a novel, long-acting β₂-adrenoreceptor agonist: characterization of pharmacological activity in vitro and in vivo. Br J Pharmacol 1991; 104:665–671.

68. Gross NJ. Ipratropium bromide. N Engl J Med 1988; 319:486–494.

69. Ullah MI, Newman GB, Saunders KB. Influence of age on response to ipratropium and salbutamol in asthma. Thorax 1981; 36:523–529.

70. Ward MJ, Macfarlane JT, Davies D. A place for ipratropium bromide in the treatment of severe acute asthma. Br J Dis Chest 1985; 79:374–378.

71. Rebuck AS, Chapman KR, Abboud R, Pare PD, Kreisman H, Wolkove N, Vickerson F. Nebulized anticholinergic and sympathomimetic treatment of asthma and chronic obstructive airways disease in the emergency room. Am J Med 1987; 82:59–64.

72. O'Driscoll BR, Taylor RJ, Horsley MG, Chambers DK, Bernstein A. Nebulised salbutamol with and without ipratropium bromide in acute airflow obstruction. Lancet 1989; 1:1418–1420.

73. Flint K, Hockley B, Johnson NM. Salbutamol versus duovent (a combination of fenoterol and ipratropium bromide) in asthma. Eur J Respir Dis 1983; 128(suppl): 548–550.

74. Svedmyr K. β_2-Adrenoceptor stimulants and theophylline in asthma therapy. Eur J Respir Dis 1981; 116(suppl):1–48.

75. Barclay J, Whiting B, Addis GJ. The influence of theophylline on maximal response to salbutamol in severe chronic obstructive pulmonary disease. Eur J Clin Pharmacol 1982; 22:389–393.

76. Chaieb J, Belcher N, Rees PJ. Maximum achievable bronchodilatation in asthma. Respir Med 1989; 83:497–502.

77. Littenberg B. Aminophylline treatment in severe, acute asthma. A meta-analysis. JAMA 1988; 259:1678–1684.

78. Murphy DG, McDermott MF, Rydman RJ, Sloan EP, Zalenski RJ. Aminophylline in the treatment of acute asthma with acute β_2-adrenergics and steroids are provided. Arch Intern Med 1993; 153:1784–17888.

79. Huang D, O'Brien RG, Harman E, Aull A, Reents S, Visser J, Shieh G, Hendeles L. Does aminophylline benefit adults admitted to the hospital for an acute exacerbation of asthma? Ann Intern Med 1993; 119:1155–1160.

80. Ellul-Micallef R, Fenech FE. Effect of intravenous prednisolone in asthmatics with diminished adrenergic responsiveness. Lancet 1975; 2:1269–1271.

81. Brodde OE, Howe U, Egerszegi S, Konietzko N, Michel MC. Effect of prednisolone and ketotifen on β_2-adrenoreceptors in asthmatic patients receiving bronchodilators. Eur J Clin Pharmacol 1988; 34:145–150.

82. Molema J, Lammers JWJ, van Herwaarden CLA, Folgering HTM. Effects of inhaled beclomethasone dipropionate on β_2-receptor function in the airways and adrenal responsiveness in bronchial asthma. Eur J Clin Pharmacol 1988; 34:577–583.

83. Derom EY, Pauwels RA. Time course of bronchodilating effect of inhaled formoterol, a potent and long acting sympathomimetic. Thorax 1992; 47:30–33.

Discussion

DIRKJE S. POSTMA

University Hospital, Groningen, The Netherlands

A. β-Agonists: More Than Bronchodilators Only

Many studies have been performed on the bronchodilator effects of inhaled β-agonists. They mostly address patients with asthma, where β-agonists are the most effective bronchodilators. Professor Löfdahl has shown in this meeting that there is a clear dose-response effect in the bronchodilator properties of β-agonists in asthmatic individuals. Generally, FEV_1 is the parameter used as an outcome measurement for the effectiveness of bronchodilators. And indeed this is the most frequently used lung function parameter in clinical practice as well. In this way, β-agonists are the most potent bronchodilators in asthma, whereas their effect in patients with COPD is small or minimal (1).

But β-agonists have more effects besides lung function improvement. I will not address their effects on hyperresponsiveness or allergen inhalation, since these have been covered by others. β-Agonists also improve symptoms, and especially long-acting ones improve nocturnal symptoms of wheeze and breathlessness and improve the quality of life in patients with asthma (2,3). Their effectiveness can be extended to patients with COPD as well (4,5). Ulrik recently investigated the use of inhaled salmeterol in 63 symptomatic current smokers with cough and phlegm and an FEV_1 <60% predicted (4). All patients had less than 15% improvement above baseline FEV_1 or a <300 ml increase in FEV_1 after inhalation of 400 μg salbutamol. Patients received placebo and twice-daily 50 μg salmeterol in a randomized order for 4 weeks. This study showed that indeed FEV_1 did not improve during salmeterol treatment. However, morning PEF as well as diurnal variation in PEF improved significantly as did morning and nighttime symptoms. Even though differences were small, the difference in morning PEF was comparable to those found in asthmatic individuals with inhaled corticosteroids, and differences were statistically significant. Jones and co-workers have published in a recent abstract that 50 μg of salmeterol twice daily improved FEV_1 to a small extent and the quality of life to a large extent (Table D–1) (6). The symptomatic benefit stresses the fact that even without or with little improvement in FEV_1 patients may gain symptomatic improvement, which was supported by the preference of the patients in the study by Ulrik for the salmeterol period above the placebo period (4).

One other study has shown that even when no benefit of long-acting β-agonists can be found on spirometric variables in patients with COPD, there is some benefit in effort-independent measures of airway diameter, like Raw

Table D–1 Improvement of Quality of Life by Salmeterol in COPD Patients

	Placebo	SM 50 μg
FEV_1, ml	27	117[a]
SGRQ impact	0	–8.0[a]
SGRQ total	–1.4	–6.8[a]
SF-36 Physical	–2.9	10.2[a]
SF-36 Energy	–0.9	3.8

[a]Significantly different from placebo.
SGRQ, St. George's Respiratory Questionnaire; SF-36, Short Form-36 questionnaire.
Source: From Ref. 6.

(airway resistance) (7). This has been found by many other investigators as well for short-acting β-agonists.

The role for bronchodilators in the long-term management of asthma and COPD may thus be enhanced when future studies do not only include spirometry as an end parameter. They should search for benefits in effort-independent lung function parameters, symptomatic benefit, and improvement in disease-specific measures of the quality of life. This appears specifically of importance in patients with COPD.

References

1. Ziment I. The β-agonist controversy. Impact in COPD. Chest 1995; 107:S198–S205.
2. Juniper EF, Johnston PR, Borkhoff CM, Guyatt GYH, Boulet L-P, Haukioja A. Quality of life in asthma clinical trials: comparison of salmeterol and salbutamol. Am J Respir Crit Care Medicine 1995; 151:66–70.
3. Rutten-van Mölken MPMH, Custers F, Van Doorslaar EKA, Jansen CCM, Heurman L, Maesen FPV, Smeets JJ, Bommer AM, Raaymakers JAM. Comparison of performance of four instruments in evaluating the effects of salmeterol on asthma quality of life. Eur Respir J 1995; 8:888–898.
4. Ulrik CS. Efficacy of inhaled salmeterol in the management of smoker with chronic obstructive pulmonary disease: A single centre randomised, double blind, placebo controlled crossover study. Thorax 1995; 50:750–754.
5. Cazzola M, Matera MG, Santangelo G, Vinciguerra A, Rossi F, D'Amato G. Salmeterol and formoterol in partially reversible severe chronic obstructive pulmonary disease: a dose response study. Respir Med 1995; 89:357–623.
6. Jones PW, Bosh TK. Improvement of quality of life in COPD patients treated with salmeterol. Am J Respir Crit Care Med 1995; 151:A464.
7. Del Torre L, Melica EV, Del Torre M. Effectiveness of salmeterol in patients with emphysema. Curr Ther Res 1992; 52:888–898.

8

Effects of Beta$_2$-Agonists on Airway Responsiveness and Allergen-Induced Responses

PAUL M. O'BYRNE

McMaster University
Hamilton, Ontario, Canada

I. Introduction

For more than 30 years, inhaled beta$_2$-agonists have been used for the treatment of asthma. Indeed, since the mid-1960s their regular use has been advocated as the first-line therapy for the treatment of regular symptoms in patients with asthma (1). This is because inhaled β_2-agonists provide rapid bronchodilation, in large part as a result of their ability to relax constricted airway smooth muscle, and thereby provide rapid improvement of symptoms. Also, inhaled β_2-agonists can protect against stimuli which cause bronchoconstriction and symptoms in asthmatics, such as exercise (2), allergen (3), or inhalation of cold, dry air (4). This ability to protect against these stimuli is known as functional antagonism. β_2-Agonists have the ability to inhibit mediator release from cells such as mast cells when studied in vitro (5). For these reasons, in many (possibly most) countries, inhaled β_2-agonists are the most widely prescribed and used drug in the treatment of asthma, and their regular use is still regarded by many physicians as the initial treatment option for asthma.

The first widely used inhaled β_2-agonists, such as isoproterenol, were very short acting and not selective for activity on β_2-receptors. Subsequent members of this class, such as terbutaline, salbutamol, and fenoterol, are very selective for β_2-receptors and have durations of action as bronchodilators of up to 6 hr (6,7), and as such are considered short-acting β_2-agonists. More recently, β_2-agonists with substantially longer durations of action of up to 12 hr or more have been developed (8,9), and they are considered long-acting inhaled β_2-agonists.

II. Airway Hyperresponsiveness in Asthma

Airway responsiveness is a term which describes the ability of the airways to narrow after exposure to constrictor agonists; airway hyperresponsiveness is an increased ability to develop this response, and it consists both of an increased sensitivity of the airways to constrictor agonists, as indicated by a smaller concentration of a constrictor agonist needed to initiate the bronchoconstrictor response (10), as well as a greater maximal response to the agonist (11) (Fig. 1).

The initial observation that bronchoconstriction occurs more readily in asthmatics when compared with nonasthmatics after exposure to a constrictor

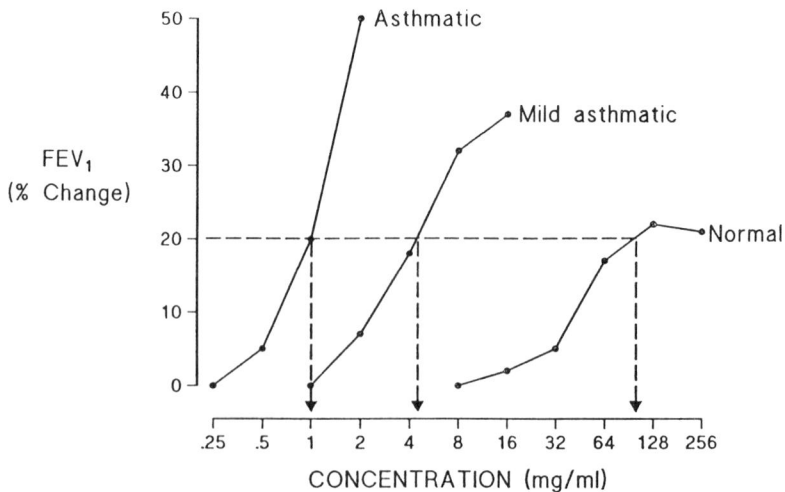

Figure 1 Airway responses as measured by changes in FEV_1 from baseline after inhalation of a bronchoconstrictor mediator from subjects with current symptomatic asthma, mild asymptomatic asthma, and a nonasthmatic subject. Subjects with asthma have an increased responsiveness to the agonist as demonstrated by a leftward shift in the dose-response curve and an increased maximal response.

agonist was made by Alexander and Paddock (12) in 1921, who demonstrated an "asthmatic breathing" in asthmatic subjects, but not normal subjects, after subcutaneous administration of the cholinergic agonist pilocarpine. This observation was confirmed subsequently by Weiss et al. (13), who reported in 1932 that asthmatic subjects, but not normal subjects, developed bronchoconstriction, as measured by changes in the vital capacity, after being given intravenous histamine. Later, Curry (14) noted that this increased bronchoconstrictive response to histamine occurred with intramuscular, intravenous, and nebulized histamine; again only in asthmatic subjects.

It is now known that in asthmatic subjects airway hyperresponsiveness is present to many chemical or physical stimuli such as histamine (15); the cholinergic agonists acetylcholine (16), methacholine (15), and carbachol (17); the peptide leukotrienes (18); prostaglandin D_2 (19) and prostaglandin $F_{2\alpha}$ ($PGF_{2\alpha}$) (20); adenosine (21); as well as to physical stimuli such as exercise (22), hyperventilation of cold, dry air (23), and both hypotonic and hypertonic solutions (24). Inhalation challenges with airway constrictor agonists, such as histamine or methacholine, are widely used in both clinical and research laboratories to measure airway responsiveness. In populations of asthmatic patients, the severity of airway hyperresponsiveness correlates with the severity of asthma (25) and with the amount of treatment needed to control symptoms (26). Research in this area has examined a variety of methods of measuring airway responsiveness, the clinical significance and the effects of antiasthma medications on these measurements, and the pathophysiology and pathogenesis of airway hyperresponsiveness in asthmatic patients. As a result of this research, the methods of its measurement have been standardized and are widely accepted.

III. Effects of Inhaled β₂-Agonists on Airway Responsiveness

A. Short-Acting Inhaled β₂-Agonists

As a result of their effect on airway smooth muscle, inhaled β₂-agonists acutely improve airway responsiveness to pharmacological stimuli. Typically, inhaled β₂-agonists will improve airway responsiveness to inhaled bronchoconstrictors such as methacholine or histamine by 10- to 15-fold (27). Inhaled β₂-agonists will also attenuate the bronchoconstriction caused by physical stimuli, such as exercise (28), and cold air hyperventilation (4); however, the magnitude of this protection is more difficult to evaluate, as these stimuli are generally not delivered in a dose-response fashion, and therefore the magnitude of shift in a dose-response curve cannot be calculated. The duration of this effect is transient, lasting usually less than 4 hr. There is a dose-response for this effect. For example, inhaled salbutamol will improve methacholine airway responsiveness in a dose-response fashion with an EC_{50} of approximately 100 μg and the maximal response of a shift of 10-fold observed at 400 μg (29). There is also individual variability in the maximal response obtained.

B. Long-Acting Inhaled β_2-Agonists

The effects of the long-acting inhaled β_2-agonists salmeterol and formoterol on airway responsiveness have also been studied. These compounds are more potent β_2-agonists, and they also may be more effective in acutely improving airway responsiveness than the short-acting compounds (30). In addition, they have a much longer duration of effect (30,31). Formoterol has been shown to increase methacholine PC_{20} for longer than 12 hr, whereas in the same subjects, salbutamol lasted less than 4 hr (31) (Fig. 2). Indeed, in some individuals, the improvement in methacholine airway responsiveness may last more than 24 hr (32). The duration of salmeterol's effect on methacholine airway responsiveness has also been reported to be greater than 12 but less than 24 hr.

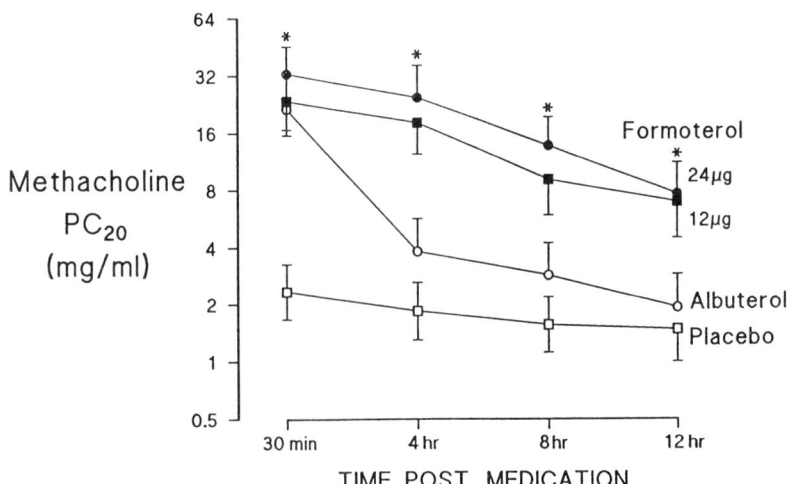

Figure 2 Comparison of the protective effect of two doses of formoterol and albuterol with placebo on methacholine airway responsiveness as measured by the provocative concentration of methacholine required to cause a 20% fall in FEV_1 (PC_{20}). Closed circles, formoterol 24 μg; closed squares, 12 μg formoterol; open circles, albuterol 200 μg; open squares, placebo. Formoterol provided significantly longer protection against methacholine-induced bronchoconstriction. (From Ref. 31.)

IV. Allergen-Induced Airway Responses

A. Early Asthmatic Responses

Inhalation of allergens by sensitized subjects results in airway narrowing which develops within 10 min of the inhalation, reaches a maximum within 30 min, and generally resolves within 1–3 hr. This airway narrowing is called the early or immediate asthmatic response. The early response is caused by mediators released from activated mast cells causing bronchoconstriction. The most important bronchoconstrictor mediators causing the early response are the cysteinyl leukotrienes (LTs) C_4, D_4, and E_4 (33). The early asthmatic response can be self-limiting, and in 40–50% of subjects, it is an isolated response with no sequelae beyond its 2- to 3-hr duration (Fig. 3, upper panel).

B. Late Asthmatic Responses

In some subjects who develop an early asthmatic response, the airway narrowing persists and either does not return to baseline values or recurs after 3–4 hr and reaches a maximum over the next few hours (see Fig. 3, lower panel). This airway narrowing may last 24 hr or more and is called the late asthmatic response (34). Furthermore, the late asthmatic response need not necessarily be

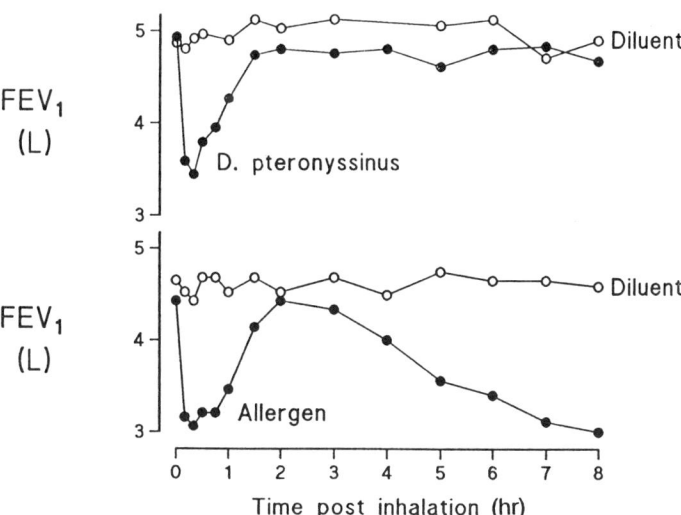

Figure 3 (Upper panel) Allergen-induced isolated early asthmatic response in a subject sensitized to house dust mite. (Lower panel) Allergen induced early followed by late asthmatic responses in another subject sensitized to house dust mite.

preceded by a clinically evident early response. Thus, in a subset of sensitized subjects, the inhaled antigen does not cause a measurable early response but is followed 3–8 hr later by a late asthmatic response. This is called an isolated late response. The late response is usually followed by increases in airway responsiveness and airway inflammation.

C. Allergen-Induced Airway Hyperresponsiveness

Increases in airway responsiveness have been associated with the development of late responses after inhaled allergen (35). This has been described for a variety of bronchoconstrictor agonists, including histamine and methacholine (36,37). The increases in airway responsiveness usually last less than 3 days but can occasionally last several weeks (36).

D. Allergen-Induced Airway Inflammation

Allergen-induced late asthmatic responses were initially shown to be associated with the development of an increase in eosinophils in bronchoalveolar lavage (BAL) fluid by De Monchy et al. (38), and this observation has been confirmed in airway biopsies (39) and in induced sputum (40). The eosinophils are activated, as indicated by an increase in eosinophil cationic protein (ECP) in BAL (39), an increase in EG2+ (a monoclonal antibody directed against cleaved ECP) eosinophils (39), and an increase in degranulated eosinophils in airway biopsies (41). The influx of eosinophils into the airways after allergen inhalation is maximal within 24 hr and has resolved within 7 days (42). Allergen-induced late responses are also associated with an increase in metachromatic cells (likely mast cells) in the airways, which is maximal within 7–24 hr after allergen inhalation and has resolved by 3 days (42).

The increases in eosinophils and metachromatic cells in the airways during and following the late response are also reflected by increases of eosinophils and basophils in the blood and by increases in the progenitor cells (colony-forming units) for eosinophils and basophils (Eo/B CFU) in the blood, which are maximal 24 hr after allergen inhalation (43), and only occur in subjects with allergen-induced late responses (43). Taken together, these results suggest that allergen-induced late asthmatic responses are the physiological manifestation of increases in asthmatic inflammation in the airways caused by inhaled allergen.

V. Effects of β_2-Agonists on Allergen-Induced Responses

Pretreatment with inhaled β_2-agonists immediately prior to the inhalation of allergen markedly attenuate allergen-induced early asthmatic responses, which is consistent with their action as functional antagonists (3) (Fig. 4). However, this effect has also been interpreted as indicating an effect of β_2-agonists inhibiting mast cell mediator release, as has been demonstrated to occur in vitro (5). The effect of inhaled β_2-agonists on the early response has been demonstrated for both short-acting (3) and long-acting compounds (32,44).

In contrast to the effects of inhaled corticosteroids and cromoglycate, pretreatment with short-acting inhaled β_2-agonists immediately prior to the inhalation of allergen have little or no effect on the late response (3) (see Fig. 4). In addition, short-acting inhaled β_2-agonists administered during the late response generally do not fully reverse the airway narrowing that occurs during the late response. Furthermore, inhaled β_2-agonists do not prevent the airway hyperresponsiveness associated with the late response (3).

In contrast to the lack of effect of the short-acting inhaled β_2-agonists on allergen-induced late responses and airway hyperresponsiveness, the long-acting compounds, salmeterol and formoterol, administered immediately prior to the inhalation of allergen, markedly attenuate the late response (32,44) and airway hyperresponsiveness, measured up to 34 hr after allergen inhalation (44). This prolonged action of salmeterol on allergen-induced responses, which appears longer than their activity as functional antagonists, has been

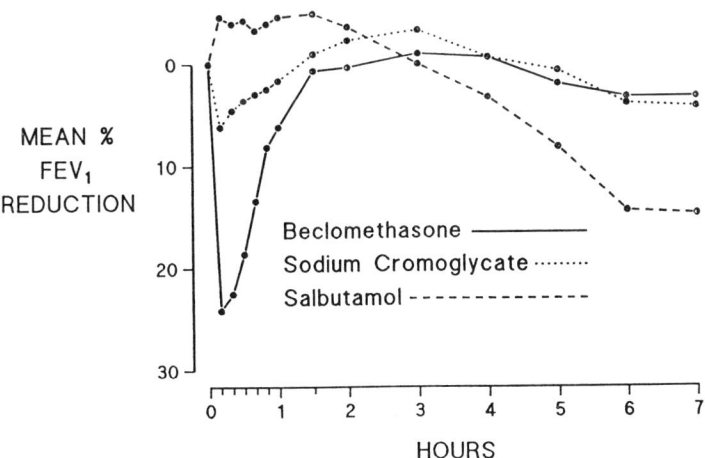

Figure 4 Effect of pretreatment with inhaled albuterol, beclomethasone, or cromoglycate or allergen-induced early and late asthmatic responses. Inhaled albuterol attenuated the early, but not the late, response. Inhaled beclomethasone attenuated the late, but not the early, response. Inhaled cromoglycate attenuated both early and late responses. (From Ref. 3.)

suggested to indicate an effect other than functional antagonist (44), perhaps through inhibiting mediator release or allergen-induced airway inflammation. However, subsequent studies using both salmeterol and formoterol measured inflammatory changes in blood and sputum and demonstrated no significant inhibitory effect. These studies also have demonstrated that when an appropriate control is used to account for the prolonged bronchodilation of these compounds in asthmatic subjects, a significant late response does occur from a newly established baseline caused by the bronchodilator effect (32,45). These studies indicate that the prolonged effect of the long-acting inhaled β_2-agonists on allergen-induced responses is due to prolonged bronchodilation and functional antagonism (32,45,46).

VI. Effects of Regular Use of Inhaled β_2-Agonists

A. Airway Responsiveness

In contrast to the acute improvement in airway responsiveness during the duration of pharmacological action of β_2-agonists, the regular use of inhaled β_2-agonists, using conventional doses four times daily for as little as 2 weeks, causes increasing airway hyperresponsiveness in asthmatic subjects. This effect has been demonstrated for all currently available short-acting inhaled β_2-agonists (47,48). The magnitude of the increase in airway responsiveness is small, being less than a doubling concentration of the inhaled agonist (48), and in most asthmatic patients, this increase may not appear to be of any clinical relevance. However, patients with the most severe asthma tend to have the most severely increased airway hyperresponsiveness. In these patients, who tend to overuse β_2-agonists, even a small increase in airway hyperresponsiveness may have important clinical consequences. In addition to the effect on regular inhaled β_2-agonists on airway responsiveness as measured by the shift of the agonist-dose response curve (as demonstrated by a decrease in PC_{20}), regular use increases the slope of the dose-response curve to the agonist and does not reduce the maximal bronchoconstrictor response (27). The mechanisms, and duration of the rebound increases in airway responsiveness after stopping regular treatment with inhaled β_2-agonists are not yet known.

B. Allergen-Induced Responses

The regular use of inhaled salbutamol, four times daily for 2 weeks, caused increasing airway hyperresponsiveness to inhaled allergen in asthmatic subjects as measured by a decrease in the provocative concentration of allergen needed to cause a 20% fall in FEV_1 (1-sec forced expiratory volume) (49). Also, treatment with salbutamol for a similar amount of time significantly increased, almost doubling, the magnitude of allergen-induced late responses

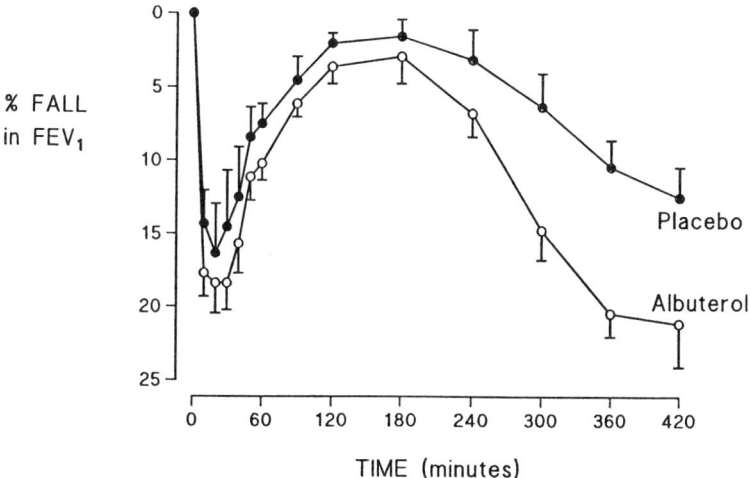

Figure 5 Mean percent change in FEV_1 versus time for allergen-induced airway responses after 1 week of treatment with placebo (open circles) and 1 week of treatment with inhaled albuterol 200 μg four times daily (closed circles). (From Ref. 50.)

(50) (Fig. 5). Regular treatment with terbutaline has been shown to diminish the protective effect of inhaled corticosteroids on allergen-induced responses (51). Last, regular salbutamol treatment for 1 week significantly increased allergen-induced blood eosinophilia (52). These studies suggest that the regular use of inhaled β_2-agonists may magnify allergen-induced inflammatory responses and reduce the ability of inhaled corticosteroids to attenuate these responses.

VII. Tachyphylaxis to Functional Antagonism

The protection provided by both short- and long-acting inhaled β_2-agonists during the duration of functional antagonist against bronchoconstrictor mediators has been shown to diminish with the regular use of these agents. This has been demonstrated for bronchoconstrictor mediators, such as methacholine (53), as well as stimuli that act through mediator release in the airways, such as adenosine monophosphate (54) and allergen (49). In addition, a recent study has shown that the regular use of inhaled salbutamol for 1 week significantly increases the magnitude of exercise-induced bronchoconstriction, when exercise is performed 12 hr after the last dose of salbutamol, and results in significantly less protection after pretreatment immediately prior to exercise

(55). Also, the protection afforded by inhaled salmeterol against exercise-induced bronchoconstriction is reduced with regular use (56). The implication of these results is that the protection that inhaled β_2-agonists give against clinically important stimuli, where pretreatment with inhaled β_2-agonists has been recommended for asthma control, such as exercise or allergen-induced bronchoconstriction, is reduced with their regular use.

VIII. Conclusions

Inhaled β_2-agonists are potent and effective functional antagonists against all bronchoconstrictor stimuli, including stimuli which likely cause bronchoconstriction through an action directly on airway smooth muscle, such as histamine and methacholine, and stimuli which cause bronchoconstriction through mediator release, such as allergen and exercise. This antagonism lasts less than 4 hr for the short-acting β_2-agonists but lasts at least 12 hr and maybe up to 24 hr for the long-acting β_2-agonists.

In contrast to the acute effect of the short-acting compounds, regular use of these drugs causes rebound airway hyperresponsiveness after their duration of functional antagonism has worn off. This has not been demonstrated for the long-acting compounds. In addition, in contrast to their ability as bronchodilators, the efficacy of both short- and long-acting compounds as functional antagonists is diminished with regular use, and regular use worsens allergen-induced responses.

Taken together, these studies suggest that the intermittent use of short-acting inhaled β_2-agonists to provide protection against clinically important bronchoconstrictor stimuli, such as exercise or allergen-induced bronchoconstriction, should continue to be recommended to asthmatic patients, as there are no other drugs that are as effective in this regard. However, the regular use of these drugs to achieve this clinical benefit should be avoided. The use of the long-acting inhaled β_2-agonists should be decided on clinical grounds other than to provide long-lasting functional antagonism.

References

1. Rebuck AS, Chapman KR. Asthma: Trends in pharmacological therapy. Can Med Assoc J 1987p; 136:483–488.
2. Anderson S, Seale JP, Ferris L, Schoeffel R, Lindsay DA. An evaluation of pharmacotherapy for exercise-induced asthma. J Allergy Clin Immunol 1979; 674:612–624.
3. Cockcroft DW, Murdock KY. Protective effect of inhaled albuterol, cromolyn, beclomethasone and placebo on allergen-induced early asthmatic responses, late asthmatic responses and allergen-induced increases in bronchial responsiveness to inhaled histamine. J Allergy Clin Immunol 1987; 79:734–740.

4. O'Byrne PM, Morris M, Roberts R, Hargreave FE. Inhibition of the bronchial response to respiratory heat exchange by increasing doses of terbutaline sulphate. Thorax 1982; 37:913–917.

5. Befus AD, Dyck N, Goodacre R, Bienenstock J. Mast cells from the human intestinal lamina propria. Isolation, histochemical subtypes, and functional characterization. J Immunol 1987; 138:2604–2610.

6. Neville A, Palmer JBD, Gaddie J, May CS, Palmer KNV, Murchison LE. Metabolic effects of salbutamol: comparison of aerosol and intravenous administration. Br Med J 1977; 1:413–414.

7. Scheinin M, Koulu M, Laurikainen E, Allonen H. Hypokalaemia and other non-bronchial effects of inhaled fenoterol and salbutamol: a placebo-controlled dose-response study in healthy volunteers. Br J Clin Pharmacol 1987; 24:645–653.

8. Lofdhal C-G, Svedmyr N. Formoterol fumarate, a new $β_2$-adrenoreceptor agonist. Allergy 1989; 44:264–271.

9. Ullman A, Svedmyr N. Salmeterol, a new long acting inhaled beta 2 adrenoceptor agonist: comparison with salbutamol in adult asthmatic patients. Thorax 1988; 43: 674–678.

10. Hargreave FE, Ryan G, Thomson NC, O'Byrne PM, Latimer K, Juniper EF, Dolovich J. Bronchial responsiveness to histamine or methacholine in asthma: measurement and clinical significance. J Allergy Clin Immunol 1981; 68:347–355.

11. Woolcock AJ, Salome CM, Yan K. The shape of the dose-response curve to histamine in asthmatic and normal subjects. Am Rev Respir Dis 1984; 130:71–75.

12. Alexander HL, Paddock R. Bronchial asthma: Response to pilocarpine and epinephrine. Arch Intern Med 1921; 27:184–191.

13. Weiss S, Robb GP, Ellis LB. The systemic effects of histamine in man. Arch Intern Med 1932; 49:360–396.

14. Curry JJ. The action of histamine on the respiratory tract in normal and asthmatic subjects. J Clin Invest 1946; 25:785–791.

15. Juniper EF, Frith PA, Dunnett C, Cockcroft DW, Hargreave FE. Reproducibility and comparison of responses to inhaled histamine and methacholine. Thorax 1978; 33:705–710.

16. Manning PJ, O'Byrne PM. Histamine bronchoconstriction reduces airway responsiveness in asthmatic subjects. Am Rev Respir Dis 1988; 137:1323–1325.

17. Sotomayor H, Badier M, Vervloet D, Orehek J. Seasonal increase of carbachol airway responsiveness in patients allergic to grass pollen. Am Rev Respir Dis 1984; 130:56–58.

18. Adelroth E, Morris MM, Hargreave FE, O'Byrne PM. Airway responsiveness to leukotrienes C4 and D4 and to methacloline in patients with asthma and normal controls. N Engl J Med 1986; 315:480–484.

19. Hardy CC, Robinson C, Tattersfield AE, Holgate ST. The bronchoconstrictor effect of inhaled prostaglandin D2 in normal and asthmatic men. N Engl J Med 1984; 311:209–213.

20. Thomson NC, Roberts R, Bandouvakis J, Newball H, Hargreave FE. Comparison of bronchial responses to prostaglandin F2a and methacholine. J Allergy Clin Immunol 1981; 68:392–398.

21. Mann JS, Holgate ST, Renwick AG, Cushley MJ. Airway effects of purine nucleo-sides and nucleotides and release with bronchial provocation in asthma. J Appl Physiol 1986; 62:1667–1676.
22. Anderson SD, Silverman M, Godfrey S, Konig P. Exercise-induced asthma: a re-view. Br J Dis Chest 1975; 69:1–39.
23. O'Byrne PM, Ryan G, Morris M, McCormack D, Jones NL, Morse JLC, Hargreave FE. Asthma induced by cold air and its relation to nonspecific bronchial respon-siveness to methacholine. Am Rev Respir Dis 1982; 125:281–285.
24. Anderson S, Schoeffel R, Finney M. Evaluation of ultrasonically nebulized solu-tions for provocative testing in patients with asthma. Thorax 1983; 38:284–291.
25. Cockcroft DW, Killian DN, Mellon JJA, Hargreave FE. Bronchial reactivity of inhaled histamine: a method and clinical survey. Clin Allergy 1977; 7:235–243.
26. Juniper EF, Frith PA, Hargreave FE. Airway responsiveness to histamine and methacholine: relationship to minimum treatment to control symptoms of asthma. Thorax 1981; 36:575–579.
27. Bel EH, Zwinderman AH, Timmers MC, Dijkman JH, Sterk PJ. The protective effect of a beta 2 agonist against excessive airway narrowing in response to bron-choconstrictor stimuli in asthma and chronic obstructive lung disease. Thorax 1991; 46:9–14.
28. Anderson S, Seale JP, Ferris L, Schoeffel R, Lindsay DA. An evaluation of phar-macotherapy for exercise-induced asthma. J Allergy Clin Immunol 1979; 64:612–624.
29. Wong A, O'Byrne PM, Lindbladt C, Stahl E, Hargreave FE. The dose-response protective effect of salbutamol pressurized metered dose inhaler on methacholine airway responsiveness. Am J Resp Crit Care Med 1996; 135:A65.
30. Gongora HC, Wisniewski AF, Tattersfield AE. A single-dose comparison of in-haled albuterol and two formulations of salmeterol on airway reactivity in asth-matic subjects. Am Rev Respir Dis 1991; 144:626–629.
31. Ramsdale EH, Otis J, Klein P, Hargreave FE, O'Byrne PM. The effect of long acting β_2-adrenoceptor agonist, formoterol, on methacholine airway responsive-ness in asthmatic subjects. Am Rev Respir Dis 1991; 143:998–1001.
32. Wond BJ, Dolovich J, Ramsdale EH, O'Byrne PM, Gontovnick L, Denburg JA, Hargreave FE. Formoterol compared to beclomethasone and placebo on aller-gen-induced asthmatic responses. Am Rev Respir Dis 1992; 146:1156–1160.
33. Taylor IK, O'Shaughnessy KM, Fuller RW, Dollery CT. Effect of a cysteinylleuk-otriene receptor antagonist, ICI 204-219 on allergen-induced bronchoconstriction and airway hyperreactivity in atopic subjects. Lancet 19??; 337:690–694.
34. O'Byrne PM, Dolovich J, Hargreave FE. State of the art: late asthmatic responses. Am Rev Respir Dis 1987; 136:740–751.
35. Cockcroft DW, Ruffin RE, Dolovich J, Hargreave FE. Allergen-induced increase in non-allergic bronchial reactivity. Clin Allergy 1977; 7:503–513.
36. Cartier A, Thomson NC, Frith PA, Roberts R, Hargreave FE. Allergen-induced increase in bronchial responsiveness to histamine: relationship to the late asth-matic response and change in airway caliber. J Allergy Clinical Immunol 1982; 70: 170–177.

37. Freitag A, Watson RW, Matsos G, Eastwood C, O'Byrne PM. The effect of a platelet activating factor antagonist, WEB 2086, on allergen-induced asthmatic responses. Thorax 1993; 48:594–598.
38. De Monchy JGR, Kauffman HF, Venge Per, Koeter GH, Jansen HM, Sluiter HJ, deVries K. Bronchoalveolar eosinophilia during allergen-induced late asthmatic reaction. Am Rev Respir Dis 1985; 131:373–376.
39. Woolley KL, Adelroth E, Woolley MJ, Ellis R, Jordana M, O'Byrne PM. Effects of allergen challenge on eosinophils, eosinophil cationic protein and granulocyte-macrophage colony-stimulating factor in mild asthma. Am J Respir Crit Care Med 1995; 151:1915–1924.
40. Pin I, Freitag AP, O'Byrne PM, Girgis-Gabardo A, Watson RM, Dolovich J, Denberg JA, Hargreave FE. Changes in the cellular profile of induced-sputum after allergen-induced asthmatic responses. Am Rev Respir Dis 1992; 145:1265–1269.
41. Gizycki MJ, Rogers AV, Ådelroth E, O'Byrne PM, Jeffery PK. Inflammatory cells during allergen-induced late phase reactions: an electron microscopy study of bronchial biopsies. Eur Respir J 1995; 8:168S.
42. Choudry NB, Watson R, Hargreave FE, O'Byrne PM. Time course of inflammatory cells in sputum after allergen inhalation in asthmatic subjects. J Allergy Clin Immunol 1993; 91:64A.
43. Pin I, Freitag AP, O'Byrne PM, Girgis-Gabardo A, Watson RM, Dolovich J, Denberg JA, Hargreave FE. Changes in the cellular profile of induced-sputum after allergen-induced asthmatic responses. Am Rev Respir Dis 1992; 145:1265–1269.
44. Twentyman OP, Finnerty J, Harris A, Palmer J, Holgate S. Protection against allergen-induced asthma by salmeterol. Lancet 1990; 336:1338–1342.
45. Weersink EJ, Aalbers R, Koeter GH, Kauffman HF, De Monchy JG, Postma DS. Partial inhibition of the early and late asthmatic response by a single dose of salmeterol. Am J Respir Crit Care Med 1994; 150:1262–1267.
46. Soler M, Joos L, Bolliger CT, Elsasser S, Perruchoud AP. Bronchoprotection by salmeterol: cell stabilization or functional antagonism? Comparative effects on histamine- and AMP-induced bronchoconstriction. Eur Respir J 1994; 7:1973–1977.
47. Kraan J, Koeter GH, v.d. Mark TW, Sluiter HJ, de Vries K. Changes in bronchial hyperreactivity induced by 4 weeks of treatment with antiasthmatic drugs in patients with allergic asthma: a comparison between budesonide and terbutaline. J Allergy Clin Immunol 1985; 76:628–636.
48. Vathenen AS, Knox AJ, Higgins BG, Britton JR, Tattersfield AE. Rebound increase in bronchial responsiveness after treatment with inhaled terbutaline. Lancet 1988; 1:554–558.
49. Cockcroft DW, McParland CP, Britto SA, Swystun VA, Rutherford BC. Regular inhaled salbutamol and airway responsiveness to allergen. Lancet 1993; 342:833–837.
50. Cockcroft DW, O'Byrne PM, Swystun VA, Bhagat R. Salbutamol inhaled regularly and the allergen-induced late asthmatic response. J Allergy Clin Immunol 1995; 95:44–49.
51. Wong CS, Wahedna I, Pavord ID, Tattersfield AE. Effect of regular terbutaline and budesonide on bronchial reactivity to allergen challenge. Am J Respir Crit Care Med 1994; 150:1268–1273.

52. Gauvreau GM, Watson RM, Jordana M, Cockcroft D, O'Byrne PM. The effect of regular inhaled salbutamol on allergen-induced airway responses and inflammatory cells in blood and sputum. Am J Resp Crit Care Med 1995; 151:A39.

53. Cheung D, Timmers MC, Zwinderman AH, Bel EH, Dijkman JH, Sterk PJ. Long-term effects of a long acting β_2-adrenoceptor agonist, salmeterol, on airway hyper-responsiveness in patients with mild asthma. N Engl J Med 1992; 327:1198–1203.

54. O'Connor BJ, Aikman SL, Barnes PJ. Tolerance to the nonbronchodilator effects of inhaled β_2-agonists in asthma. N Engl J Med 1992; 327:1204–1208.

55. Inman M, O'Byrne PM. The effect of regular inhaled albuterol on exercise-induced bronchoconstriction. Am J Respir Crit Care Med 1996; 153:65–69.

56. Ramage L, Lipworth BJ, Ingram CG, Cree IA, Dhillon DP. Reduced protection against exercise induced bronchoconstriction after chronic dosing with salmeterol. Respir Med 1994; 88:363–368.

Discussion

ERIC DEROM

University Hospital, Ghent, Belgium

It is generally accepted that both the protective and bronchodilating actions of β_2-agonists result from functional antagonism. Indeed, β_2-agonists inhibit or reverse the contractile response of airway smooth muscle irrespective of the origin of the constricting stimulus (1). This property is of particular importance in asthma, since several spasmogens, such as leukotriene D_4, histamine, acetylcholine, and bradykinine, are likely to be involved in bronchoconstriction. It has been claimed that a β_2-agonist might exert part of its protective effect in vivo through an additional non–smooth muscle action (2). Further studies are needed to determine the exact clinical relevance of this effect, which, if present, appears to be small (2).

The association between the frequent use of β_2-agonists, a decrease in asthma control, and an increase in morbidity and mortality has been attributed to the detrimental effects of their regular use (3,4), such that intermittent use of inhaled short-acting β_2-agonists is now currently prescribed to patients with asthma. However, the clinical relevance of β_2-agonist–induced tolerance to bronchodilation and protection against several bronchoconstrictive agents remains a matter of debate (5,6). In this context, mention should be made of a carefully conducted trial by de Jong et al. (7), who were unable to confirm the appearance of a rebound airway responsiveness in asthmatic patients 2 weeks after cessation of regular treatment of inhaled terbutaline. Nevertheless, they did observe a very small decrease in baseline FEV_1, which could be prevented by regular treatment with budesonide. Interestingly, comparison of their data with those of others indicate that the way data are expressed may critically affect the outcome of treatment as well as the conclusion of a given study (7). The whole issue of regular versus intermittent use of short-acting β_2-agonists will remain unanswered unless a large prospective, randomized, double-blind, and placebo-controlled study is conducted in which sensitive outcome markers of morbidity are used and the amount of inhaled puffs is the primary variable.

It is well established that the duration of the protective action of a given dose of a short-acting β_2-agonist lasts usually for less than 4 hr. Conversely, the duration of the bronchodilating effects is usually longer and averages 6 hr. This difference in duration has been unequivocally demonstrated in a well-designed, randomized, placebo-controlled study in which six asthmatic patients were involved (8). Inhalation of aerosolized metaproterenol resulted in a substantial bronchodilating effect, which persisted for at least 4 hr compared with placebo. Conversely, the protective effect of metaproterenol against methacholine had completely disappeared at that time point (8). Further evidence for the discrepancy between the duration of the bronchodilating effect and the protective action of short-acting β_2-agonists is provided by studies demonstrating that 500 μg of inhaled terbutaline did not protect against exercise-induced bronchoconstriction for more than 2 hr (9), whereas it is well known its bronchodilating effect lasts for more than 4 hr (10).

It is beyond any doubt that the aforementioned differences between the duration of the protective and the bronchodilating effects of short-acting β_2-agonists is of clinical relevance. Interestingly, such a difference has not been observed in a randomized, placebo-controlled, crossover trial, in which Rabe et al. investigated both the protective and bronchodilating effect of two long-acting β_2-agonists (11). They administered single, equipotent doses of inhaled salmeterol and formoterol to 12 patients with mild asthma. Both 12 μg of formoterol and 50 μg of salmeterol increased FEV_1 and PC_{20} for methacholine for 24 hr, compared with placebo. Active treatment resulted in an upward, parallel shift of the time course of both the FEV_1 and the PC_{20}, but it did not alter the phase and amplitude of their circadian variation (11).

Maximum bronchodilatation occurs 1 hr after inhalation of salbutamol (13), whereas the protective effect of short-acting β_2-agonists against exercise-induced bronchoconstriction occurs within 30 min (9). Current data indicate that the rate of onset of action of the bronchodilating effect is slower with salmeterol than with salbutamol (12,13) and formoterol (14). With the former drug, mean peak bronchodilation is achieved 5 hr after inhalation. Whether these differences between long- and short-acting β_2-agonists also exist in terms of the onset of their protective activity against various stimuli may be derived from recently published data. Indeed, in a randomized, crossover study in 12 mild asthmatic patients, the protection against methacholine of 50 μg of inhaled salmeterol and 200 μg of inhaled salbutamol was similar in magnitude after 1 hr (15). Moreover, Kemp et al., who compared the protective effects of 42 μg of inhaled salmeterol and 180 μg of inhaled albuterol (salbutamol) in a randomized, placebo-controlled study (16), showed that both salmeterol and salbutamol protected 80% of subjects with asthma susceptible to exercise-induced bronchoconstriction already 30 min after inhalation. This almost immediate protective effect of salmeterol contrasts with the delay observed in the studies in which the bronchodilating action of salmeterol was assessed.

References

1. Torphy TJ, Rinard GA, Rietola MG, Mayer SE. Functional antagonism in canine tracheal smooth muscle: inhibition by methacholine of the mechanical and biochemical responses to isoproterenol. J Pharmacol Exp Ther 1983; 227:694–699.
2. O'Connor BJ, Fuller RW, Barnes PJ. Nonbronchodilator effects of inhaled β_2-agonists. Greater protection against adenosine monophosphate- than methacholine-induced bronchoconstriction in asthma. Am J Respir Crit Care Med 1994; 150: 381–387.
3. van Schayck CP, Domperling E, van Herwaarden CL, Folgering H, Verbeek AL. Bronchodilator treatment in moderate asthma or chronic bronchitis: continuous or on demand? A randomized controlled trial. Br Med J 1991; 303:1426–1431.
4. Sears MR, Taylor DR, Print CG, Lake DC, Li QQ, Flannery EM, Yates DM, Lucas MK, Herbison GP. Regular inhaled beta-agonist treatment in bronchial asthma. Lancet 1990; 336:1391–1396.
5. Wanner A. Is the routine use of inhaled β-adrenergic agonists appropriate in asthma treatment? Yes. Am J Respir Crit Care Med 1995; 151:597–599.
6. Sears MR. Is the routine use of inhaled β-adrenergic agonists appropriate in asthma treatment? No. Am J Respir Crit Care Med 1995; 151:600–601.
7. de Jong JW, van der Mark TW, Koëter GH, Postma DS. Rebound airway obstruction and responsiveness after cessation of terbutaline: effects of budesonide. Am J Respir Crit Care Med 1996; 153:70–75.
8. Ahrens RC, Bonham AC, Maxwell GA, Weinberger MM. A method for comparing the peak intensity and duration of action of aerosolized bronchodilators using bronchoprovocation with methacholine. Am Rev Respir Dis 1984; 129:903–906.
9. Wooley M, Anderson SD, Quigley BM. Duration of the protective effect of terbutaline sulphate and cromolyn sodium alone and in combination on exercise-induced asthma. Chest 1990; 97:39–45.
10. Borgström L, Derom E, Ståhl E, Wåhlin-Boll E, Pauwels R. The inhalation device influences the pulmonary deposition and bronchodilating effect of terbutaline. Am J Respir Crit Care Med 1996; 153:1636–1640.
11. Rabe KF, Jörres R, Nowak D, Behr N, Magnussen H. Comparison of the effects of salmeterol and formoterol on airway tone and responsiveness over 24 hours in bronchial asthma. Am Rev Respir Dis 1993; 147:1436–1441.

12. Anderson GP, Lindén A, Rabe KF. Why are long-acting beta-adrenoreceptor agonists long-acting? Eur Respir J 1994; 569–578.
13. Dahl R. Comparative studies of inhaled salmeterol with other bronchodilators. Eur Respir Rev 1995; 5:27, 138–141.
14. Derom EY, Pauwels RA. Time course of the bronchodilating effect of inhaled formoterol, a potent and long acting sympathomimetic. Thorax 1992; 47:30–33.
15. Derom EY, Pauwels RA, Van Der Straeten MEF. The effect of inhaled salmeterol on methacholine responsiveness in subjects with asthma up to 12 hours. J Allergy Clin Immunol 1992; 89:811–815.
16. Kemp JP, Dockhorn RJ, Busse WW, Bleecker ER, Van As A. Prolonged effect of inhaled salmeterol against exercise-induced bronchospasm. Am J Respir Crit Care Med 1994; 150:1612–1615.

9

Effect of Beta-Adrenergic Agonists on Cough and Mucociliary Clearance

KIAN FAN CHUNG

National Heart and Lung Institute
Imperial College School of Medicine
London, England

I. Cough

Cough is a common symptom of asthma and may occur in different settings. In general, it may be considered to be a protective and defensive act that can be under voluntary or involuntary control for the removal of mucus, noxious substances, and foreign particles from the larynx, trachea, and larger bronchi. The act of coughing functions as a clearance mechanism for the respiratory tract in addition to mucociliary clearance, and this may also be beneficial in asthma, particularly in exacerbations, when excess mucus is being produced. On the other hand, excessive and persistent cough in the absence of excessive mucus production and without the obvious need for mucus clearance or for protecting the airways may be harmful to the asthmatic by interfering with breathing and impairing cardiac activity and even exacerbating bronchoconstriction (1).

A. Pathways for the Cough Reflex

The current knowledge of the afferent and efferent neural pathways has been the subject of recent reviews (2–4). The cough reflex depends on vagal afferent pathways arising from the trachea and intrapulmonary airways and also on the larynx whose afferent nerves pass into the superior laryngeal nerves. Cough-sensitive nerves in the lower airways extend to the division of segmental bronchi (5,6) and probably beyond, with the most important tussive zones being at the level of the larynx and trachea, especially in the region around the carina. Sensory nerve fibers presumed to mediate cough are present in the airway epithelium and have been observed under the electron microscope (7,8).

The afferent pathways are carried to the medulla in the brain stem. Studies concerning the interaction of a "cough center" with respiratory brain stem neuronal activity have not provided definitive answers (9), although some pharmacological studies indicate that cough may be modified independently of breathing (10,11). Neurotransmitters such as 5-hydroxytryptamine (5-HT) and γ-aminobutyric acid (GABA) have been implicated, and the antitussive effects of opiates may be mediated through an effect on these neurotransmitters (12,13). Whether there is an abnormality of these central pathways in chronic persistent dry cough has not been explored.

Afferent nerve endings of the tracheobronchial tree can be divided into four types: slow-adapting pulmonary stretch receptors (SARs), rapidly adapting pulmonary stretch or irritant receptors (RARs), pulmonary C-fibers or J-receptors, and bronchial C-fibers (14). The rapidly adapting stretch receptors with small-diameter, thick myelinated Aδ-fibers that innervate the airway mucosa are in the carinal region. These receptors were named cough receptors as they elicited cough by a very light touch of the larynx and carinal mucosa (15,16). Mechanical and chemical stimuli that induce cough also stimulate the rapidly adapting pulmonary stretch receptors (14), and many nonmyelinated fibers are connected to myelinated fibers in vagal trunks.

There is substantial evidence implicating the bronchial C-fiber receptor in the induction of cough despite the fact that direct and selective stimulation of C-fiber receptors in animals does not induce cough (4). In humans, cough and intense retrosternal burning sensations have been described within the pulmonary circulation time when lobeline, which is known to stimulate pulmonary C-fibers, was injected into the pulmonary artery (17). Nonmyelinated C-fibers can be selectively stimulated by capsaicin, bradykinin, and prostaglandins when administered via the vasculature; these same agents are known to induce cough in animals and humans when administered by aerosol (18–21). However, these agents can also stimulate rapidly adapting stretch receptors. Light mechanical stimuli applied to the mucosal surface were found to be effective in eliciting bursts of impulses from bronchial C-fibers located in the main stem bronchus (22). Such fibers are also present in the lower trachea and extrapulmonary bronchi, which are highly tussigenic areas (23). Capsaicin pretreatment of guinea pigs, in which substance P–containing C-fiber afferents of the respiratory tract have degenerated, resulted in a reduction of the cough reflex induced by citric acid and capsaicin but not that due to nicotine and mechanical stimulation. It has been argued that citric acid and capsaicin acted via C-fiber receptor stimulation and that nicotine and mechanical stimulation via rapidly adapting stretch receptors (24,25). On the other hand, pulmonary and bronchial C-fibers have also been proposed as inhibitors of the cough reflex (26,27).

It is likely that most of the known categories of airway afferent receptors participate in the cough reflex, with the primary mechanism being activation of irritant receptors and of bronchial C-fibers.

B. Tussive Stimuli

Various tussive agents such as citric acid, capsaicin, and low-chloride content solutions are used to test the cough reflex, and although some of the stimuli have been used as specific stimulants of certain afferent nerve endings, the evidence that they are selective for one type of receptor (e.g., irritant receptors vs bronchial C-fibers) is circumstantial in humans.

Capsaicin is specific in evoking discharges from airway C-fibers and not from $A\delta$-fibers (28), and in the guinea pig, capsazepine inhibits cough induced by capsaicin but not the cough induced by hypertonic saline (29), which excites rapidly adapting receptors (30). In humans, capsaicin induces cough reproducibly, an effect associated with transient bronchoconstriction (19,31). Intravenous administration of capsaicin in one of three subjects produced paroxysmal coughing (32), and the cough response of heart-lung transplant recipients to capsaicin is blunted (33). The cough response to citric acid is profoundly tachyphylactic in humans (34), but it may activate similar cough receptors as capsaicin (24).

Solutions lacking in chloride anions induce cough, which is an effect not associated with bronchoconstriction (35,36). Low-chloride content solutions are stimulators of rapidly adapting stretch receptors when applied to the laryngeal or tracheal mucosa (37,38). In the isolated guinea pig trachea, there is a significant population of $A\delta$- and C-fibers in the larynx and trachea mediating low-chloride–evoked cough. The observation that frusemide inhibits low-chloride solution–induced cough in normal subjects (39) has led to the suggestion that inhibition of Na^+-K^+-$2Cl^-$ cotransport mechanisms by frusemide in the tracheal epithelium could alter levels of chloride within the epithelium close to sensory nerve endings such that the depolarized response to a low-chloride stimulus is reduced. Frusemide has been shown to inhibit the stimulation of $A\delta$- and C-fibers induced by low-chloride content solutions in the guinea pig trachea and dog larynx (30,40).

C. Enhanced Cough Reflex

Although cough can be induced directly by airway secretions and irritants, persistent cough may also result from an increase in the sensitivity of the cough receptor. Patients with a nonproductive persistent cough secondary to a range of causes such as following viral upper respiratory tract infections and treatment with angiotensin-converting enzyme inhibitors possess an enhanced cough reflex to capsaicin when compared with healthy noncoughing subjects (41). Successful treatment of the primary condition underlying the chronic cough often leads to a normalization of the cough reflex (42). In contrast, patients with a productive cough such as in bronchiectasis and chronic bronchitis do not demonstrate an enhanced cough reflex. Thus, excessive production of mucus itself does not lead to an enhanced cough reflex. In general, the cough reflex in asthma is not enhanced, but there are subgroups of asthmatics in which it is, particularly those who complain of a persistent dry cough even in the presence of clinically stable asthma (42–44).

Several mediators known to be released in asthma may be implicated in the enhanced cough reflex found in asthma. Prostaglandin E_2 (PGE_2) and $PGF_{2\alpha}$ induce tracheal irritation and cough (45,46) in addition to causing an enhancement of the cough reflex to capsaicin in normal volunteers (47,48). Although $PGF_{2\alpha}$ is a more potent enhancer of the capsaicin cough response than PGE_2, only $PGF_{2\alpha}$ at an equivalent tussive concentration as PGE_2 enhanced the cough response to low-chloride content solutions (49). In the guinea pig, bradykinin, a selective activator of bronchial C-fibers (28,50), augments the tussive response to citric acid. In addition, chronic treatment with an angiotensin-converting enzyme enhanced the cough response to citric acid, an effect that was inhibited by a bradykinin receptor antagonist, HOE140 (51). Because the citric acid cough response is inhibited by a neurokinin-2 receptor antagonist (52) and bradykinin induces the release of tachykinins (53,54), the role of tachykinins in the induction and in the sensitization of the cough reflex has been raised. Neither substance P (SP) nor neurokinin A appear to induce cough when administered by aerosol in normal subjects or in asthmatics (55). However, SP induces cough during an upper respiratory tract infection (56,57). Whether bradykinin or tachykinins, which have been implicated in asthma, can enhance the cough reflex in humans is not known.

D. Cough and Bronchoconstriction

Salem and Aviado (11) observed that the bronchodilators ephedrine and isoprenaline were effective in inhibiting cough and postulated that cough could be stimulated by the process of bronchoconstriction. The degree of induced bronchoconstriction by methacholine and histamine in normal volunteers has been reported to be closely related to the degree of induced cough (58). In rabbits, intravenous histamine caused increased firing of the rapidly adapting receptors and bronchoconstriction (59) and isoprenaline abolished histamine-induced bronchoconstriction with a marked reduction in receptor excitation.

However, in studies in the anesthetized, paralyzed, and ventilated dog, iso-prenaline prevented the increase in tracheal pressure but not the activity of rapidly adapting receptors induced by aerosols of histamine (60). For a given increase in airways resistance, histamine was found to produce a greater receptor discharge than acetylcholine (60,61). Thus, there was a direct effect of histamine on the rapidly adapting receptor, an effect that was not inhibited by isoprenaline irrespective of bronchial smooth muscle contraction. However, local smooth muscle contraction could also either sensitize the cough receptors to the action of constrictors or intensify its direct effects on them.

Although there may be a link between cough and bronchoconstriction, there is enough evidence to support the notion that these are subserved by different pathways (4). Cough very often occurs independently of bronchocon-striction. For example, low-chloride content solutions cause cough without bronchoconstriction (35,36). The cough induced by distilled water is inhibited by lignocaine, which does not inhibit the bronchoconstriction; on the other hand, sodium cromoglycate inhibits bronchoconstriction but not the cough (62). Although cough and bronchoconstrictor reflexes are closely related and can potentiate each other, neither is dependent on the other for its actions.

E. Cough in Asthma

Chronic dry cough may occur in asthma in different clinical settings. Asthmat-ics may present predominantly with cough, often nocturnal, and the diagnosis is often supported by the presence of reversible airflow limitation and bron-chial hyperresponsiveness (63). This condition is often referred to as "cough-variant" asthma, which is a common type of asthma in children. Elderly asth-matics may give a history of chronic cough prior to a diagnosis of asthma made on the basis of episodic wheeze (64). Cough may also occur as a sign of wors-ening of asthma, usually presenting first at night, and associated with other symptoms such as wheeze and shortness of breath with falls in early morning peak expiratory flow rates (65). On the other hand, some patients with asthma develop a persistent dry cough despite good control of their asthma with an-tiasthma therapy. There may be other associated causes for the cough such as postnasal drip or gastroesophageal reflux that may occur concomitantly with asthma.

24–hour ambulatory monitoring of cough events in a group of asthmatic patients with relatively well-controlled disease but complaining of a persistent dry cough reveal a wide range of cough counts (45–1577 coughs in 24 hr), with very few coughs occurring during the sleeping hours (Fig. 1) (43). Using re-cording of cough in a child's own bedroom with a voice-activated cough recorder, peak coughing times of 1900–2100 and 0600–0800 hr, with a maxi-mum cough rate in the first 2 hr in bed (1900–2100) were observed (66). These

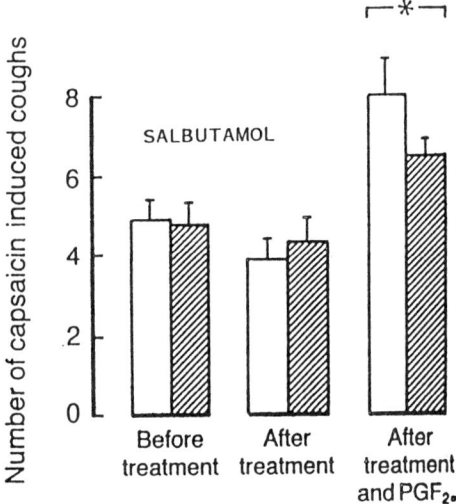

Figure 1 Effect of salbutamol (200 μg aerosol) on $PGF_{2\alpha}$ enhancement of capsaicin-induced cough. Open bars indicate measurement of cough numbers on placebo day and hatched bars on salbutamol day. $PGF_{2\alpha}$ caused an enhancement of capsaicin-induced cough that was inhibited by salbutamol. Data shown as mean ± SEM. *$p < .05$. (Data adapted from Ref. 47.)

studies indicate that the persistent dry cough of some asthmatics is at its lowest during the sleeping hours.

Patients with asthma do not usually have an enhanced cough reflex, although a subgroup with a persistent cough may do so (41,43). In 57 asthmatic patients who do not experience cough, 11 were reported to have an enhanced cough response to inhaled acetic acid (44). In these patients, cough receptors may be sensitized by inflammatory mediators such as bradykinin, tachykinins, and prostaglandins. Induction of sputum by inhalation of hypertonic saline often reveals a predominance of eosinophils, and bronchial hyperresponsiveness is invariably present. A condition of eosinophilic bronchitis in patients with chronic productive cough associated with eosinophils in sputum but without bronchial hyperresponsiveness has been described (67). However, the cough and sputum production is responsive to steroids. It is not clear whether this condition is associated with an enhanced cough reflex.

When mucociliary transport fails or is overwhelmed as in acute severe asthma, cough assumes an important role as a back-up defense system that removes retained respiratory secretions. It is unclear to what extent excessive airway mucus contributes to the cough of the patient with bronchial asthma, as the cough reflex may be triggered by inflammatory changes of the epithelium. The relationship between the quantity and the rheological properties of airway mucus and the cough frequency and efficiency has not been determined.

F. β-Adrenergic Agonists in Cough in Asthma

Very little is known about the distribution of beta-adrenergic receptors on cough receptors and whether β_2-adrenergic receptor activation results in a direct effect on cough receptor firing. The intermediary contribution of changes in airway smooth muscle tone resulting from β_2-adrenergic receptor activation in modulating cough receptor activity cannot be ruled out. β_2-Adrenergic agonists inhibit airway smooth muscle contractile responses mediated by nonadrenergic noncholinergic pathways through modulation of capsaicin-sensitive sensory neurons in the guinea pig (68,69). β_2-Adrenergic agonists may inhibit the release of prejunctional neurotransmitters such as tachykinins involved in neurally induced airway microvascular leakage (70), and such inhibition could be relevant to the effect of β_2-adrenergic agonists on activation of nonmyelinated C-fibers.

A number of studies have examined the direct effect of β_2-adrenergic agonists on the cough response to various tussive agents. In the conscious guinea pig, isoprenaline administered intraperitoneally and other bronchodilators such as theophylline and papaverine inhibited citric acid–induced cough, suggesting that the relaxant response of airway smooth muscle to these agents dictated the reduced cough response to citric acid (71). On the other hand, inhaled terbutaline did not have a significant effect on citric acid–induced cough in the conscious guinea pig (29), but only one dose was studied. The effects of ipratropium bromide and salbutamol on the cough response to citric acid were studied in normal and asthmatic subjects (72). The cough response in the two groups was not significantly different. However, both drugs reduced cough in asthmatics but had no effect in normal subjects. In a group of normal subjects, both aerosolized fenoterol (400 μg) and ipratropium bromide (40 μg) inhibited cough induced by low-chloride content solutions (73). These studies would support the notion that the antitussive effect of these bronchodilator drugs was secondary to their bronchodilator effects.

Other evidence, however, points to an inhibitory effect irrespective of the relaxant effect of β_2-adrenergic effects. Thus, in a group of normal volunteers, salbutamol (200 μg) had a small but significant effect in inhibiting $PGF_{2\alpha}$-induced cough, whereas ipratropium bromide (40 μg) had no effect (Fig. 2). Of greater interest is the inhibitory effect of salbutamol, but not of ipratropium bromide, on the enhanced cough reflex after $PGF_{2\alpha}$ (47). These cough

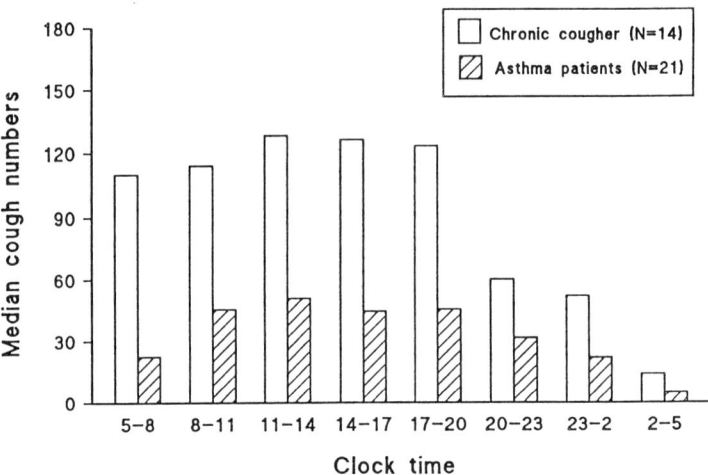

Figure 2 Median cough numbers obtained over a 24-hr period by recording cough sounds and electromyographic activity of lower respiratory muscles on an ambulatory recorder in patients with a chronic cough with no cause found (open bars) and with asthma on adequate antiasthma therapy (hatched bars). During the sleeping hours, the cough count was at its lowest. (From Ref. 43.)

responses were not accompanied by changes in total respiratory resistance measured by the forced oscillation technique. β-Adrenergic agonists may directly inhibit the cough receptors or sensitization of the cough receptors stimulated by $PGF_{2\alpha}$. Alternatively, by increasing intracellular cyclic adenosine monophosphate (cAMP) accumulation, β-adrenergic agonists may reduce the access of $PGF_{2\alpha}$ or citric acid to epithelial paracellular spaces where cough receptors are situated (74). Other effects may be mediated through epithelial transport systems and on secretory processes in the airway glands and epithelium (75,76). More studies are needed on the effect of β-adrenergic agonists on the *heightened* cough reflex.

    In a group of asthmatic patients presenting with cough, bronchodilator therapy abolished the cough in most patients (77). Similarly, in patients presenting with cough but with no symptoms of dyspnea or wheeze but with mild reversible airflow obstruction, oral terbutaline reduced cough significantly without an improvement in peak expiratory peak flow rates (78). Inhaled fenoterol inhibited cough following a fiberoptic bronchoscopic procedure in nonasthmatic patients (79). Other studies have not demonstrated such beneficial effects. Bronchodilator medication did not influence cough events in asthmatic children and only temporarily inhibited coughing attacks (66). In the study of

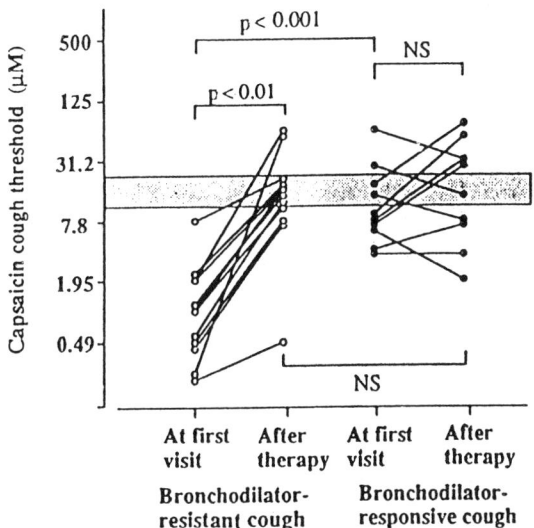

Figure 3 Airway cough receptor sensitivity to inhaled capsaicin at first visit and after therapy in patients with β_2-agonist–resistant cough (n=12; open circles) and β_2-agonist–responsive cough (n=11; closed circles). The β_2-agonist–resistant coughers had a lower starting capsaicin cough threshold and responded to treatment with azelastine and steroids. The shaded area shows 95% confidence interval of the mean value for 43 volunteers. The β_2-agonist used was oral clenbuterol (10 μg, 4 times per day for 1 week). (From Ref. 80.)

Hsu et al. (43), all asthmatic patients complained of a persistent cough despite using regular treatment with inhaled β_2-adrenergic agonists. A recent study indicates that patients presenting with a chronic dry cough with bronchial hyperresponsiveness but with a normal capsaicin cough reflex respond to a β-adrenergic agonist, whereas those with normal bronchial responsiveness but with an enhanced capsaicin cough reflex do not respond to β-adrenergic agonist therapy (Fig. 3) (80,81). The cough in the latter group, however, responded to azelastine and steroid therapy. These studies dissociate the chronic dry coughers into two distinct categories in terms of bronchial responsiveness and of cough sensitivity.

II. Mucociliary Clearance

Mucociliary clearance is an important nonspecific host defense mechanism that operates from the terminal bronchioles to the larynx, whereas cough is the main clearing mechanism acting centrally from the trachea to the seventh or eighth generation (82,83). The overall effect of mucociliary clearance depends on three essential components; namely, cilia, mucus, and the coupling of cilia and mucus. Human ciliated cells are present from the tracheal level down to terminal bronchioles and each ciliated cell has approximately 200 cilia. Each cilium consists of a shaft, basal body, and roots. The shaft consists of central microtubules made of contractile protein or tubulin and of outer fibrils composed of adenosine triphosphate (ATPase). At the ciliary tip, a crown of claws is present which grips the overlying mucus and helps in propulsion. Any mucus produced floats on an underlying layer of periciliary fluid, with the cilia beating within a watery sol layer enabling the ciliary tips to propel the underside of the overlying secretion layer in a cephalad direction. Ciliary beat frequency in the proximal airways is about 13 Hz with a range of 8–15 Hz, and mucus is propelled at a rate of 2–20 mm/min with slower rates in the more distal airways (84). This rate of mucus flow decreases toward the periphery of the lung down to one-fortieth to one-twentieth that of the trachea in the terminal bronchioles (85). The effectiveness of mucociliary clearance is influenced by ciliary motion, secretion of mucins and other macromolecules, and fluid secretions.

Mucus from the conducting airways forms a major component of lung secretions. Lung secretions consist of mucus produced by mucous and serous submucosal glands and goblet cells, and tissue fluid and their daily volume in healthy individuals amounts to 2–10 ml. The submucosal glands and goblet cells produce mucous glycoproteins. Active water, sodium, and chloride transport and protein transport across the airway epithelium also contribute to the composition of mucus and modify its viscoelastic properties. The efficiency of particle transport depends on the presence of mucus, particularly on its rheological properties rather than on its biochemical characteristics, although these two properties may be linked (86,87). The efficiency of mucociliary interaction is influenced by factors such as the thickness of the sol layer, its viscosity, and the elasticity of the gel layer.

A. Measurement of Mucociliary Clearance

Mucociliary transport in the lungs has been measured mainly in two ways. Mucus velocities in the trachea and main bronchi have been assessed by timing the movement of markers placed on mucus such as Teflon discs over a given distance. Linear velocity of mucus flow can thus be determined (88,89). The other approach involves inhalation of a radioactive aerosol and subsequent monitoring of radioactivity by external scintillation gamma counters. From the reduction in radioactivity observed over a period of hours and after correcting for the physical decay of the radionuclide, the rate of the removal of the tracer particles from the lungs can be determined. Counting the remaining radioactivity in the lungs 24 hr later gives the proportion of tracer particles that has deposited beyond the ciliated airways and therefore not available for mucus clearance. This alveolar deposition is subtracted to give the tracheobronchial clearance curve of the deposited particles (90).

B. Mucociliary Clearance in Asthma

Airway inflammation accompanied by increased tracheobronchial secretions is a characteristic feature of asthma. Mucous plugs in chronic asthma causing atelectasis is well-recognized in addition to the widespread mucous plugging in status asthmaticus contributing to deaths in asthmatics (91). Several studies now point to a decrease in lung mucociliary clearance in asthma. In serial studies of asthmatic patients admitted with exacerbations, severe impairment of mucociliary clearance was observed, improving as the patient recovered (92). Marked slowing of the tracheal mucus velocity has been reported in asthmatic patients with normal spirometry (93,94). Mucociliary clearance has been reported to be reduced in stable asthmatics (95–97) when compared with normal volunteers. In patients in remission, clearance was either normal or only slightly impaired (95,96,98–100). However, the measurement of mucociliary clearance is complicated by the central airway retention of radioactivity after 24 hr in more obstructed asthmatics and by the frequent number of coughs experienced by these patients during the period of observation. In patients with severe chronic airways obstruction, mucociliary clearance was also found to be impaired (101), whereas in another study where allowance for differences in the initial deposition of aerosol in asthmatics was not made, no differences in mucociliary clearance was shown (99). In a study where the initial deposition patterns were matched between patients by using a ^{133}Xe ventilation scan rather than using a subtraction of 24-hr retention, asthmatics with tidal flow limitation as assessed by the relationship between the tidal flow–volume loop and the maximal expiratory flow volume curve demonstrated significant slowing of mucociliary clearance in the central airways (102). However, those that had no tidal flow limitation, had normal mucociliary clearance. This study also showed a wide range of mucociliary clearance observed in their 17 asthmatic patients who were on a wide range of antiasthma medication, including bronchodilators and corticosteroids.

C. Mechanisms of Reduced Mucociliary Clearance in Asthma

The impairment of mucociliary clearance in asthma may be the result of several factors, including an abnormality of ciliary function, changes in rheological properties, or an increase in the quantity of mucus and narrowing of the airways leading to inspissation of mucus within. Although epithelial denudation may contribute to the decrease in mucociliary clearance during asthma exacerbations, it is unlikely to be so in stable asthma. The contribution of inflammatory mediators to mucociliary clearance has been studied. Thus, following ragweed challenge in ragweed-sensitive asthmatics, a fall in tracheal mucus velocity was observed independently of the degree of induced bronchoconstriction, an effect prevented by prior treatment with an antagonist of slow-reacting substance (SRS-A), FPL55712 (94). Similar results were found in studies in dogs (103). Leukotriene D_4 decreased tracheal mucus velocity in conscious sheep (104), whereas histamine increased it in dogs (103). However, most mediators, including histamine, leukotrienes C_4 and D_4, and prostaglandins E_1 and E_2, increase ciliary beat frequency in vitro (105,106), but platelet-activating factor decreases it (105). Eosinophils activated by platelet-activating factor may contribute to slowing of ciliary beating by causing epithelial detachment through the release of eosinophil proteins and reactive oxygen species (107). Sputum obtained from patients with asthma caused impairment of ciliary beat frequency in a bronchial explant, with a more pronounced cilioinhibitory effect of sputum obtained during clinical exacerbations of asthma (108).

Changes in airway mucus that could affect its rheology have been reported in asthma with increased concentrations of polysaccharides and cross binding between transudated serum protein and secretory IgA (109–111). Sputum from patients with asthma is more viscous than that from those with other obstructive airway disease (112). Various mediators may stimulate glycoprotein secretion, particularly products of arachidonic acid such as leukotrienes (113,114) and also histamine (115). A major proportion of the mucous plugs found in asthma consists of plasma proteins that have leaked across the vascular endothelial barrier (116). Plasma constituents induce sputum production and also markedly enhance the viscosity of mucus (117–119). Finally, net absorption of water from the luminal side followed by a transient increase of water flux toward the lumen may lead to alterations in the thickness of the sol phase of periciliary fluid induced, as observed following allergen challenge (120).

Thus, the reduction in mucociliary clearance observed in asthma may result from multiple factors such as the direct effect of chemical mediators on epithelial integrity and ciliary action and on the biochemistry and rheology of airway secretions and periciliary fluid.

D. Effect of β-Adrenergic Agonists on Ciliary Activity

β-Adrenergic agonists through stimulation of surface β-receptors (121,122) stimulate ciliary beat frequency of airway epithelial cells (123–129). For example, on cultured human bronchial cells, ciliary beat frequency was increased from a mean of 8.6 to 9.6 Hz by the $β_2$-adrenergic agonist salbutamol at 10^{-4} M and from 9.2 to 10.9 Hz by the long-acting β_2-adrenergic agonist salmeterol (129). The effect of salmeterol lasted for up to 24 hr. The stimulatory effects of salbutamol, but not that of salmeterol, were inhibited by the β-receptor antagonist propranolol. Stimulation of intracellular cAMP by these adrenergic agonists was demonstrated in these cells. cAMP appears to mediate the effect of β-adrenergic agonists, since cAMP analogues such as dibutyryl cAMP significantly increased ciliary beat frequency (130–132). In addition, the phosphodiesterase inhibitor 3-isobutyl-1-methylxanthine and the adenylate cyclase stimulator forskolin augmented ciliary beat frequency (131). Preincubation with a cAMP-dependent protein kinase inhibitor blocked a dibutyryl cAMP–induced increase in ciliary beat frequency in human nasal epithelium (130). Inhibition of adenylate cyclase by adenosine has been shown to reduce ciliary beat frequency in rabbit tracheal epithelium (132). cAMP may control ciliary activity by regulating the availability or use of adenosine triphosphate (ATP) by the ciliary axomere (133).

Further evidence implicating the activation of adenylate cyclase in mediating changes in ciliary beat frequency comes from the effect of β-adrenergic agonists in preventing impairment of ciliary beat frequency. Pyocyanin, a pigment produced by the bacteria *Pseudomonas aeruginosa*, which can colonize airways of patients with chronic airways obstruction, potently impairs human nasal ciliary beat frequency (134). Salmeterol and isoprenaline attenuate a pyocyanin-induced reduction in ciliary beat frequency, which is an effect blocked by a specific β_2-antagonist (135). Pyocyanin-induced slowing of ciliary beat frequency was associated with a fall in intracellular cAMP accumulation, which is an effect reversed by incubation with salmeterol (135). In addition, this was prevented by dibutyryl cAMP and forskolin (136). There is no available data as to whether β-adrenergic agonists can prevent ciliary slowing induced by inflammatory mediators.

E. Effect of β-Adrenergic Agonists on Airway Secretions

β-Adrenergic agonists stimulate the transport of chloride ions and water toward the lumen through cAMP-dependent Cl^- channel (76,137,138), thereby creating an optimal depth of the periciliary layer (sol) and hydration of the mucous (gel) layer. It is also clear that stimulation of chloride transport also occurs with mediators implicated in asthma such as $PGF_{2\alpha}$, PGE_1, PGE_2, leukotrienes, substance P, eosinophil major basic protein, and bradykinin (139–143). The mode of action of these agents is likely to be through stimulation of cAMP (139,144,145). β-Adrenergic agonists stimulate mucus glycoprotein secretion from mucous glands rather than serous cells of submucosal glands (75, 146,147), although others have found no effect (148,149). This increase in mucus secretion may also contribute to an increase in mucociliary clearance.

β-Adrenergic agonists may also prevent airway microvascular leakage and therefore alter the composition of airway secretions in asthma. Stimulation of endothelial β_2-receptors reduces plasma exudative effects induced by a variety of mediators, including histamine, platelet-activating factor, and allergen in the guinea pig (150–154). There is indirect evidence to support a protective effect of β-adrenergic agonists against the exudative effects of inhaled platelet-activating factor in humans (155).

F. Effect of β-Adrenergic Agonists on Mucociliary Clearance

β-Adrenergic agonists stimulate ciliary clearance in normal subjects (84, 156–163) and in patients with asthma (99,100,160). In normal subjects, the stimulatory effect of a single dose of oral β-agonist together with theophylline was lost after 1 week of treatment (163). Not all studies in asthma have shown positive results (98,164–166) even when a bronchodilator effect was observed (98). The negative studies have been performed with doses of β_2-agonists corresponding to doses less than 1 mg of terbutaline by a metered-dose inhaler or with oral doses of salbutamol (98,164). Interestingly, there was no effect of terbutaline (1 mg) in increasing mucociliary clearance in asthmatics when it was delivered from a dry-powder inhaler (Turbuhaler, Astra Draco, Lund, Sweden) compared with delivery from a metered-dose inhaler despite achieving a similar degree of bronchodilation (Fig. 4) (160). In one study, terbutaline (2 mg) from a metered-dose inhaler improved lung mucociliary clearance in the asthmatics with more severe initial impairment, whereas terbutaline (0.25 mg) administered subcutaneously improved mucociliary clearance from predominantly distal ciliated airways of the asthmatics with more severe initial impairment (160).

An increase in mucociliary clearance induced by β-adrenergic agonists has also been observed in chronic bronchitis (93,159,167–169). In one study, no effect was found following chronic treatment with inhaled terbutaline (170), which could have resulted from the development of tolerance. In cystic fibrosis, terbutaline did not increase mucociliary clearance (171,172), which is consistent with the lack of β-adrenergic modulation of Cl⁻ transport (137,173) and therefore lack of rehydration of dry mucus in cystic fibrosis.

There is also evidence that β-adrenergic agonists may increase the effectiveness of mucus clearance by coughing. Thus, terbutaline increased radioaerosol clearance following chest physiotherapy in patients with bronchiectasis (174), which is an effect that may be attributed to improved hydration of mucus either directly or through β-adrenergic stimulation of ion and water transport leading to an enhancement of the mucus-clearing effectiveness of forced expirations. Terbutaline also induced bronchodilation, but this did not appear to diminish the effectiveness of cough clearance. Such an effect in bronchiectasis

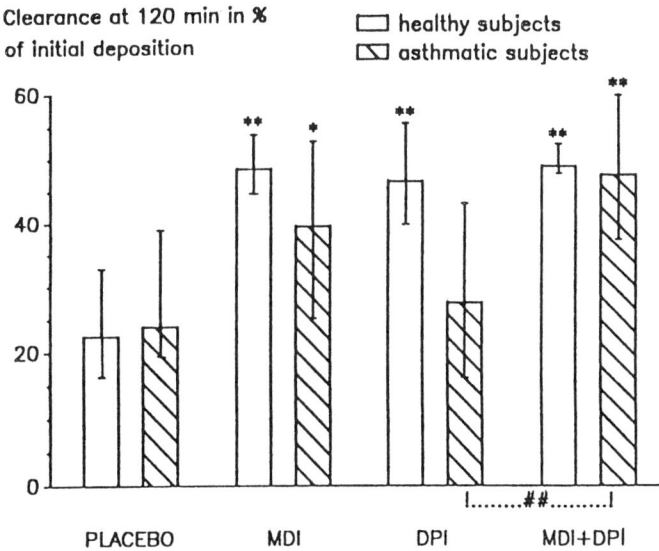

Figure 4 Effect of β₂-adrenergic agonist in mucociliary clearance expressed as clearance at 120 min of the percentage of initial deposition of ^{99m}Tc in normal and asthmatic subjects. Terbutaline (1 mg) inhaled from a metered-dose inhaler (MDI) significantly increased clearance in both groups, whereas terbutaline (1 mg) inhaled from a dry-powder inhaler (DPI; Turbuhaler) increased clearance in normal subjects only. Inhalation of terbutaline from MDI (1 mg) and DPI (12 mg) increased clearance in both groups. *$P < .05$; **$P < .01$ compared with placebo; ## $P < .01$ between terbutaline treatments; bars are median, upper and lower quartiles. (From Ref. 160.)

may be relevant to the use of β-adrenergic agonists in the clearing of mucous plugs from the airways of patients with acute severe asthma.

III. Conclusions

β-Adrenergic agonists improve not only airway caliber by causing airway smooth muscle relaxation but also have beneficial effects on mucociliary clearance, which is impaired in asthma, and may control cough, particularly when associated with bronchoconstriction. Both mucociliary clearance and cough are defensive mechanisms for clearing the airways of mucus and foreign particles. These potential benefits of β-adrenergic agonists result from a number of effects on ciliary activity, mucus production, water and chloride secretion, and cough receptors. Much remains to be elucidated about the mechanisms by which β-adrenergic agonists influence and modulate these factors, particularly in the airways of asthmatic patients. The pharmacological aspects of the actions of β-adrenergic agonists need further exploration, in particular the potential for tolerance with repeated administration. Maximization of the beneficial effects of β-adrenergic agonists may enhance the therapeutic benefits on mucociliary clearance and cough. The use of β-adrenergic agonists in various types of cough associated with asthma has not been fully assessed.

Acknowledgment

I thank Dr. Duncan Rogers for his critical review of this chapter and for his suggestions.

References

1. Stanescu DC, Teculescu DB. Exercise- and cough-induced asthma. Respiration 1970; 27:377–383.
2. Chung KF. Cough. In: Crystal RG, West JB, Weibel ER, Barnes PJ, eds. The Lung: Scientific Foundations. New York: Raven Press, 1995.
3. Widdicombe JG. Neurophysiology of the cough reflex. Eur Respir Dis 1995; 8: 1193–1202.
4. Karlsson J, Sant'Ambrogio G, Widdicombe J. Afferent neural pathways in cough and reflex bronchoconstriction. J Appl Physiol 1988; 65:1007–1023.
5. Larsell O, Burget GE. The effects of mechanical and chemical stimulation of the tracheobronchial mucous membrane. J Physiol (Lond) 1924; 70:311–321.
6. Widdicombe JG. Receptors in the trachea and bronchi of the cat. J Physiol (Lond) 1954; 123:71–104.
7. Laitinen L. Detailed analysis of the neural elements in human airways. In: Kaliner M, Barnes PJ, eds. Neural Regulation of the Airways in Health and Disease. New York: Marcel Dekker, 1986:35–36.
8. Das RM, Jeffery PK, Widdicombe JG. The epithelial innervation of the lower respiratory tract of the cat. J Anat 1978; 126:123–131.
9. David-Milner MS, Lara JP, Milan A, Gonzalez-Baron S. Activity of inspiratory neurons of the ambiguus complex during cough in the spontaneously breathing decerebrate cat. Exp Physiol 1993; 78:835–838.
10. May AJ, Widdicombe JG. Depression of the cough reflex by pentobarbitone and some opium derivatives. Br J Pharmacol 1954; 9:335–340.
11. Salem H, Aviado DM. Antitussive drugs with special reference to a new theory for the initiation of the cough reflex and the influence of bronchodilators. Am J Med Sci 1964; 247:586–600.
12. Bolser DC, Aziz SM, Degennaro FC. Antitussive effects of GABA agonists in the cat and guinea-pig. Br J Pharmacol 1993; 110:491–495.
13. Kamei J, Hosokawa T, Yanaura S, Hukuhara T. Involvement of central serotonergic mechanisms in the cough reflex. Jpn J Pharmacol 1986; 42:531–538.

14. Coleridge HM, Coleridge JCG. Reflexes Evoked from Tracheobronchial Trees and Lungs. In: Cherniack NS, Widdicombe JG, eds. Handbook of Physiology, The Respiratory System II, Part I. Control of Breathing. Baltimore: Williams & Wilkins, 1986:395–429.

15. Widdicombe JG. Defensive mechanisms of the respiratory system. In: Widdicombe JG, ed. International Review of Physiology: Respiratory Physiology II. Baltimore: University Park Press, 1977:291–315.

16. Sant'Ambrogio G, Sant'Ambrogio FB, Davies A. Airway receptors in cough. Clin Respir Physiol 1984; 20:43–47.

17. Jain SK, Subramanian S, Julka DB, Guz A. Search for evidence of lung chemoreflexes in man: study of respiratory and circulatory effect of phenyldiguanide and lobeline. Clin Sci 1972; 42:163–177.

18. Forsberg K, Karlsson J. Cough induced by stimulation of capsaicin-sensitive sensory neurons in conscious guinea-pigs. Acta Physiol Scand 1986; 128:319–320.

19. Collier JG, Fuller RW. Capsaicin inhalation in man and the effects of sodium cromoglycate. Br J Pharmacol 1984; 81:113–117.

20. Fuller RW, Dixon CMS, Cuss FMC, Barnes PJ. Bradykinin-induced bronchoconstriction in man: mode of action. Am Rev Respir Dis 1987; 135:176–180.

21. Simonsson BG, Skoogh BE, Berg NP, Andersson BR, Svedmyr N. In vivo and in vitro effect of bradykinin on bronchial motor tone in normal subjects and patients with airway obstruction. Respiration 1973; 30:378–388.

22. Coleridge JCG, Coleridge HM. Afferent vagal C fibre innervation of the lungs and airways and its functional significance. Rev Physiol Biochem Pharmacol 1984; 99:1–110.

23. Coleridge HM, Coleridge JCG, Roberts AM. Rapid shallow breathing evoked by selective stimulation of airway C fibres in dogs. J Physiol (Lond) 1983; 340:415–433.

24. Forsberg K, Karlsson J, Theodorosson E, Lundberg JM, Persson CGA. Cough and bronchoconstriction mediated by capsaicin-sensitive sensory neurons in guinea-pigs. Pulm Pharmacol 1988; 1:33–39.

25. Karlsson JA. A role for capsaicin positive, tachykinin containing nerves in chronic coughing and sneezing, but not in asthma: a hypothesis. Thorax 1993; 48:396–400.

26. Jackson DM, Norris AA, Eady RP. Nedocromil sodium and sensory nerves in the dog lung. Pulm Pharmacol 1989; 2:179–184.

27. Tatar M, Webber SE, Widdicombe JG. Lung C-fibre receptor activation and defensive reflexes in anaesthetised cats. J Physiol (Lond) 1988; 402:411–420.

28. Fox AJ, Barnes PJ, Urban L, Dray A. An in vitro study of the properties of single vagal afferents innervating guinea-pig airways. J Physiol (Lond) 1993; 469:21–35.

29. Lalloo UG, Fox AJ, Belvisi MG, Chung KF, Barnes PJ. Inhibition by capsazepine of cough induced by capsaicin and citric acid, but not by hypertonic saline in awake guinea-pigs. J Appl Physiol 1995; 79:1082–1087.

30. Fox AJ, Barnes PJ, Dray A. Stimulation of guinea-pig tracheal afferent fibres by non-osmotic and low-chloride solutions and the effect of frusemide. J Physiol (Lond) 1995; 482:179–187.

31. Fuller RW, Dixon CMS, Barnes PJ. The bronchoconstrictor response to inhaled capsaicin in humans. J Appl Physiol 1985; 85:1080–1084.

32. Winning AJ, Hamilton RD, Shea SA, Guz A. Respiratory and cardiovascular effects of central and peripheral intravenous injections of capsaicin in man: evidence for pulmonary chemosensitivity. Clin Sci 1986; 71:519–526.

33. Hathaway TJ, Higenbottam TW, Morrison JF, Clelland CA, Wallwork J. Effects of inhaled capsaicin in heart-lung transplant patients and asthmatic sub. Amer Rev Respir Dis 1993; 148:1233–1237.

34. Midgren B, Hansson L, Karlsson JA, Simonsson BG, Persson CG. Capsaicin-induced cough in humans. Am Rev Respir Dis 1992; 146:347–351.

35. Eschenbacher WL, Boushey HA, Sheppard D. Alteration in osmolariaty of inhaled aerosols cause bronchoconstriction and coug absence of a permeant anion causes cough alone. Am Rev Respir Dis 1984; 129:211–215.

36. Godden DJ, Borland C, Lowry R, Higenbottam TW. Chemical specificity of coughing in man. Clin Sci 1986; 70:301–306.

37. Anderson JW, Sant'Ambrogio FB, Mathew OP, Sant'Ambrogio G. Water-responsive laryngeal receptors in the dog are not specialized endings. Respir Physiol 1990; 79:33–44.

38. Lee BP, Sant'Ambrogio G, Sant'Ambrogio FB. Afferent innervation and receptors of the canine extrathoracic trachea. Respir Physiol 1992; 90:55–65.

39. Ventresca P, Nichol GM, Barnes PJ, Chung KF. Inhaled furosemide inhibits cough induced by low chloride content solutions and not by capsaicin. Am Rev Respir Dis 1990; 142:143–146.

40. Sant'Ambrogio FB, Sant'Ambrogio G, Anderson JW. Effect of frusemide on the response of laryngeal receptors to low-chloride solutions. Eur Respir J 1993; 6: 1151–1155.

41. Choudry NB, Fuller RW. Sensitivity of the cough reflex in patients with chronic cough. Eur Respir J 1992; 5:295–300.

42. O'Connell F, Thomas VE, Pride NB, Fuller RW. Capsaicin cough sensitivity decreases with successful treatment of chronic cough. Am J Respir Crit Care Med 1994; 150:374–380.

43. Hsu J, Stone RA, Logan-Sinclair R, Worsdell M, Busst C, Chung KF. Coughing frequency in patients with persistent cough using a 24-hour ambulatory recorder. Eur Respir J 1994; 7:1246–1253.

44. Mitsuhashi M, Mochizuki H, Tokuyama K, Morikawa A, Kuroume T. Hyperresponsiveness of cough receptors in patients with bronchial asthma. Pediatrics 1985; 75:855–858.

45. Costello JF, Dunlop LS, Gardiner PJ. Characteristics of prostaglandin-induced cough. Br J Clin Pharm 1985; 20:355–359.

46. Kawakami Y, Uchiyama K, Irie T, Murao M. Evaluation of aerosols of prostaglandins E1 and E2 as bronchodilators. Eur J Clin Pharmacol 1973; 6:127–132.

47. Nichol GM, Nix A, Barnes PJ, Chung KF. Enhancement of capsaicin-induced cough by inhaled prostaglandin F2α: modulation by beta-adrenergic agonist and anticholinergic agent. Thorax 1990; 45:694–699.

48. Choudry NB, Fuller RW, Pride NB. Sensitivity of the human cough reflex: effect of inflammatory mediators prostaglandin E2, bradykinin, and histamine. Am Rev Respir Dis 1989; 140:137–141.

49. Stone R, Barnes PJ, Fuller RW. Contrasting effects of prostaglandins E2 and F2α on sensitivity of the human cough reflex. J Appl Physiol 1992; 73:649–653.
50. Kaufman MP, Coleridge HM, Coleridge JCG, Baker DG. Bradykinin stimulates afferent vagal C-fibers in intrapulmonary airways of dogs. J Appl Physiol 1980; 48: 511–517.
51. Lalloo UG, Fox AJ, Bernareggi M, Belvisi MG, Chung KF, Barnes PJ. Bradykinin and captopril-induced cough in guinea-pigs. Nature Medicine 1996; 2:814–817.
52. Advenier C, Giraud V, Naline E, Villain P, Emonds-Alt X. Antitussive effect of SR 48968, a non-peptide tachykinin NK2 receptor antagonist. Eur J Pharmacol 1992; 250:169–173.
53. Ichinose M, Nakajima N, Takahashi T, Yamauchi H, Inoue H, Takishima T. Protection against bradykinin-induced bronchoconstriction in asthmatic patients by neurokinin receptor antagonist. Lancet 1992; 340:1248–1251.
54. Saria A, Martling C, Yan Z, Theodorsson-Norheim E, Gamse R, Lundberg JM. Release of multiple tachykinins from capsaicin-sensitive sensory nerves in the lung by bradykinin, histamine, dimethylphenyl piperazinium, and vagal nerve stimulation. Am Rev Respir Dis 1988; 137:1330–1335.
55. Joos G, Pauwels R, van der Straeten M. The effect of inhaled substance P and neurokinin A on the airways of normal and asthmatic subjects. Thorax 1987; 42: 779–783.
56. Katsumata U, Sekizawa K, Inoue H, Sasaki H, Takishima T. Inhibitory actions of procaterol, a beta-2 stimulant, on substance P–induced cough in normal subjects during upper respiratory tract infection. Tohoku J Exp Med 1989; 158:105–106.
57. Yoshihawa S, Kanno N, Ando T, Fukuda N, Abe T, Ishimura T, Yamaihara N. Involvement of substance P in the paroxysmal cough of pertussis. Regul Peptides 1993; 46:238–240.
58. Chausow AM, Banner AS. Comparison of the tussive effects of histamine and methacholine in humans. J Appl Physiol 1983; 55:541–546.
59. Mills JE, Sellick H, Widdicombe JG. Activity of lung irritant receptors in pulmonary microembolism, anaphylaxis and drug-induced bronchoconstriction. J Physiol (Lond) 1969; 203:337–357.
60. Vidruk EH, Hahn HL, Nadel JA, Sampson SR. Mechanisms by which histamine stimulates rapidly adapting receptors in dog lungs. J Appl Physiol 1977; 43:397–402.
61. Dixon M, Jackson DM, Richards IM. The effects of histamine, acetylcholine and 5-hydroxytryptamine on lung mechanics and irritant receptors in the dog. J Physiol (Lond) 1979; 287:393–403.
62. Sheppard D, Rizk NN, Boushey HA, Bethel RA. Mechanism of cough and bronchoconstriction induced by distilled water aerosol. Amer Rev Respir Dis 1983; 127:691–694.
63. Carrao WM, Braman SS, Irwin RS. Chronic cough as the sole presenting manifestation of bronchial asthma. N Engl J Med 1979; 300:633–637.
64. Burrows B, Lebowitz MD, Barbee RA, Cline MG. Findings before diagnoses of asthma among the elderly in a longitudinal study of a general population sample. J Allergy Clin Immunol 1991; 88:870–877.
65. McFadden ER. Exertional dyspnea and cough as preludes to acute attacks of bronchial asthma. N Engl J Med 1975; 292:555–559.

66. Thomson AH, Pratt C, Simpson H. Nocturnal cough in asthma. Arch Dis Child 1987; 62:1001–1004.
67. Gibson PG, Dolovich J, Denburgh J, Ramsdale EH, Hargreave FE. Chronic cough: eosinophilic bronchitis without asthma. Lancet 1989; 1:1246–1247.
68. Kamikawa Y, Shimo Y. Inhibitory effects of catecholamines on cholinergically and non-cholinergically mediated contractions of guinea-pig isolated bronchial muscle. J Pharm Pharmacol 1990; 42:131–134.
69. Verleden GM, Belvisi MG, Rabe KF, Miura M, Barnes PJ. Beta 2-adrenoceptor agonists inhibit NANC neural bronchoconstrictor responses in vitro. J Appl Physiol 1993; 74:1195–1199.
70. Hui JP, Vantresca P, Brown AC, Barnes PJ, Chung KF. Modulation of neurally-mediated airway microvascular leakage in guinea-pig airways by β2-adrenoceptor agonists. Agents Actions 1992; 3629–3633.
71. Clay TP, Thompson MA. Irritant induced cough as a model of intrapulmonary airway reactivity. Lung 1985; 163:183–191.
72. Pounsford JC, Birch MJ, Saunders KB. Effect of bronchodilators on the cough response to inhaled citric acid in normal and asthmatic subjects. Thorax 1985; 40:662–667.
73. Lowry R, Higenbottam T, Johnson T, Godden D. Inhibition of artificially induced cough in man by bronchodilators. Br J Clin Pharmacol 1987; 24:503–510.
74. Duffey ME, Hainau B, Ho S, Bentzel CJ. Regulation of epithelial tight junction permeability by cyclic AMP. Nature 1981; 294:451–453.
75. Phipps RJ, Williams IP, Richardson PS, Pell J, Pack RJ, Wright N. Sympathomimetic drugs stimulate the output of secretory glycoproteins from human bronchi in vitro. Clin Sci 1982; 63:23–28.
76. Davis B, Marin MG, Yee JW, Nadel JA. Effect of terbutaline on movement of Cl– and Na+ across the trachea of the dog in vitro. Am Rev Respir Dis 1979; 120:547–552.
77. Irwin RS, Carrao WM, Pratter MR. Chronic persistent cough in the adult: the spectrum and frequency of causes and successful outcome of specific therapy. Am Rev Respir Dis 1981; 123:413–417.
78. Ellul-Micallef R. Effect of terbutaline sulphate in chronic "allergic" cough. Br Med J 1983; 287:940–943.
79. Vesco D, Kleisbauer J, Orehek J. Attenuation of bronchifiberscopy-induced cough by an inhaled beta2-adrenergic ag fenoterol. Am Rev Respir Dis 1988; 138:805–806.
80. Fujimura M, Kamio Y, Hasimoto T, Matsuda T. Cough receptor sensitivity and bronchal responsiveness in patients with only chronic non-productive cough: in view of effect of bronchodilator therapy. J Asthma 1994; 31:463–472.
81. Fujimura M, Sakamoto S, Matsuda T. Bronchodilator-resistive cough in atopic patients: bronchial reversibility and hyperresponsiveness. Intern Med 1992; 31:447–452.
82. Wanner A. Clinical aspects of mucociliary transport (review). Am Rev Respir Dis 1977; 116:73–125.
83. Pavia D. Lung mucociliary clearance. In: Clarke SW, Pavia D, eds. Aerosols and the Lung: Clinical and Experimental Aspects. London: Butterworth, 1984:127–155.

84. Yeates DB, Aspin N, Levison H, Jones MT, Bryan AC. Mucociliary tracheal transport rates in man. J Appl Physiol 1975;. 39:487–495.

85. Yeates DB, Aspin N. A mathematical description of the airways of the human lungs. Respir Physiol 1978; 32:91–104.

86. Eliezer N, Sade J, Silberberg A, Nevo AC. The role of mucus in transport by cilia. Am Rev Respir Dis 1970; 102:48–52.

87. King M, Gilboa A, Meyer FA, Silberberg A. On the transport of mucus and its rheologic simulants in ciliated systems. Am Rev Respir Dis 1974; 110:740–745.

88. Friedman M, Stott FD, Poole DO, Dougherty R, Chapman GA, Watson H, Sackner MA. A new roentgenographic method for estimating mucous velocity in airways. Am Rev Respir Dis 1977; 115:67–72.

89. Yeates DB, Pitt BR, Spektor DM, Karron GA, Albert RE. Coordination of mucociliary transport in human trachea and intrapulmonary airways. J Appl Physiol Respir Environ Exercise Physiol 1981; 51:1057–1064.

90. Pavia D, Sutton PP, Agnew JE, Lopez-Vidriero MT, Newman SP, Clarke SW. Measurement of bronchial mucociliary clearance (review). Eur J Respir Dis 1983; 127(suppl):41–56.

91. Dunnill MS. The pathology of asthma with special reference to changes in the bronchial mucosa. J Clin Pathol 1960; 13:27–33.

92. Messina MS, O'Riordan TG, Smaldone GC. Changes in mucociliary clearance during acute exacerbations of asthma (see comments). Am Rev Respir Dis 1991; 143:993–997.

93. Santa Cruz R, Landa J, Hirsch J, Sackner MA. Tracheal mucous velocity in normal man and patients with obstructive lung disease: effects of terbutaline. Am Rev Respir Dis 1974; 109:458–463.

94. Mezey RJ, Cohn MA, Fernandez RJ, Januszkiewicz AJ, Wanner A. Mucociliary transport in allergic patients with antigen-induced bronchospasm. Am Rev Respir Dis 1978; 118:677–684.

95. Bateman JR, Pavia D, Sheahan NF, Agnew JE, Clarke SW. Impaired tracheobronchial clearance in patients with mild stable asthma. Thorax 1983; 38:463–467.

96. Pavia D, Bateman JR, Sheahan NF, Agnew JE, Clarke SW. Tracheobronchial mucociliary clearance in asthma: impairment during remission. Thorax 1985; 40: 171–175.

97. Agnew JE, Bateman JR, Pavia D, Clarke SW. Peripheral airways mucus clearance in stable asthma is improved by oral corticosteroid therapy. Bull Eur Physiopathol Respir 1984; 20:295–301.

98. Isawa T, Teshima T, Hirano T, Ebina A, Anazawa Y, Konno K. Effect of bronchodilation on the deposition and clearance of radioaerosol in bronchial asthma in remission. J Nucl Med 1987; 28:1901–1906.

99. Mossberg B, Strandberg K, Philipson K, Camner P. Tracheobronchial clearance in bronchial asthma: response to beta-adrenoceptor stimulation. Scand J Respir Dis 1976; 57:119–128.

100. Pavia D, Agnew JE, Sutton PP, Lopez-Vidriero MT, Clay MM, Killip M, Clarke SW. Effect of terbutaline administered from metered dose inhaler (2 mg) and subcutaneously (0.25 mg) on tracheobronchial clearance in mild asthma. Br J Dis Chest 1987; 81:361–370.

101. Foster WM, Langenback EG, Bergofsky EH. Lung mucociliary function in man: interdependence of bronchial and tracheal mucus transport velocities with lung clearance in bronchial asthma and healthy subjects. Ann Occup Hyg 1982; 26: 227–244.
102. O'Riordan TG, Zwang J, Smaldone GC. Mucociliary clearance in adult asthma. Am Rev Respir Dis 1992; 146:598–603.
103. Wanner A, Zarzecki S, Hirsch J, Epstein S. Tracheal mucous transport in experimental canine asthma. J Appl Physiol 1975; 39:950–957.
104. Russi EW, Abraham WM, Chapman GA, Stevenson JS, Codias E, Wanner A. Effects of leukotriene D4 on mucociliary and respiratory function in allergic and nonallergic sheep. J Appl Physiol 1985; 59:1416–1422.
105. Seybold ZV, Mariassy AT, Stroh D, Kim CS, Gazeroglu H, Wanner A. Mucociliary interaction in vitro: effects of physiological and inflammatory stimuli. J Appl Physiol 1990; 68:1421–1426.
106. Wanner A, Sielczak M, Mella JF, Abraham WM. Ciliary responsiveness in allergic and nonallergic airways. J Appl Physiol 1986; 60:1967–1971.
107. Yukawa T, Read RC, Kroegel C, Rutman A, Chung KF, Wilson R, Cole PJ, Barnes PJ. The effects of activated eosinophils and neutrophils on guinea pig airway epithelium in vitro. Am Rev Respir Cell Mol Biol 1990; 2:341–354.
108. Dulfano MJ, Luk CK. Sputum and ciliary inhibition in asthma. Thorax 1982; 37: 646–651.
109. Guirgis HA, Townley RG. Biochemical study on sputum in asthma and emphysema. J Allergy Clin Immunol 1973; 5186–190.
110. Ryley HC, Brogan TD. Variation in the composition of sputum in chronic chest diseases. Br J Exp Pathol 1968; 49:625–633.
111. Salvato G. Some histological changes in chronic bronchitis and asthma. Thorax 1968; 23:168–172.
112. Charman J, Reid L. Sputum viscosity in chronic bronchitis, bronchiectasis, asthma and cystic fibrosis. Biorheology 1972; 9;185–199.
113. Marom Z, Shelhamer JH, Kaliner M. Effects of arachidonic acid, monohydroxyeicosatetraenoic acid and prostaglandins on the release of mucous glycoproteins from human airways in vitro. J Clin Invest 1981; 67:1695–1702.
114. Marom Z, Shelhamer JH, Bach MK, Morton DR, Kaliner M. Slow-reacting substances, leukotrienes C4 and D4, increase the release of mucus from human airways in vitro. Am Rev Respir Dis 1982; 126:449–451.
115. Shelhamer JH, Marom Z, Kaliner M. Immunologic and neuropharmacologic stimulation of mucous glycoprotein release from human airways in vitro. J Clin Invest 1980; 66:1400–1408.
116. Chung KF, Rogers DF, Barnes PJ, Evans TW. The role of increased microvascular permeability and plasma exudation in asthma. Eur Respir J 1990; 3:329–337.
117. Williams IP, Rich B, Richardson PS. Action of serum on the output of secretory glycoproteins from human bronchi in vitro. Thorax 1983; 38:682–685.
118. Marriott C, Beeson MF, Brown DT. Biopolymer-induced changes in mucus viscoelasticity. Adv Exp Med Biol 1982; 144:89–92.
119. List SJ, Findlay BP, Forstner GG, Forstner JF. Enhancement of the viscosity of mucin by serum albumin. Biochem J 1978; 175:565–571.

120. Phipps RJ, Denas SM, Wanner A. Antigen stimulates glycoprotein secretion and alters ion fluxes in sheep trachea. J Appl Physiol Respir Environ Exercise Physiol 1983; 55:1593–1602.
121. Davis PB, Silski CL, Kercsmar CM, Infeld M. Beta-adrenergic receptors on human tracheal epithelial cells in primary culture. Am J Physiol 1990; 258:C71–76.
122. Carstairs JR, Nimmo AJ, Barnes PJ. Autoradiographic visualisation of beta-adrenoceptor subtype in human lung. Am Rev Respir Dis 1985; 133:541–547.
123. Iravani J, Melville GN. Mucociliary function of the respiratory tract as influenced by drugs. Respiration 1974; 31:350–357.
124. Van As A. The role of selective beta2-adrenoceptor stimulants in the control of ciliary activity. Respiration 1974; 31:146–151.
125. Hesse H, Kasparek R, Mizera W, Unterholzner C, Konietzko N. Influence of reproterol on ciliary beat frequency of human bronchial epithelium in vitro. Arzneimittelforschung 1981; 31:716–718.
126. Sanderson MJ, Lansley AB, Dirksen ER. Regulation of ciliary beat frequency in respiratory tract cells. Chest 1992; 101(suppl 3):69S–71S.
127. Verdugo P, Johnson NT, Tam PY. beta-Adrenergic stimulation of respiratory ciliary activity. J Appl Physiol Respir Environ Exercise Physiol 1980; 48:868–871.
128. Wong LB, Miller IF, Yeates DB. Stimulation of ciliary beat frequency by autonomic agonists: in vivo. J Appl Physiol 1988; 65:971–981.
129. Devalia JL, Sapsford RJ, Rusznak C, Toumbis MJ, Davies RJ. The effects of salmeterol and salbutamol on ciliary beat frequency of cultured human bronchial epithelial cells, in vitro. Pulm Pharmacol 1992; 5:257–263.
130. Di Benedetto G, Manara-Shediac FS, Mehta A. Effect of cyclic AMP on ciliary activity of human respiratory epithelium. Eur Respir J 1991; 4:789–795.
131. Tamaoki J, Kondo M, Takizawa T. Effect of cAMP on ciliary function in rabbit tracheal epithelial cells. J Appl Physiol 1989; 66:1035–1039.
132. Tamaoki J, Kondo M, Takizawa T. Adenosine-mediated cyclic AMP-dependent inhibition of ciliary activity in rabbit tracheal epithelium. Am Rev Respir Dis 1989; 139:441–445.
133. Lansley AB, Sanderson MJ, Dirksen ER. Control of the beat cycle of respiratory tract cilia by Ca^{2+} and cAMP. Am J Physiol 1992; 263:L232–L342.
134. Fick RB Jr. Pathogenesis of the pseudomonas lung lesion in cystic fibrosis (review). Chest 1989; 96:158–164.
135. Kanthakumar K, Cundell DR, Johnson M, Wills PJ, Taylor GW, Cole PJ, Wilson R. Effect of salmeterol on human nasal epithelial cell ciliary beating: inhibition of the ciliotoxin, pyocyanin. Br J Pharmacol 1994; 112:493–498.
136. Kanthakumar K, Taylor G, Tsang KW, Cundell DR, Rutman A, Smith S, Jeffery PK, Cole PJ, Wilson R. Mechanisms of action of Pseudomonas aeruginosa pyocyanin on human ciliary beat in vitro. Infect Immun 1993; 61:2848–2853.
137. Welsh MJ, Liedtke CM. Chloride and potassium channels in cystic fibrosis airway epithelia. Nature 1986; 322:467–470.
138. Boucher RC, Stutts MJ, Knowles MR, Cantley L, Gatzy JT. Na^+ transport in cystic fibrosis respiratory epithelia. Abnormal basal rate and response to adenylate cyclase activation. J Clin Invest 1986; 78:1245–1252.

139. Al-Bazzaz F, Yadava VP, Westenfelder C. Modification of Na and Cl transport in canine tracheal mucosa by prostaglandins. Am J Physiol 1981; 240:F101–F105.
140. Nathanson I, Widdicombe JH, Barnes PJ. Effect of vasoactive intestinal peptide on ion transport across dog tracheal epithelium. J Appl Physiol 1983; 55:1844–1848.
141. Leikauf GD, Ueki IF, Widdicombe JH, Nadel JA. Alteration of chloride secretion across canine tracheal epithelium by lipoxygenase products of arachidonic acid. Am J Physiol 1986; 250:F47–F53.
142. Jacoby DB, Ueki IF, Widdicombe JH, Loegering DA, Gleich GJ, Nadel JA. Effect of human eosinophil major basic protein on ion transport in dog tracheal epithelium. Am Rev Respir Dis 1988; 137:13–16.
143. Leikauf GD, Ueki IF, Nadel JA, Widdicombe JH. Bradykinin stimulates Cl secretion and prostaglandin E2 release by canine tracheal epithelium. Am J Physiol 1985; 248:F48–F55.
144. Smith PL, Welsh MJ, Stoff JS, Frizzell RA. Chloride secretion by canine tracheal epithelium: I. Role of intracellular c AMP levels. J Memb Biol 1982; 70:217–226.
145. Al-Bazzaz FJ. Role of cyclic AMP in regulation of chloride secretion by canine tracheal mucosa. Am Rev Respir Dis 1981; 123:295–298.
146. Leikauf GD, Ueki IF, Nadel JA. Autonomic regulation of viscoelasticity of cat tracheal gland secretions. J Appl Physiol Respir Environ Exercise Physiol 1984; 56:426–430.
147. Ueki I, German VF, Nadel JA. Micropipette measurement of airway submucosal gland secretion. Autonomic effects. Am Rev Respir Dis 1980; 121:351–357.
148. Sturgess J, Reid L. An organ culture study of the effect of drugs on the secretory activity of the human bronchial submucosal gland. Clin Sci 1972; 43:533–543.
149. Boat TF, Kleinerman JI. Human respiratory tract secretions. 2. Effect of cholinergic and adrenergic agents on in vitro release of protein and mucous glycoprotein. Chest 1975; 67(suppl 2):32S–34S.
150. Tokuyama K, Lötvall JO, Löfdahl C, Barnes PJ, Chung KF. Inhaled formoterol inhibits histamine-induced airflow obstruction and airway microvascular leakage. Eur J Pharmacol 1991; 193:35–39.
151. Sakamoto T, Barnes PJ, Chung KF. Effect of β2-adrenoceptor agaonists against platelet-activating factor-induced airway microvascular leakage and bronchoconstriction in the guinea-pig. Agents Actions 1993; 40:50–56.
152. Persson CGA, Ekman M, Erjefalt I. Vascular anti-permeability effect of β-receptor agonists and theophylline in the lung. Acta Pharmacol Toxicol 1979; 44:216–220.
153. Erjefalt I, Persson CGA. Pharmacologic control of plasma exudation into tracheobronchial airways. Am Rev Respir Dis 1991; 143:1008–1014.
154. Baluk P, McDonald DM. The beta 2-adrenergic receptor agonist formoterol reduces microvascular leakage by inhibiting endothelial gap formation. Am J Physiol 1994; 266:L461–L468.
155. Roca J, Félez MA, Chung KF, Barberà JA, Rotger M, Santos C, Rodriguez-Roisin R. Salbutamol inhibits pulmonary effects of platelet activating factor in man. Am J Respir Cell Mol Biol 1995; 151:1740–1744.

156. Foster WM, Bergofsky EH, Bohning DE, Lippmann M, Albert RE. Effect of adrenergic agents and their mode of action on mucociliary clearance in man. J Appl Physiol 1976; 41:146–152.
157. Konietzko N, Klopfer M, Adam WE, Matthys H. [The influence of beta-adrenergic stimulation on the mucociliary system of the human lung (author's transl)] [German]. Pneumonologie 1975; 152:203–208.
158. Camner P, Strandberg K, Philipson K. Increased mucociliary transport by adrenergic stimulation. Arch Environ Health 1976; 31:79–82.
159. Lafortuna CL, Fazio F. Acute effect of inhaled salbutamol on mucociliary clearance in health and chronic bronchitis. Respiration 1984; 45:111–123.
160. Mortensen J, Groth S, Lange P, Hermansen F. Effect of terbutaline on mucociliary clearance in asthmatic and healthy subjects after inhalation from a pressurised inhaler and a dry powder inhaler. Thorax 1991; 46:817–823.
161. Groth S, Mortensen J, Lange P, Munch EP, Sorensen PG, Rossing N. Imaging of the airways by bronchoscintigraphy for the study of mucociliary clearance. Thorax 1988; 43:360–365.
162. Mortensen J, Groth S, Lange P, Rossing N. Bronchoscintigraphic visualization of the acute effect of tobacco exposure and terbutaline on mucociliary clearance in smokers. Eur Respir J 1989; 2:721–726.
163. Perry RJ, Smaldone GC. Effect of bronchodilators on mucociliary clearance in normal adults. J Aerosol Med 1990; 31:87–96.
164. Hasani A, Agnew JE, Pavia D, Vora H, Clarke SW. Effect of oral bronchodilators on lung mucociliary clearance during sleep in patients with asthma. Thorax 1993; 48:287–289.
165. Isawa T, Teshima T, Hirano T, Anazawa Y, Miki M, Konno K, Motomiya M. Does a beta 2-stimulator really facilitate mucociliary transport in the human lungs in vivo? A study with procaterol. Am Rev Respir Dis 1990; 141:715–720.
166. Bateman JR, Pavia D, Sheahan NF, Newman SP, Clarke SW. Effects of terbutaline sulphate aerosol on bronchodilator response and lung mucociliary clearance in patients with mild stable asthma. Br J Clin Pharmacol 1983; 15:695–700.
167. Sadoul P, Puchelle E, Zahm JM, Jacquot J, Aug F, Polu JM. Effect of terbutaline on mucociliary transport and sputum properties in chronic bronchitis. Chest 1981; 80(suppl 6):885–889.
168. Weiss T, Dorow P, Felix R. Effects of a beta adrenergic drug and a secretolytic agent on regional mucociliary clearance in patients with COLD. Chest 1981; 80 (suppl 6):881–885.
169. Mossberg B, Strandberg K, Philipson K, Camner P. Tracheobronchial clearance and beta-adrenoceptor stimulation in patients with chronic bronchitis. Scand J Respir Dis 1976; 57:281–289.
170. Pavia D, Bateman JR, Sheahan NF, Clarke SW. Clearance of lung secretions in patients with chronic bronchitis: effect of terbutaline and ipratropium bromide aerosols. Eur J Respir Dis 1980; 61:245–253.
171. Mortensen J, Hansen A, Falk M, Nielsen IK, Groth S. Reduced effect of inhaled beta 2-adrenergic agonists on lung mucociliary clearance in patients with cystic fibrosis. Chest 1993; 103:805–811.

172. Kollberg H, Mossberg B, Afzelius BA, Philipson K, Camner P. Cystic fibrosis compared with the immotile-cilia syndrome. A study of mucociliary clearance, ciliary ultrastructure, clinical picture and ventilatory function. Scand J Respir Dis 1978; 59:297–306.

173. Boucher RC, Botton CU, Gatzy JT, Knowles MR, Yankaskas JR. Evidence for reduced Cl⁻ and increased Na⁺ permeability in cystic fibrosis human primary cell cultures. J Physiol (Lond) 1988; 405:77-103:77-103.

174. Sutton PP, Gemmell HG, Innes N, Davidson J, Smith FW, Legge JS, Friend JA. Use of nebulised saline and nebulised terbutaline as an adjunct to chest physiotherapy. Thorax 1988; 43:57–60.

Discussion

JAN-ANDERS KARLSSON

Bayer Yakuhin Ltd., Kyoto, Japan

A. Introduction

Cough, mucus hypersecretion, and airflow obstruction are well recognized airway defense reflexes that are also prominent symptoms in a wide range of lung diseases. Coughing as a result of viral or bacterial chest infections is often relatively trivial and self-limiting, whereas patients with chronic cough may prove a difficult problem for the primary care physician. The cough reflex is uniquely triggered by irritant agents or particulate matter exciting a defined population of sensory nerve endings in the tracheobronchial mucosa. Many of the other defense reactions can be mediated either reflexly via sensory nerves or by mediators acting directly on, for example, the smooth muscle, submucosal glands, or ciliated epithelial cell (1,2). Although being such an obvious symptom to both patient and physician, coughing carries little diagnostic value in itself, since it is present in many different airway diseases and, in addition, cough can be evoked also from extrapulmonary sites such as the tympanic membrane and the external auditory meatus. To the patient, coughing is often irritating, inconvenient, and unwanted as indicated by the substantial sales of over-the-counter (OTC)–labeled antitussive drugs.

　　Coughing can be suppressed either directly by antitussive agents acting at a cough center in the central nervous system or by agents reducing the effect of irritant mediators on the sensory nerve ending locally in the tracheobronchial tree. Local anesthetic agents which block conduction in afferent nerves also inhibit cough. β_2-Adrenoceptor agonists are widely used in the treatment of obstructive lung diseases, and it has been reported that these agents inhibit coughing in patients with asthma and upper respiratory tract infections. Consequently, they are also being prescribed to patients with cough who may not have airway obstruction, although there are little documented data to support this particular usage. In this discussion, the antitussive effect of β_2-agonists in asthma and other lung disorders is examined and possible mechanisms for this effect are considered.

B. Asthmatic Cough and β-Adrenoceptor Agonists

It is now well established that cough is an early and sometimes the only symptom of asthma (3,4). Coughing is often most prominent during nighttime, and the asthma diagnosis is supported by the presence of variable airflow limitation and bronchial hyperresponsiveness. Asthma is considered to be one of the most common causes of chronic cough in young children (5). Even though coughing can be prominent, asthmatics do not necessarily have a heightened cough reflex compared with normal subjects (6–9). The frequent use of β-agonists to reverse and prevent bronchial obstruction prompted the study of its possible antitussive effect in asthmatic patients. Ellul-Micallef (10) examined the effect of terbutaline in a double-blind, placebo-controlled study in subjects with "allergic" cough. He found that cough symptoms in all patients dminished in parallel with an improvement in lung function (measured as an increase in FEV_1), whereas during the placebo period, there were no changes in either symptoms or lung function. The effect of terbutaline on "spontaneous" cough was statistically significant. Other studies also refer to diminished symptoms (including cough) in asthmatic patients during β-agonist therapy (11,12), although some observations do not support this conclusion (13).

What is the mechanism behind the antitussive effect produced by β_2-agonists? The most obvious explanation would be a direct inhibitory effect on the cough reflex itself. However, this seems unlikely, since β_2-agonists do not inhibit cough induced by citric acid (6,14), capsaicin (15,16), or tartaric acid (17) in healthy subjects. Moreover, inhaled epinephrine (adrenaline) is without effect on capsaicin-induced cough in healthy subjects and does not potentiate the antitussive effect of an inhaled local anesthetic (18). One study reportedly found that when distilled water was used as the cough challenge, salbutamol produced a small but statistically significant reduction of the response (19). The reason for this is not known but could conceivably be due to water triggering a different set of afferent nerves in the respiratory mucosa than other cough-inducing agents.

Interestingly, in asthmatic subjects, salbutamol reduces coughing induced by citric acid (6), and one might therefore speculate that this effect is due to a direct relaxant effect of the bronchial smooth muscle. Although an attractive possibility, particularly in the light of Salem and Aviado's (20) hypothesis that both afferent neural activity and coughing is triggered by contraction of the local bronchial smooth muscle, available data indicate that the antitussive effect of β-agonists is unrelated to their bronchodilator effect (9,15). Supporting this view are studies showing that the sensitivity of the cough reflex is independent of airways tone, as investigated by the use of drugs increasing tone (methacholine) as well as decreasing it (β-agonists, anticholinergic agents [9, 17]).

β-Agonists possess a number of pharmacological properties which can contribute to the antitussive effect seen in asthmatic subjects. It is possible that either a stimulation of airway mucous secretion and ciliary beat frequency (see the part of this chapter by Chung) could have contributed to the antitussive effect. Alternatively, β-agonists are capable of modulating prostaglandin (PG) E_2 and $F_{2\alpha}$ production in the airway mucosa. Both PGE_2 and $PGF_{2\alpha}$ potentiate capsaicin-induced coughing (21,22). Nichol and colleagues (16) reported that the $PGF_{2\alpha}$-mediated enhancement of the capsaicin-induced cough reflex was inhibited by salbutamol, although it did not affect the cough reflex itself. It is tempting to speculate that the β_2-agonist act through the inhibition of the release of mediators from inflammatory cells like the mast cell, which selectively upregulate the cough reflex in chronic inflammatory lung diseases. Alternatively, a change in epithelial ion transport could perhaps alter membrane function and nerve sensitivity (7).

C. β-Agonists in Subjects with Respiratory Tract Infections

The increased awareness of cough as an early symptom of asthma has resulted in a widespread use of this class of drugs in patients with lung disorders with a possible obstructive component. The early use of β-agonists in patients with persistent coughing seems to be particularly prevalent in northern Europe and is somewhat of a puzzle, since there are no published data to support their use in respiratory tract infections. A Finnish study examined the effect of salbutamol on coadministration with dextromethorphan in subjects with cough due to acute respiratory tract infection (23). Interestingly, the combination was more effective as an inhibitor of nighttime cough than dextromethorphan alone or placebo. Unfortunately, the study did not include a group that received only salbutamol. The potentiation of the antitussive effect of dextromethorphan may be due to a facilitation of the mucociliary clearance apparatus.

In whooping cough, inhaled salbutamol has been reported to reduce the frequency and intensity of the whoop but not the cough (24), whereas oral salbutamol was found to reduce both symptoms (25).

It is well established that bronchial reactivity is increased during the common cold. Empey and coworkers (26) found enhanced bronchoconstrictor responses to histamine and citric acid in subjects with a cold, which was accompanied by a decreased cough threshold. Inhalation of isoprenaline reduced both bronchospasm and coughing, but the sensitivity did not return back to normal.

Thus, at present, there is no supportive evidence for the use of β_2-agonists for symptom control in individuals with bacterial or viral infections.

D. Chronic, Idiopathic Cough: Sensory Hyperresponsiveness

A significant proportion (about 30–35%) of patients with chronic cough referred to specialist lung clinics are diagnosed as having asthma; with chronic obstructive pulmonary disease, postnasal drip, respiratory tract infections, and gastroesophageal reflux being other common causes of cough (see Ref. 27). It is interesting to note, however, that in several recent studies, between 25 and 50% of such patients have idiopathic cough; that is, no specific cause can be identified with certainty (27,28).

Characteristically, subjects with idiopathic cough have a normal lung function and sensitivity to bronchoconstrictor agents but a very significant hyperresponsiveness to inhaled capsaicin. These subjects may have up to a 10-fold increased sensitivity to the tussive effect of capsaicin compared with age- and sex-matched healthy subjects (8,27,28). There is no evidence of an increased cellularity in bronchoalveolar lavage (27,29). However, preliminary data from bronchial biopsies obtained from these subjects indicate an increased number of inflammatory cells in the tracheobronchial mucosa which is accompanied by submucosal edema and fibrosis (27). Clearly, this airway inflammatory response is significantly different from that in asthma. Bronchi obtained from subjects with chronic cough have an increased amount of the neuropeptide calcitonin gene–related peptide (CGRP) in the mucosa relative to control biopsies (30). Tachykinin- and CGRP-containing afferent nerves are thought to constitute the afferent limb of the cough reflex, so these observations are consistent with an increased sensitivity of capsaicin-sensitive nerves in idiopathic cough. The term *sensory hyperresponsiveness* has been coined to describe this enhanced responsiveness of capsaicin-sensitive airway nerves, but it may also be applicable to other organs which can have a similarly heightened responsiveness in their afferent innervation (see Ref. 31).

Few studies of traditional antitussive drugs or antiasthma medications have been reported in this particular group of patients, but because β_2-agonists are generally used to examine the reversibility of bronchial tone and support a diagnosis of asthma, it can be presumed that bronchodilators and steroids have been tried without success (see Refs. 27 and 28). A recent study (32) observed that patients with chronic cough and bronchial hyperresponsiveness benefited from treatment with clenbuterol, whereas this β-agonist was without effect in subjects with chronic cough but having normal lung function. Although this was only an open, unblinded study, it still supports the view that β_2-agonists reduce coughing in asthma but not in patients with chronic, idiopathic cough.

E. Conclusions

β_2-Agonists are the most commonly used drugs in asthma therapy, with their popularity being due to the rapid onset of action and effective reversal of induced bronchospasm, providing good symptom control (see Chapters 8 and 12). In most patients with asthma, treatment with β_2-agonists also diminishes other symptoms of the disease such as coughing. Unfortunately, very few clinical investigations have examined this purported antitussive effect of β_2-agonists. In contrast to asthmatics, β_2-agonists do not suppress coughing in subjects with respiratory tract infections or chronic, idiopathic cough with sensory hyperresponsiveness.

β_2-Agonists do not have a direct antitussive effect; that is, they do not inhibit the irritant-induced cough reflex in healthy subjects. Furthermore, the sensitivity to the tussive effect of inhaled irritants is not altered by changes in bronchial tone, suggesting that the suppression of coughing is not secondary to a relaxation of airways tone. It therefore seems most likely that these drugs suppress coughing by reducing the release of mediators such as prostaglandins and bradykinin which trigger or facilitate the cough reflex in the asthmatic airway. It is also possible that an improvement in the mucociliary escalator or stimulation of ion and water transport across the epithelium may contribute to diminished coughing in the asthmatic (see the part of this chapter by Chung). Further studies are required to confirm the clinical efficacy and elucidate the mechanism behind the antitussive effect of β_2-agonists in asthma.

References

1. Karlsson J-A, Sant'Ambrogio G, Widdicombe J. Afferent neural pathways in cough and reflex bronchoconstriction. J Appl Physiol 1988; 65:1007–1023.
2. Widdicombe JG. Neurophysiology of the cough reflex. Eur J Respir Dis 1995; 8: 1193–1202.
3. Corrao WM, Braman SS, Irwin RS. Chronic cough as the sole presenting manifestation of bronchial asthma. N Engl J Med 1979; 300:633–637.
4. McFadden ER. Exertional dyspnea and cough as preludes to acute attacks of bronchial asthma. N Engl J Med 1975; 292:555–559.
5. Holinger LD. Chronic cough in infants and children. Laryngoscope 1986; 96:316–322.
6. Pounsford JC, Birch MJ, Saunders KB. Effect of bronchodilators on the cough response to inhaled citric acid in normal and asthmatic subjects. Thorax 1985; 40: 662–667.
7. Lowry R, Wood A, Johnson T, Higenbottam T. Antitussive properties of inhaled bronchodilators on induced cough. Chest 1988; 93:1186–1189.
8. Coudry NB, Fuller RW. Sensitivity of the cough reflex in patients with chronic cough. Eur Respir J 1992; 5:296–300.

9. Fujimura M, Sakamoto S, Kamio Y, Bando T, Kurashima K, Matsuda T. Effect of inhaled procaterol on cough receptor sensitivity to capsaicin in patients with asthma or chronic bronchitis and in normal subjects. Thorax 1993; 48:615–618.

10. Ellul-Micallef R. Effect of terbutaline sulphate in chronic "allergic" cough. Br Med J 1983; 287:940–943.

11. Irwin RS, Corrao WM, Pratter MR. Chronic persistent cough in the adult: the spectrum and frequency of causes and successful outcome of specific therapy. Am Rev Respir Dis 1981; 123:413–417.

12. Thomson AH, Pratt C, Simpson H. Nocturnal cough in asthma. Arch Dis Child 1987; 62:1001–1004.

13. Hsu J, Stone RA, Logan-Sinclair R, Worsdell M, Busst C, Chung KF. Coughing frequency in patients with persistent cough using a 24-hour ambulatory recorder. Eur Respir J 1994; 7:1246–1253.

14. Belcher N, Rees PJ. Effects of pholcodine and salbutamol on citric acid induced cough in normal subjects. Thorax 1986; 41:74–75.

15. Smith CA, Adamson DL, Coudry NB, Fuller RW. The effect of altering airway tone on the sensitivity of the cough reflex in normal volunteers. Eur Respir J 1991; 4:1076–1079.

16. Nichol GM, Nix A, Barnes PJ, Chung KF. Prostaglandin $F_{2\alpha}$ enhancement of capsaicin-induced cough in man: modulation by beta$_2$ adrenergic and anticholinergic drugs. Thorax 1990; 45:694–698.

17. Fujimura M, Sakamoto S, Kamio Y, Matsuda T. Effects of methacholine induced bronchoconstriction and procaterol induced bronchodilation on cough receptor sensitivity to inhaled capsaicin and tartaric acid. Thorax 1992; 47:441–445.

18. Hansson L, Midgren B, Karlsson J-A. Effects of inhaled lignocaine and adrenaline on capsaicin-induced cough in humans. Thorax 1994; 49:1166–1168.

19. Lowry R, Higenbottam T, Johnson T, Godden D. Inhibition of artificially induced cough in man by bronchodilators. Br J Clin Pharmacol 1987; 24:503–510.

20. Salem H, Avaido DM. Antitussive drugs with special reference to a new theory for the initiation of the cough reflex and the influence of bronchodilators. Am J Med Sci 1964; 247:586–600.

21. Coudry MB, Fuller RW, Pride NB. Sensitivity of the human cough reflex: effect of inflammatory mediators prostaglandin E_2, bradykinin, and histamine. Am Rev Respir Dis 1989; 140:137–141.

22. Stone R, Barnes PJ, Fuller RW. Contrasting effects of prostaglandins E_2 and $F_{2\alpha}$ on sensitivity of the human cough reflex. J Appl Physiol 1992; 73:649–653.

23. Tukiainen H, Karttunen P, Silvasti M, Flygare U, Korhonen R, Korhonen T, Majander R, Seuri M. The treatment of acute transient cough: a placebo-controlled comparison of dextromethorphan and dextromethorphan-beta$_2$-sympathomimetic combination. Eur J Respir Dis 1986; 69:95–99.

24. Peltola H, Michelsson K. Efficacy of salbutamol in treatment of infant pertussis demonstrated by sound spectrum analysis. Lancet 1982; 1:310–312.

25. Pavesio D, Ponzone A. Salbutamol and pertussis. Lancet 1977; 1:50–51.

26. Empey DW, Laitinen LA, Jacobs L, Gold WM, Nadel JA. Mechanisms of bronchial hyperreactivity in normal subjects after upper respiratory tract infection. Am Rev Respir Dis 1976; 113:131–139.

27. Hansson L. The Human Cough Reflex in Health and Disease. Ph.D. dissertation. University of Lund, Sweden, 1995.

28. O'Connell F, Thomas VE, Pride NB, Fuller RW. Capsaicin cough sensitivity decreases with successful treatment of chronic cough. Am J Respir Crit Care Med 1994; 150:374–380.

29. Boulet L-P, Milot J, Boutet M, St. Georges F, Laviolette M. Airway inflammation in non-asthmatic subjects with chronic cough. Am J Respir Crit Care Med 1994; 149:482–489.

30. O'Connell F, Springall DR, Moradoghli-Haftvani A, Krausz T, Price D, Fuller RW, Polak JM, Pride NB. Abnormal intraaepithelial airway nerves in persistent unexplained cough? Am J Respir Crit Care Med 1995; 152:2068–2075.

31. Karlsson J-A. Sensory hyperresponsiveness—a role for capsaicin-sensitive nerves in the airways. In: Pauwels R, Advenier C, O'Byrne PM, eds. Progress in Basic and Clinical Pharmacology. In press.

32. Fujimura M, Kamio Y, Hashimoto T, Matsuda T. Cough receptor sensitivity and bronchial responsiveness in patients with only chronic nonproductive cough: in view of effect of bronchodilator therapy. J Asthma 1994; 31:463–472.

10

Inhalation Technique and Inhalation Devices

MYRNA DOLOVICH

McMaster University
Hamilton, Ontario, Canada

I. Introduction

Aerosols for therapy are produced by three basic systems: pneumatic and ultrasonic nebulizers, and pressurized metered-dose inhalers (pMDIs), which can be used alone or with a variety of spacer devices and dry-powder inhalers (DPIs). A major difference among these types of delivery systems is the means of generating the aerosol. For the pMDI, the most widely used delivery system for therapeutic aerosols, and the nebulizer, the power sources are an integral part of the system. In the MDI, chlorofluorocarbon (CFC) propellants or the alternative, more environmentally friendly hydrofluoroalkane (HFA) propellants are used. In jet or pneumatic nebulizers, compressed air or oxygen supplied by a tank or compressor is used. The ultrasonic nebulizer is operated from a battery pack or wall electrical outlet. By contrast, DPIs are breath-actuated devices. Current designs rely on the inspiratory effort of the patient to provide sufficient energy for dispensing the powder from the inhaler. The inhalation technique practiced by the patient is necessarily different for these different types of aerosol-delivery systems. Usually passive, tidal breathing is recommended for nebulizers and inspiratory or vital capacity inhalations at flow rates of somewhat less than 1 L sec^{-1} for pressurized aerosols and powders, with the former requiring synchronization of actuation with inhalation.

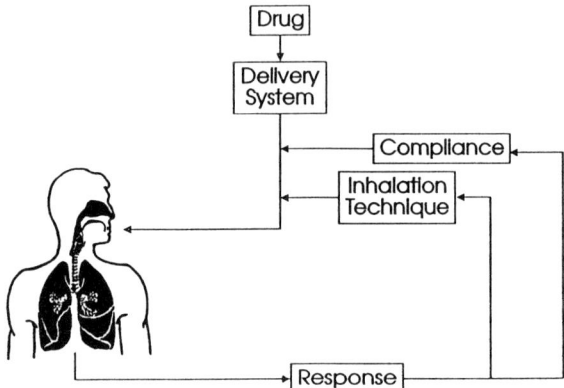

Figure 1   Diagram showing the interrelationship between the drug, drug delivery system, administration or inhalation of the aerosol, and the clinical outcome. Inhalation technique affects the dose of aerosolized drug reaching the lung and consequently the response. Improvements in response are likely to stimulate a favorable adaptation of technique. Compliance may depend on the patient's perception that the drug is providing relief.

The links between the drug formulation, the aerosol-delivery system, the administration of or inhalation technique used for the drug, and the clinical response effected are illustrated in Figure 1. In general, the benefit from the medication is proportional to the dose of aerosolized drug inhaled into the lungs. The dose inhaled, in turn, is directly related to the ability of the patient to execute the inhalation maneuvre properly.

In adults and in children, the efficiency for depositing aerosolized drug in the lung is less than 30% of the nominal or prescribed dose for all types of delivery systems even under favorable breathing conditions and near normal lung function. Figures ranging from 1 to 15%, representing deposition values for a variety of jet nebulizers, obtained with normal subjects and with patients have been published in the literature (1–4). The cost of newer medications, which use the lung as the entry port to the systemic circulation, are more expensive than drugs used to treat asthma. Therefore, it is important to maximize delivery either through improved designs of existing aerosol-generating systems or by ensuring that the inhalation technique for inhaling the medication from any of the systems is one that will promote maximum delivery of drug to the lower respiratory tract. Reduced clinical response due to poor delivery of aerosol or poor inhalation technique has been demonstrated in a number of studies. It is important to recognize that even a well-designed delivery system depends on the patient's ability to be able to use the system and inhale the medication to derive clinical benefit.

II. Physical Characteristics of Aerosols

Therapeutic aerosols are heterodisperse and consist of droplets or particles with a range of physical diameters and shapes. Deposition is mainly due to the combined action of inertial impaction, sedimentation due to gravity, and diffusion, all of which are predominantly dependent on the size of the particle or droplet (d) (Table 1). The larger the particle, the more readily it will be influenced by gravity and removed from the airstream. Large particles ($>6 \mu m$) impact in the oropharyngeal area and upper airways, whereas particles $<6 \mu m$ deposit by sedimentation and diffusion on successively smaller airways as the size of the aerosol particles decreases (5,6). Impaction of inhaled particles in the mouth, throat, and onto central airways also increases with increasing inspiratory flow rate (Q) (5), whereas sedimentation is proportional to the time (t) spent within the airway (see Table 1). Delivery to more peripheral airway surfaces can be increased by inhaling the aerosol at a low flow rate, and, in general, deposition can be further augmented by following the inhalation with a prolonged breath hold to allow greater time for sedimentation and diffusion to occur (6). In addition, any reduction in airway caliber due to disease will alter the airflow pattern in the lung and affect the deposition of inhaled aerosol (6).

The site of deposition of an aerosol can be predicted from its particle size distribution and specifically from the median diameter of the mass distribution (MMD) of the aerosol (5–7). Instruments that classify aerosols and obtain this measurement in terms of aerodynamic diameter normalize for differences in density between drug formulations and particle shape. Most therapeutic aerosols contain droplets or particles within the size range of 1–10 μm mass median aerodynamic diameter (MMAD). These different sized particles will deposit in the lung with varying degrees of efficiency when inhaled at a particular flow rate.

Table 1 Deposition Mechanisms: Factors Affecting Delivery in the Lung

Parameter	Probability of deposition
Sedimentation	$\propto d^2_{ae}t$
Impaction	$\propto d^2_{ae}Q$
Diffusional	$\propto (t/d_{te})^{1/2}$
Electrostatic	$\propto \{(ne)^2/d\}^{1/3}$

Estimates of the lung deposition fractions for stable, nonhygroscopic particles of varying aerodynamic size have been made by many investigators using a variety of geometrical models of the respiratory tract (1,6,8). For example, predictors from the size-deposition equations of Yu and colleagues, indicate that the deposition fraction for particles of 6 μm aerodynamic diameter (dae), inhaled through the mouth, will be 30% to the pulmonary region of the lung and approximately 20% to airways comprising the first 16 generations (8). Above 6 μm, more particles deposit on airway surfaces and less in the peripheral lung, whereas below 6 μm, the opposite occurs. For particles 3 μm in size, maximum deposition is obtained in the pulmonary region. This decreases to a minimum of approximately 15% for 0.5 μm particles. However, less than 5% of a submicronic 0.5 μm aerosol is deposited and retained on the airways. Thus, particular sizes of aerosol can be used to target specific regions in the lung.

Most predictions of deposition fractions are calculated for normal lung geometries and low inspiratory flow rates. In the presence of reduced airway caliber and/or high inspiratory flows, a shift in the deposition distribution within the lung toward more proximal airways will occur (9,10). In patients with airways disease, inhalation at lower flow rates may not entirely improve the delivery of the drug to the peripheral lung (11), but a low-flow technique will promote better bronchodilatation (12).

Deposition patterns also differ with age. Theoretical calculations show that in children under 5 years of age, total as well as airway deposition is increased compared with adults, but delivery to the peripheral lung is reduced (13), reflecting both the increased respiratory rate of young children and the reduction in the total number of alveoli in the immature lung.

III. Components of the Inhalation Technique

Delivery of drugs to the lower respiratory tract is dependent on the pattern of breathing and primarily on the inspiratory flow rate (IFR). The relative importance of variables associated with the inhalation maneuvre (Table 2) may differ for different drug-delivery systems; for example, breath-actuated systems may require higher inspiratory flow rates than inhalation from a spacer used with a pMDI, whereas a breath hold at end inspiration to increase deposition by gravitational settling may be relevant when inhaling pMDI aerosols but not for pMDIs used with spacers.

Assessment of the inhalation maneuvre can be made using scoring systems, inhalation of radiolabeled aerosols to measure drug delivery to the lung and the distribution of the inhaled drug within the lung, pharmacokinetic measurements, and spirometry. The ability of each of these methods to detect the effects of changes in the inhalation technique varies, but all have been used

Table 2 Important Components of the
Inhalation Technique

Position of aerosol device/mouth
Inspiratory volume
Inspiratory flow rate[a]
Synchronization[a]
Breath hold[a]

[a]Critical to outcome.

successfully in a number of studies, not only for comparing the effects of inhalation variables on drug delivery but also for comparing the in vivo performance of inhalation devices (14–17). It is advantageous to measure deposition and clinical effects in the same subjects, as this can provide a correlation between current methodologies and perhaps broaden the interpretation of the findings (18).

A. Position of Inhaler Device

The open-mouth versus the closed-mouth technique for inhaling pMDI aerosols is still somewhat controversial. In the closed-mouth technique, the pMDI is placed in the mouth, with the lips closed around the mouthpiece, whereas in the open-mouth method, the pMDI is held 4 cm outside the wide open mouth. This distance provides "space" in which the aerosol can decelerate and lose propellant, which in turn reduces the particle size of the aerosol, a function performed by pMDI spacer devices (19). Measurement of deposition and response have demonstrated benefit when the open-mouth technique was used. In normal persons, deposition increased twofold as the inhaler was moved 4 cm out of the mouth (Fig. 2) (20), whereas spirometry significantly improved in a group of 18 asthmatic patients using the open-mouth technique with fenoterol pMDI (21). More recently, Hindle and Chrystyn measured higher plasma salbutamol concentrations at 30 min with the open-mouth technique compared with the conventional closed-mouth pMDI technique (22). However, it may be difficult for patients to practice the open-mouth technique, as they must synchronize actuation with inhalation while maintaining proper orientation of the pMDI in front of the mouth.

Facemasks attached to nebulizers and to spacer devices also need to be positioned correctly against the face for effective treatment. A series of in vitro measurements of cromoglycate delivered from a jet nebulizer positioned up to 2 cm away from the "face" clearly showed an 80% decrease in the amount of drug deposited in the lung model (23). Thus, it is important to secure the

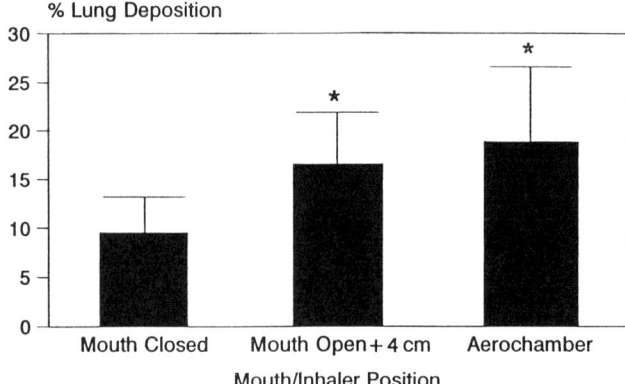

Figure 2 Bar graph illustrating the effect on delivery of a pMDI aerosol to the lung (mean ± sd) with a change in position of the pMDI in relation to the mouth. Lung deposition increased twofold ($P < .001$) when the pMDI was actuated 4 cm in front of the wide open mouth (MO+4 cm) compared with inhalation of a pMDI dose released into the closed mouth (MC). The benefit of using a valved holding chamber with the pMDI is evident from the comparable deposition values obtained with the Aerochamber® (Monaghan Medical, Syracuse, NY) and the MO+4 cm position. n = 10 normals; $^{99m}TcO_4^-$ solution placebo pMDI; V_i @ FRC, Q @ 45 L/min. % lung deposition corrected for tissue attenuation. *$P < .001$ compared with MC. (From Refs. 11 and 20.)

facemask against the face, particularly when treating children, to ensure sufficient inhalation of drug.

B. Inspiratory Volume

The lung volume from which inhalation begins when taking a pMDI aerosol does not appear to be as important a determinant of lung deposition as the inspiratory flow rate (20,24) provided the aerosol is given during inhalation. Actuating the pMDI at residual volume before commencement of inhalation or at total lung capacity when the breath was completed significantly reduced the amount deposited in the lung and the response to bronchodilator (20,24). With nebulizers, the lung dose obtained is related to the minute ventilation; as the inspiratory volume or number of breaths taken increases, the dose inhaled increases (25,26). Increasing the flow rate, however, will reduce the inhaled dose and distribute the aerosol preferentially to the central airways (1). A low inspiratory volume combined with a rapid inspiratory rate, such as in a crying infant, will markedly reduce delivery of aerosol to the lung (27). Improved dosing can be obtained when the child is sleeping, as tidal volumes will be increased and flow rates reduced (27).

Table 3 Errors Observed During Inhalation of a pMDI Aerosol

Timing
    actuation of pMDI before inhalation
    actuation of pMDI at the end of inhalation
    actuation of pMDI during exhalation
    actuation of pMDI ends inhalation
    multiple actuations of pMDI during inhalation
Inhalation
    rapid inhalation
    inhalation through nose
    no breath hold at end inhalation
Others
    failure to remove dust cap on pMDI mouthpiece
    failure to shake pMDI
    less than 30-sec wait between actuations of pMDI

C. Synchronization

Inhalation of pMDI aerosols requires the patient to coordinate actuation of the pMDI with inhalation of the aerosol. This is difficult for approximately 30% of adult patients and all children (28). The aerosol released from the pMDI has a forward velocity of approximately 15 m sec^{-1} (29). Within 0.1–0.2 sec, the cloud produced will have dissipated and will no longer be available for inhalation. Thus, the ability to synchronize the two actions is critical to inhaling the pMDI drug aerosol to derive clinical benefit from it. Of all the errors in pMDI technique observed during the inhalation maneuvre (Table 3), failure to synchronize properly the generation of the aerosol with the breathing maneuvre were the most prevalent (28,30,31).

D. Inspiratory Flow Rate

The effects on lung deposition and response of changes in inspiratory flow rate, inhaled lung volume, and length of breath hold following inhalation of a drug aerosol from a pressurized metered-dose inhaler have demonstrated the importance of these factors in providing drug to the lung (20,24,32). In general, high flow rates (>1 L sec^{-1}), a short or no breath hold at end inspiration and the inability to synchronize actuation of the pMDI with inhalation result in less drug delivered to the lung, deposition mainly on central or more proximal airways, and reduced response. Figure 3 illustrates data from two separate investigations of the effect of varying inspiratory flow rate on lung deposition

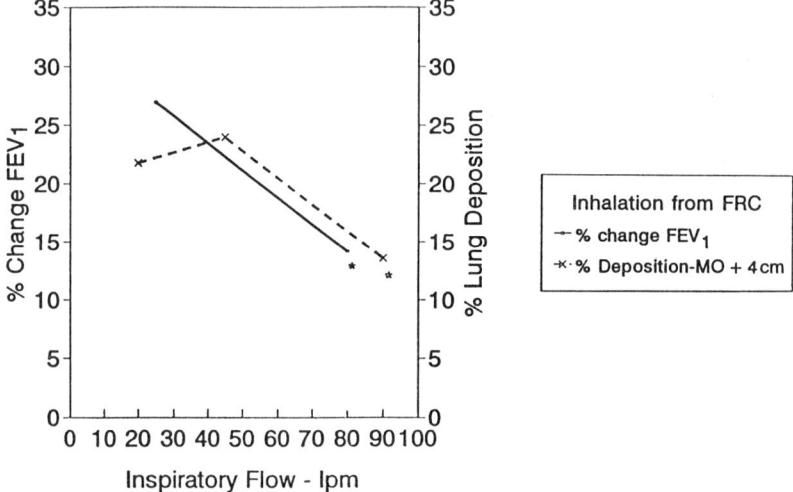

Figure 3 Graph showing the effect of inspiratory flow rate (IFR) on lung deposition and response. High IFRs (>60 L min^{-1}) resulted in poor delivery of aerosol
and a reduced FEV$_1$ response. IFRs of <60 L min^{-1} are recommended to derive
optimal benefit from a pMDI aerosol. *$P < .05$ compared with lower flows. Lung
deposition values corrected for tissue attenuation. (From Refs. 20 and 32.)

and response. Both these outcomes are significantly reduced at IFRs >1 L
sec^{-1}, confirming that the poorer clinical response resulted from less drug deposited in the lung.

To demonstrate the influence of the inhalation technique on response,
Lindgren and coworkers (33) devised a system to control the pattern of breathing and the time at which the dose from a pMDI was introduced into the
airstream. They demonstrated that poor inhalation technique resulted in suboptimal bronchodilator responses compared with responses when variables of
the technique were optimized. Changes in spirometry were measured in 23
asthmatic patients following inhalation of a pMDI bronchodilator aerosol in
which patients used their own routine for inhaling the aerosol. These were
compared with their responses following a repeat inhalation under controlled
conditions of inspiratory flow rate, the lung volume at which the drug was
given, and the length of breath hold. Patients who were observed to have a
poor, spontaneous inhalation technique had a significant improvement in flow
rates following the controlled inhalation, whereas those patients with good
technique showed similar bronchodilator responses for controlled and uncontrolled inhalations.

Varying the inhalation flow rate affects not only the response to pMDI bronchodilator aerosols but also to bronchodilator and bronchoconstrictor challenge aerosols inhaled from jet nebulizers (34–36). As mentioned earlier, increasing the IFR reduces the dose of aerosol inhaled and preferentially deposits aerosol on central airways. Responses may change with this altered deposition pattern (14,34–36), but there is still uncertainty as to the importance of the topographical distribution of aerosolized drug to the clinical response (18).

Other factors such as drug formulation and pMDI actuator design also influence drug-delivery efficiency. Highly concentrated pMDI formulations produce coarser aerosols, with reduced respirable fractions and lower lung deposition efficiencies (37–39). With these formulations, absolute doses delivered to the mouth may be higher, but these pMDIs might not be cost efficient (39). A redesigned pMDI actuator containing a baffle in the mouthpiece caused the forward velocity of the aerosol to be reduced. Compared with the pMDI used with the original standard actuator, the built-in baffle decreased the oropharyngeal deposition by approximately 50% while maintaining whole lung deposition and elicited a similar bronchodilator response (40). However, extrapulmonary effects were greater from the aerosol produced by the new actuator, suggesting changes to the aerosol that gave rise to an enhanced absorption from the lung.

IV. Methods to Improve Inhalation Technique

The optimal conditions for inhaling a pMDI aerosol are outlined in Table 4. Performing all the steps correctly results in greater deposition of drug in the lower respiratory tract (20) (Figure 2) and better therapeutic response to the medication (32). Poor technique consisting of some or all of the following—inhalation of aerosol with high IFRs, actuation of the pMDI at end inspiration, lack of coordination between actuation of the pMDI and inhalation, and no breath hold at end inspiration—needs to be corrected so that optimum benefit can be derived from the pMDI therapy.

Table 4 Optimal Inhalation Technique for pMDIs

Mouth–pMDI distance = 4 cm
Starting lung volume = FRC
Actuation of pMDI at start of inhalation
Inspiratory flow rate <60 L min^{-1}
Breath hold at end inspiration = 10 sec

FRC, functional residual capacity.

Table 5 Steps to Improve Inhalation Technique

Instruction
Spacers for pMDIs
Breath-actuated devices
valved spacers for pMDIs
AutoHaler for pMDIs
DPIs
dose-metered nebulizers
dosimeter
flow interrupter switch in air line

Improving performance of the inhalation technique can be achieved through reinforced instruction to patients and the use of spacer devices with pressurized metered-dose inhalers and breath-actuated devices (Table 5). The latter include valved spacers, the Autohaler (3M Co., St. Paul, MN) for MDIs and dry-powder inhalers. Breath-actuated, dose-metering nebulizers increase the overall delivery of aerosol to the lung by reducing wastage of drug during the expiratory phase of the breathing cycle (41). Some newer designs of nebulizers contain a series of one-way valves to eliminate entrainment of air through the nebulizer during exhalation (42). The production of aerosol is reduced during this part of the breathing cycle as output becomes a function of the jet airflow only.

A. Spacers

Spacers attached to pMDIs have been used successfully to improve the inhalation technique for pMDIs. Spacers with valves eliminate the need to coordinate actuation with inhalation. Open-tube spacers and reverse-flow designs, in which the drug is fired into the device away from the mouth, require the patient to synchronize inhalation with actuation (Fig. 4). Failure to coordinate reduces the drug available for deposition in the lung by approximately 50% (43,44) compared with that from a valved holding-chamber device (Fig. 5 and Table 6).

The particle size characteristics of aerosols released from spacers with the three types of design are similar. The aerosols from a number of pMDI drugs tested with a variety of spacers are finer, with an approximately 25% decrease in the mass median aerodynamic diameter (37,45). As well, the fine particle fraction ($\% < 5.8\,\mu m$) of the aerosol provided at the exit of the spacer is increased compared with the original aerosol, with the increase differing among the drug formulations (37,46,47). The distribution within the lung of

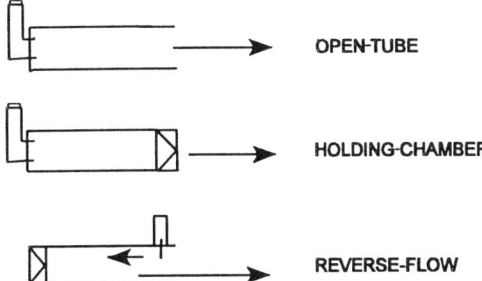

Figure 4 Schematic illustration of three current designs of spacer devices: (1) open tube; (2) holding chamber with a one-way valve placed between the chamber and the mouthpiece allowing the aerosol to be contained in the chamber after firing the pMDI; and (3) the reverse-flow design. This latter device contains a built-in actuator orifice for the pMDI. The one-way valve in the distal wall remains closed during actuation of the pMDI, opening to allow air entry on inhalation.

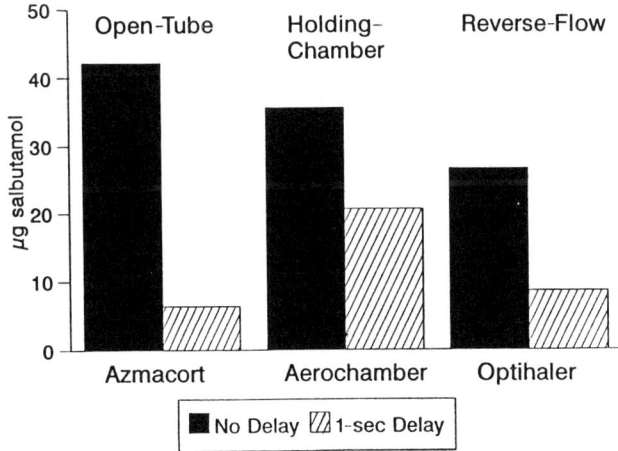

Figure 5 In vitro measurements of Ventulin pMDI doses available from three types of spacer devices. Differences in the dose of salbutamol available were measured between the different spacers. Differences were also present when "inhalation" occurred 1 sec after actuation of the pMDI into the spacers. Loss of drug occurred for all three designs with the delay with approximately 60% of the dose available from the holding chamber device compared with 15% from the open-tube device and 32% from the reverse-flow design when actuation was not synchronized with inhalation.

Table 6 Aerosol Delivery Through the Azma-
cort Tube Spacer:[1] Inhalation *After* Actuation of
$^{99m}TcO_4^-$– Triamcinolone Acetonide MDI (n = 8
normal, nonsmokers)

	Deposition (mean ± sd)
Lungs	5.2 ± 1.23%[a]
Oropharynx	2.3 ± 1.30%[a]
Stomach	0.7 ± 0.50%[a]
Tube spacer	49.9 ± 8.40%

[1]Rhone-Poulenc Rorer, Collegeville, Pennsylvania.
[a]Multiply by 1.90 to correct for tissue attenuation.
Source: From Ref. 43.

this finer aerosol is more uniform in the normal lung, with increased delivery to the peripheral airways (11). In the patient with airways obstruction, however, distribution of aerosol appears to be unchanged (11,48).

With the use of spacers, the aerosols provided are also slower moving and undergo less impaction of drug in the oropharyngeal area (11,43,48,49). The use of spacers results in similar or enhanced delivery of drug to the lung, which is a finding demonstrated through gamma scintigraphy (11,48,49) and pharmacokinetic studies (22). Other considerations concerning spacers used with pMDIs include the actuation of multiple doses into the spacer and the time interval between spraying into the spacer and taking a breath. If more than one drug dose is placed into the spacer or there is too long a delay prior to performing the inhalation, both the total dose and respirable dose of drug available for inhalation are reduced (43,44,50). The extent of these losses will also vary for different drugs and spacer designs (45,47). Attention to the physical properties of the delivery system along with the details for performing a good inhalation maneuvre are thus important in providing successful therapy.

There have been several studies investigating the effects on the bronchodilator response when varying the components of the inhalation maneuvre for pMDIs used with spacers compared with using the pMDI alone. Results have shown that a slow inhalation through an open-tube spacer gives an increased response compared with a fast inhalation (51). However, neither the lung volume at which the inhalation was initiated nor the completion of the inhalation with a breath hold appeared to have had an effect on the pulmonary function response in the asthmatic children tested. Studies have also shown that children can derive similar benefit from multiple breaths with tidal breathing through a valved spacer (aerosol holding chamber) fitted with a facemask, as with a full inspiratory breath (52). This inhalation method is easier to perform, particularly when the volume of the spacer device is greater than the inspiratory capacity of the child (39,53). It may also be a useful practice in the emergency room for adults, when breathing rates are increased owing to acute shortness of breath (54). The loss of aerosol to the walls of the spacer will still occur between tidal breaths, but it appears that sufficient drug is obtained to provide a bronchodilator effect (55).

B. Dry-Powder Inhalers

All dry-powder inhaler (DPIs) designs require the patient to dispense the powder from the device on initiation of the inspiratory breath. This necessitates inhalation at flows varying from 30 to 120 L min^{-1}, depending on the design of the DPI (16,17,56,57). The resistance of the DPI determines how easily it is for the patient to inhale from the device (58,59). If the "optimal" inspiratory flow rate for a device is not achieved, the drug dose obtained is reduced (60) with resulting decreased clinical efficacy (57,61–63). Using pulmonary function tests, side effects, and plasma concentrations of terbutaline as outcomes, Engel and coworkers demonstrated the influence of the variables of the inhalation technique for Turbuhaler (Astra Draco, Lund, Sweden) (64) in adult asthmatics. Their findings illustrate that although plasma levels of terbutaline were significantly lower following inhalation at 34 L min^{-1}, similar bronchodilator responses were obtained with IFRs from 34 to 88 L min^{-1}. There appeared to be no advantage to starting the inhalation from residual volume, whereas a poorer response to the drug resulted if the subject exhaled into the device prior to inhalation. An earlier study by Pedersen and colleagues showed that during an acute exacerbation of asthma, most 4–5 year olds tested had difficulty generated flow rates of 28 L min^{-1}, whereas in children with stable asthma, bronchodilatation did not diminish until the IFR through Turbuhaler decreased below this level (62). Other studies of Pedersen, also conducted in children, have shown similar effects of IFR on response for different DPI designs (57, 65).

Depending on the DPI design, inhalation at higher IFRs can deliver more drug to the lung (Table 7). Data obtained with Turbuhaler, in both asthmatic and normal subjects, have demonstrated that lung deposition, but not response, is increased with IFRs of 60 L min^{-1} compared with 30 L min^{-1} (61,66). Similar deposition findings were noted for the Pulvinal DPI (Chiesi Farmaceutici S.p.A, Parma, Italy) in healthy normals (67). The IFR that can be drawn through a DPI to obtain maximum deposition, and the response will vary with the DPI design. High-resistance DPIs decrease the ability to draw air through the device (58,59,68), which may be a problem for patients with acute asthma. However, they appear to deliver a greater percentage of drug to the lung than DPIs which offer low resistance to inhalation (37). A likely

Table 7 DPI Radiolabeled Deposition Studies: Effect of Inspiratory Flow Rate

Reference	DPI	Subjects (n = 10 each study)	Drug	IFR[1] (1 min⁻¹)	Lung deposition— % emitted dose (mean [sd])	P
61	Turbuhaler (Astra Draco, Lund, Sweden)	Asthmatics	Terbutaline sulfate	28 57	9.1 (4.74) 16.8 (8.22)	.01
73	Spinhaler (Fisons, Loughborough, UK)	Normals	Sodium cromoglycate	60 120	5.5 (1.6–9.7)[2] 13.1 (3.7–22.1)	.001
66	Turbuhaler (Astra Draco, Lund, Sweden)	Normals	Budesonide	36 58	14.8 (3.3) 27.7 (9.5)	.01
67	Pulvinal (Chiesa, Parma, Italy)	Normals	Salbutamol	27 46	11.7 (2.3) 14.1 (3.2)	.05
72	Spiros (Dura, San Diego, CA)	Normals	Albuterol sulfate	16 58	37.4 (12.0) 24.9 (9.1)	.023

[1]IFR = Inspiratory flow rate.
[2]Mean (range).

explanation is that the high-pressure drop across the device more readily deaggregates the powder in the device and also from the lactose or glucose carrier, if present, providing a finer more "respirable" cloud of powder for inhalation (69). A recent, interesting study by Svartengren and colleagues conducted in asthmatic patients has demonstrated that the delivery of radiolabeled Teflon particles to the lung can markedly increase with the addition of an external resistance (70), supporting the use of high-resistance DPIs even though patients may find it difficult to achieve the optimal target IFR for that design.

Several lung deposition studies using radiolabeled powders have been performed recently for new DPI designs. One of these, a device manufactured by Leiras Oy (Turku, Finland) shows comparable delivery at 30 L min^{-1} to that from Turbuhaler at 60 L min^{-1} (71). Preliminary data in healthy normal individuals using the Spiros (Dura Pharmaceuticals, San Diego, CA), a DPI with a specific resistance comparable to Turbuhaler, indicates a mean lung dose of 25.8% of the nominal dose or 37.4% of the emitted dose at an inspiratory flow rate of 15 L min^{-1} (see Table 7; Fig. 6) (72). Thus, a device with high resistance which can be used with a low IFR and not compromise the amount of drug delivered to the lung would be an obvious benefit for patients, particularly when they are experiencing respiratory symptoms.

Other factors may influence the response to a DPI. The importance of initiating and maintaining a breath hold at end inspiration when inhaling a DPI dose needs to be further investigated. Although a breath hold did not appear to provide a better clinical response (65) or improve lung deposition (73), it is not known what the effect would be for DPIs of more recent designs. The time in the inspiratory cycle at which the powder is made available for inhalation has been studied using the Easyhaler DPI (Orion Farmos Kuopio, Finland). Metering the dose from the bulk powder reservoir prior to initiation of the breath appeared to provide similar bronchodilatation to having the patient "actuate" the DPI during inspiration (74). The risk of losing the dose because of an inadvertent exhalation into the DPI may make the former maneuver less desirable, whereas synchronization in the latter may be problematic for some patients.

C. Other Types of Breath-Actuated Devices

The means of controlling the release of aerosol from a delivery system can be accomplished by using integrated triggering devices. The Autohaler (3M Pharmaceuticals, St. Paul, MN) delivers a dose from a pMDI at the time of inhalation after the patient activates a simple spring mechanism built into the device. The pMDI is placed in the mouth and the spring is released with initiation of a low-flow inhalation of at least 0.5 L min^{-1}, which automatically fires the pMDI. Thus, the need to synchronize actuation with inhalation is eliminated. Deposition to the lung and oropharyngeal region appears to be similar to the

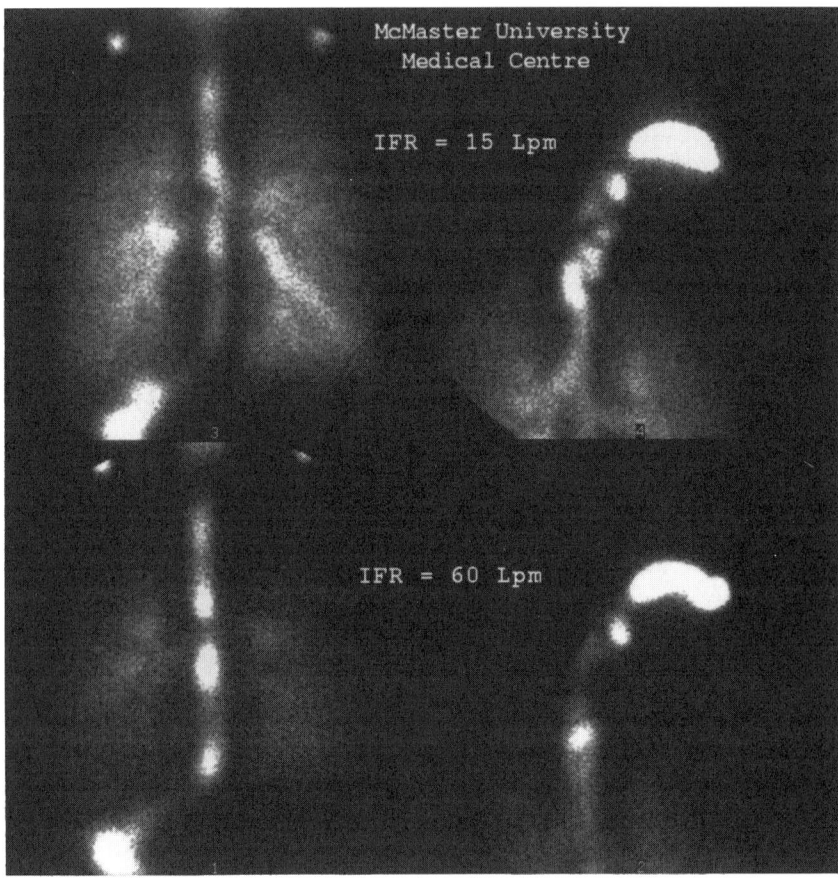

Figure 6   Deposition scans from one normal subject inhaling a $^{99m}TcO_4^-$-labeled powder from the Dryhaler at an IFR of 15 L min^{-1} on 1 day and 60 L min^{-1} on a second study day. At the higher IFR, total dose to the lung was reduced with less radiolabeled aerosol deposited in the lung periphery.

pMDI for those patients who use their inhalers correctly and enhanced in those who experience difficulty using the pMDI alone (75). Similar clinical benefit compared with that from the unaided pMDI has been observed in both children (76) and adults (77). In a recent study conducted in elderly patients, five times as many patients unfamiliar with pMDIs were able to use the Autohaler correctly after minimal instruction as were successful with the pMDI. Seventy-one percent preferred the Autohaler compared with 19% for the pMDI alone

(78). Although the Autohaler can improve pMDI inhalation technique for those who tend to have faulty technique, such as the elderly and children, there is the risk that the high oropharyngeal dose may induce more side effects from steroid pMDIs. The use of a spacer with the Autohaler should reduce the oropharyngeal dose while maintaining the same lung dose (11).

The BI-Neb is a hand-held device under development by Boehringer Ingelheim (Ingelheim, Germany) that provides a dose of aerosolized drug over a fixed period of time of approximately 1–2 sec, by pressing a button on the side of the nebulizer. The aerosol is released as a gentle cloud, with a low forward velocity, enabling the patient to inhale the aerosol using a single low-flow inhalation. Deposition studies using radiolabeled drug solutions have demonstrated high delivery efficiencies to the lower respiratory tract (79) similar to that obtained in asthmatics inhaling methacholine aerosol via the Rosenthal-French dosimeter (80). The BI-Neb may be an alternative, easy-to-use, portable drug-delivery system for patients provided the device can also be used to aerosolize drug suspensions.

The inhalation technique can also affect the dose delivered to the lung and the response to challenge aerosols (35). These aerosols are usually inhaled by tidal breathing or several consecutive high IFR breaths (80). Both methods use jet nebulizers to produce the aerosol, but in the latter technique, the nebulizer is coupled to a breath-actuated dosimeter. The higher inspiratory flow rates required to trigger the dosimeter resulted in a similar lung dose, but more aerosol was deposited in the oropharynx and central airways than when inhaling the aerosol by tidal breathing (80). Despite this difference, equal responses to methacholine were obtained when the dosimeter technique was compared with the Wright nebulizer tidal breathing method (80). These findings are in contrast to those of Ruffin et al., who demonstrated a 20% reduction in FEV_1 with one-tenth the dose of histamine deposited in central airways that was achieved by using a high rather than a low IFR (34). The latter inhalation technique placed the aerosol in the peripheral airways distributed over a wider surface area. More drug, therefore, was needed to effect the same response as when the histamine was targeted to central airways. Depositing equal doses of methacholine aerosol either in central or peripheral airways, accomplished by inhaling a large- or a small-particle aerosol, also elicited different responses in lung mechanics but not ventilation/perfusion relationships (81). This discrepancy in outcomes was attributed to the initial differences in the site of deposition and the intrinsic differences in the rate of absorption of methacholine from the peripheral versus central regions of the lung. A recent study comparing responses to pMDI and nebulizer-generated bronchodilator aerosols, assessed using bronchoconstrictor aerosols, further confirms the importance of the influence of the inhalation technique on the clinical response (82).

Table 8 Factors to Be Considered for
Successful Aerosol Therapy

Suitable drug
Appropriate delivery system
Correct inhalation technique
Disease state
Compliance
Monitoring
Effective drug dose
Minimal or no side effects

V. Patient Instruction in the Use of Inhalers

It is recognized that patients need proper and repeated instruction to learn how to self-administer their therapy using the optimal inhalation technique for whatever aerosol-delivery device has been prescribed by their physician. Even children as young as 4 years of age can be taught to use inhalers properly if sufficient time is spent in training them (83). However, those in a position to teach patients do not always know or fully understand the basics of aerosol therapy nor are totally familiar with the correct inhalation technique to be followed for a particular inhaler to ensure optimal delivery of therapy (84–86). A number of recent studies have shown that healthcare workers need to be educated about inhaler devices and receive proper instruction in their use to demonstrate these procedures effectively to their patients (87,88).

VI. Conclusions

Issues to be considered when implementing aerosol therapy are listed in Table 8. The inhalation technique used is of prime importance, as this governs the dose of medication received by the patient and hence the clinical response. Proper attention to the details for the correct administration of the aerosol will provide beneficial and effective therapy.

References

1. Dolovich MB, Newhouse MT. Aerosols: generation, methods of administration and therapeutic applications in asthma. In: Middleton E Jr, Reed CE, Ellis EF,

Adkinson NF Jr, Yunginger JW, Busse WW, eds. Allergy: Principles and Practice. 4th ed. St. Louis: Mosby, 1993, pp. 712–739.

2. Newman SP, Pitcairn GR, Hooper G, Knoch M. Efficient drug delivery to the lungs from a continuously operated open-vent nebulizer and low pressure compressor system. Eur Respir J 1994; 7:1177–1181.

3. Fok TF, Monkman S, Dolovich M, Gray S, Coates G, Paes B, Rashid F, Newhouse M, Kirpalani H. Efficiency of aerosol medication delivery from a metered dose inhaler versus jet nebulizer in infants with bronchopulmonary dysplasia. Pediatr Pulmon 1996; 21:301–309.

4. Fuller HD, Dolovich MB, Posmituck G, Wong Pack W, Newhouse MT. Pressurized aerosol versus jet aerosol delivery to mechanically ventilated patients: comparison of dose to the lungs. Am Rev Respir Dis 1990; 141:440–444.

5. Lippmann M. Regional deposition of particles in the human respiratory tract. In: Lee DHK, Falk HL, Murphy SD, eds. Handbook of Physiology—Section 9: Reactions to Environmental Agents. Bethesda, MD: American Physiological Society, 1977: 213–232.

6. Heyder J, Gebbart J, Rudolf G, Stahlhofen W. Physical factors determining particle deposition in the human respiratory tract. J Aerosol Sci 1980; 11:505–515.

7. Morrow PE. Aerosol characterization and deposition. Am Rev Respir Dis 1974; 110(part 2):88–99.

8. Yu CP, Nicolaides P, Soong TT. Effect of random airway sizes on aerosol deposition. Am Ind Hyg Assoc J 1979; 40:999–1005.

9. Gerrity T. Pathophysiological and disease constraints on aerosol delivery. In: Byron PR, ed. Respiratory Drug Delivery. Boca Raton, FL: CRC Press, 1990:1–38.

10. Dolovich M, Sanchis J, Rossman C, Newhouse MT. Aerosol penetrance: a sensitive index of peripheral airways obstruction. J Appl Physiol 1976; 40:468–471.

11. Dolovich M, Ruffin R, Corr D, Newhouse MT. Clinical evaluation of a simple demand inhalation MDI aerosol delivery device. Chest 1983; 84:36–41.

12. Lawford P, McKenzie D. Pressurized aerosol inhaler technique: how important are inhalation from residual volume, inspiratory flowrate and the time interval between puffs? Br J Dis Chest 1983; 77:276–281.

13. Xu JB, Yu CP. The effects of age on deposition of inhaled aerosols in the human lung. Aerosol Sci Technol 1986; 5:349–357.

14. Zainudin BMZ, Biddiscombe M, Tolfree SEJ, Short M, Spiro SG. Comparison of bronchodilator responses and deposition patterns of salbutamol inhaled from a pressurized metered dose inhaler, as a dry powder, and as a nebulised solution. Thorax 1990; 45:469–473.

15. Hindle M, Newton DAG, Chrystyn H. Investigations of an optimal inhaler technique with the use of urinary salbutamol excretion as a measure of relative bioavailability to the lung. Thorax 1993; 48:607–610.

16. Newman SP. A comparison of lung deposition patterns between different asthma inhalers. J Aerosol Med 1995; 8(suppl 3):S21–S27.

17. Borgstrom L, Derom E, Stahl E, Wahlin-Boll E, Pauwels R. The inhalation technique influences lung deposition and bronchodilating effect of terbutaline. Am J Respir Crit Care Med 1996; 153:1636–1640.

18. Dolovich M. Lung dose, distribution and clinical response to therapeutic aerosols. Aerosol Sci Technol 1994; 18:230–240.
19. Corr D, Dolovich M, McCormack D, Ruffin R, Obminski G, Newhouse M. Design and characteristics of a portable breath-actuated particle size selective medical aerosol inhaler. J Aerosol Sci 1982; 13:1–7.
20. Dolovich M, Ruffin RE, Roberts R, Newhouse MT. Optimal delivery of aerosols from metered dose inhalers. Chest 1981; 80:S911–S915.
21. Thomas P, Williams T, Reilly PA, Bradley D. Modifying delivery technique of fenoterol from a metered dose inhaler. Ann Allergy 1984; 52:279–281.
22. Hindle M, Chrystyn H. Relative bioavailability of salbutamol to the lung following inhalation using metered dose inhalation methods and spacer devices. Thorax 1994; 49:549–553.
23. Everard ML, Clark AR, Milner AD. Drug delivery from jet nebulizers. Arch Dis Child 1992; 67:586–591.
24. Newman SP, Pavia D, Garland N, Clarke SW. Effects of various inhalation modes on the deposition of radioactive pressurized aerosols. Eur J Respir Dis 1982; 63 (suppl 119):57–65.
25. Pavia D, Thomson ML, Clarke SW, Shannon HS. Effect of lung function and mode of inhalation on penetration of aerosol into the human lung. Thorax 1977; 32: 194–197.
26. Fraser I, Duvall A, Dolovich M, Newhouse M. Therapeutic aerosol delivery in a ventilator system. Am Rev Respir Dis 1981; 123(part 2):107.
27. Murakami G, Igarashi T, Adachi Y, Matsuno M, Abachi Y, Sawai M, Yoshizumi A, Okada T. Measurement of bronchial hyperreactivity in infants and preschool children using a new method. Ann Allergy 1990; 64:383–387.
28. Cromptom GK. Problems patients have using pressurized aerosol inhalers. Eur J Respir Dis 1982; 63(suppl 119):101–104.
29. Dhand R, Malik SK, Balakrishnan M, Verma SR. High speed photographic analysis of aerosol produced by metered dose inhalers. J Pharm Pharmacol 1988; 49: 429–430.
30. Epstein SW, Parsons JE, Corey PN, Worsley GH, Reilly PA. A comparison of three means of pressurized aerosol inhaler use. Am Rev Respir Dis 1983; 128:253–255.
31. De Blaquiere P, Christensen DP, Carter WB, Martin TR. Use and misuse of metered-dose inhalers by patients with chronic lung disease. Am Rev Respir Dis 1989; 140:910–916.
32. Newman SP, Pavia D, Clarke SW. How should a pressurized beta adrenergic bronchodilator be inhaled. Eur J Respir Dis 1981; 62:3–20.
33. Lindgren S, Bake B, Larsson S. Clinical consequences of inadequate inhalation technique in asthma therapy. Eur J Respir Dis 1987; 70:93–98.
34. Ruffin RE, Dolovich MB, Wolff RK, Newhouse MT. The effect of preferential deposition of histamine in the human airway. Am Rev Respir Dis 1978; 117:485–592.
35. Ryan G, Dolovich M, Obminski G, Cockcroft D, Juniper E, Hargreave F, Newhouse M. Standardization of inhalation provocation tests: influence of nebulizer output, particle size and method of inhalation. J Allergy Clin Immunol 1981; 67: 156–161.

36. Ruffin R, Dolovich M, Oldenburg FA Jr, Newhouse M. Preferential deposition of inhaled isoproterenol and propranolol in asthmatic patients Chest 1981; 80:S904–S907.
37. Dolovich M. Characterization of medical aerosols: physical and clinical requirements for new inhalers. Aerosol Sci Technol 1995; 22:392–399.
38. Newman SP, Clark AR, Talaee N, Clarke SW. Lung deposition of 5 mg Intal from a pressurized metered dose inhaler assessed by radiotracer technique. Int J Pharm 1991; 74:203–208.
39. Everard ML, Clark AR, Milnar AD. Drug delivery from holding chambers with attached facemask. Arch Dis Child 1992; 67:580–585.
40. Newman SP, Clarke SW. Bronchodilator delivery from Gentlehaler, a new low-velocity pressurized aerosol inhaler. Chest 1993; 103:1442–1446.
41. Clay MM, Clarke SW. Wastage of drug from nebulizers: a review. J R Soc Med 1987; 80:38–39.
42. Newnham DM, Lipworth BJ. Nebuliser performance, pharmacokinetics, airways and systemic effects of salbutamol given via a novel nebuliser delivery system ("Ventstream"). Thorax 1994; 49:762–770.
43. Dolovich M, Chambers C, Girard L, Newhouse M. Aerosol delivery through an open tube spacer: importance of inhalation technique. Am Rev Respir Dis 1989; 139:A144.
44. Dolovich M, Chambers C. Effect of a pause prior to inhaling a MDI aerosol on drug availability through an open tube spacer. J Allergy Clin Immunol 1994; 93 (part 2):169.
45. Dolovich M, Chambers C, Mazza M, Newhouse MT. Relative efficiency of four metered dose inhaler (MDI) holding chambers (HC) compared to albuterol MDI. J Aerosol Med 1992; 5:307.
46. O'Callaghan C, Lynch J, Cant M, Robertson C. Improvement in sodium cromoglycate delivery from a spacer device by use of an antistatic lining, immediate inhalation, and avoiding multiple actuations of drug. Thorax 1993; 48:603–606.
47. Ahrens R, Lux C, Bahl T, Han S-H. Choosing the metered-dose inhaler spacer or holding chamber that matches the patient's need: evidence that the specific drug being delivered is an important consideration. J Allergy Clin Immunol 1995; 96:288–294.
48. Newman SP, Talaee N, Clarke SW. Salbutamol aerosol delivery in man with the Rondo spacer. Acta Ther 1991; 17:49–58.
49. Vidgren MT, Paronen TP, Kärkkäinen A, Karjalainen P. Effect of extension devices on the drug deposition from inhalation aerosols. Int J Pharm 1987; 39:107–112.
50. Barry PW, O'Callaghan C. Multiple actuations of salbutamol MDI reduce the amount of drug recovered in the respirable range. Eur Respir J 1994; 7:1707–1709.
51. Pedersen S. Optimal use of tube spacer aerosols in asthmatic children. Clin Allergy 1985; 15:473–478.
52. Bâ M, Spier S, Lapiere G, Lamarre A. Wet nebulizer versus spacer and metered dose inhaler via tidal breathing. J Asthma 1989; 26:355–358.

53. Campbell R, Dolovich M, Chambers C, Newhouse MT. Holding chamber volume/ salbutamol dose delivered through an endotracheal tube at low tidal volumes. J Aerosol Med 1992; 5:304.

54. Gervais A, Bégin P. Bronchodilatation with a metered-dose inhaler plus an extension, using tidal breathing vs jet nebulization. Chest 1987; 92:822–824.

55. Gleeson JGA, Price JF. Nebuhaler technique. Br J Dis Chest 1988; 82:172–174.

56. Auty RM, Brown K, Neale MG, Snashall P. Respiratory tract deposition of sodium cromoglycate is highly dependent upon technique of inhalation using the spinhaler. Br J Dis Chest 1987; 81:371–380.

57. Pedersen S. How to use a rotahaler. Arch Dis Child 1986; 61:11–14.

58. Clark AR, Hollingworth A. The relationship between powder inhaler resistance and peak inspiratory conditions in healthy volunteers—implications for *in vitro* testing. J Aerosol Med 1993; 6:99–110.

59. Timsina MP, Martin GP, Marriott C, Ganderton D, Yianneskis M. Drug delivery to the respiratory tract using dry powder inhalers. Int J Pharm 1994; 101:1–13.

60. Kim CS, Garcia L. Delivery characteristics of albuterol powder aerosol by rotahaler. J Aerosol Med 1993; 6:199–211.

61. Newman SP, Moren F, Trofast E, Talaee N, Clarke SW. Terbutaline sulphate Turbuhaler: effect of inhaled flow rate on drug deposition and efficacy. Int J Pharm 1991; 74:209–213.

62. Pedersen S, Hansen OR, Fuglsgang G. Influence of inspiratory flow rate upon the effect of a Turbuhaler. Arch Dis Child 1990; 65:308–310.

63. Dolovich MB, Vanzieleghem H, Hidinger K-G, Newhouse MT. Influence of inspiratory flow rate on the response to terbutaline inhaled via the Turbuhaler. Am Rev Respir Dis 1988; 137:433.

64. Engel T, Scharling B, Skovsted B, Heinig JH. Effects, side effects and plasma concentrations of terbutaline in adult asthmatics after inhaling from a dry powder inhaler device at different inhalation flows and volumes. Br J Clin Pharmacol 1992; 33:439–444.

65. Pedersen S, Steffensen G. Fenoterol powder inhaler technique in children: influence of inspiratory flow rate and breath-holding. Eur J Respir Dis 1986; 68:207–214.

66. Borgström L, Bondesson E, Morén F, Trofast E, Newman SP. Lung deposition of budesonide inhaled via the Turbuhaler: a comparison with terbutaline sulphate in normal subjects. Eur Respir J 1994; 7:69–73.

67. Pictairn G, Lunghetti G, Ventura P, Newman S. A comparison of the lung deposition of salbutamol inhaled from a new dry powder inhaler at two inhaled flow rates. Int J Pharm 1994; 102:11–18.

68. Clark AR. Effect of powder inhaler resistance upon inspiratory profiles in health and disease. Proc Respir Drug Deliv IV, Interpharm Press, Florida, 1994:117–123.

69. Olsson B, Asking L. Critical aspects of the function of inspiratory flow driven inhalers. J Aerosol Med 1994; 7(suppl 1):S43–S47.

70. Svartengren K. Lindestad P-Å, Svartengren M, Philipson K, Bilin G, Camner P. Added external resistance reduces oropharyngeal deposition and increases lung deposition of aerosol particles in asthmatics. Am J Respir Crit Care Med 1995; 152:32–37.

71. Pitcairn GR, Lankinen T, Valkila E, Newman SP. Lung deposition of salbutamol from the Leiras metered dose powder inhaler. J Aerosol Med 1995; 8:307–311.

72. Dolovich M, Rhem R, Rashid F, Bowen B, Coates G, Hill M. Lung deposition of albuterol sulphate from the Dura Dryhaler®. Amer J Respir Crit Care Med 1996; 153(part 2):A62.

73. Newman SP, Hollingworth A, Clark AR. Effect of different modes of inhalation on drug delivery from a dry powder inhaler. Int J Pharm 1994; 102:127–132.

74. Haahtela T, Vidgren M, Nyberg A, Korhonen P, Laurikainen K, Silvasti M. A novel multiple dose powder and aerosol give equal bronchodilation with equal doses. Ann Allergy 1994; 72:178–182.

75. Newman SP, Weisz AWB, Talaee N, Clarke SW. Improvement of drug delivery with a breath actuated pressurized aerosol for patients with poor inhaler technique. Thorax 1991; 46:712–716.

76. Ruggins NR, Milner AD, Swarbrick A. An assessment of a new breath actuated inhaler device in acutely wheezy children. Thorax 1993; 68:477–480.

77. Schecker MH, Wilson AF, Mukai DS, Hahn M, Crook D, Novey H. A device for overcoming discoordination with metered-dose inhalers. J Allergy Clin Immunol 1993; 92:783–789.

78. Chapman KR, Love L, Brubaker H. A comparison of breath-actuated and conventional metered dose inhaler inhalation techniques in elderly subjects. Chest 1993; 104:1332–1337.

79. Steed KP, Freund B, Towse L, Newman SP. High lung deposition of fenoterol from BI-Neb®, a novel multiple dose nebulizer device. Eur Respir J 1995; 8:204s.

80. Ryan G, Dolovich M, Roberts RS, Frith PA, Hargreave FE, Newhouse MT. Standardization of inhalation provocation tests: two techniques of aerosol generation and inhalation compared. Am Rev Respir Dis 1981; 123:195–199.

81. Schmekel B, Hedenström H, Kämpe M, Lagerstrand L, Stålenheim G, Wollmer P, Hedenstierna G. The bronchial response, but not the pulmonary response to inhaled methacholine is dependent on the aerosol deposition pattern. Chest 1994; 106:1781–1787.

82. Blake KV, Hoppe M, Harman E, Hendeles L. Relative amount of albuterol delivered to lung receptors from a metered-dose inhaler and nebulizer solution. Chest 1992; 101:309–315.

83. Faurisson F, Contrpois A, Grosskopf C. Aerosol inhalation before reading age. Lancet 1995; 346:1298.

84. Kelling JS, Strohl KP, Smith RL, Altose MD. Physician knowledge in the use of canister nebulizers. Chest 1983; 83:612–614.

85. Kesten S, Zive K, Chapman KR. Pharmacist knowledge and ability to use inhaled medication delivery systems. Chest 1993; 104:1737–1742.

86. Hanania NA, Wittman R, Kesten S, Chapman KR. Medical personnel's knowledge of and ability to use inhaling devices. Chest 1994; 105:111–116.

87. Amirav I, Goren A, Pawlowski NA. What do pediatricians in training know about the correct use of inhalers and spacer devices? J Allergy Clin Immunol 1994; 94: 669–675.

88. Thompson J, Irvine T, Grathwohl K, Roth B. Misuse of metered-dose inhalers in hospitalized patients. Chest 1994; 94:715–717.

Discussion

LARS BORGSTRÖM

Astra Draco AB, Lund, Sweden

A. Variability in Lung Deposition

Inhalation systems for the administration of aerosolized drug are traditionally evaluated by in vitro analysis to ascertain the quality of the manufactured product. The evaluations include analyses of the absolute amount of drug leaving the inhaler and of the dose reproducibility. The in vitro analysis is designed with the quality-control aspect in mind but also with an eye to the in vivo situation. Thus, dry-powder inhalers are tested at a flow that is relevant for the clinical use of the inhaler in question.

It is well known that Turbuhaler, a dry-powder inhaler, shows a greater variability in the delivered dose in the in vitro analysis than does the corresponding pMDI. Turbuhaler, and dry-powder inhalers in general, are easier to use than pMDIs, as the need for a hand-lung coordination is unnecessary. Thus, it was of interest to investigate if the in vitro variability in delivered dose was reflected in a corresponding in vivo variability in lung deposition. In a crossover and randomized study in 12 healthy volunteers, the inter- and intravariability in lung deposition after inhalation of terbutaline sulfate from Turbuhaler and a pMDI was evaluated (Table D–1) (1). To mimic a patient situation, each subject was instructed in the use of the inhaler by a study nurse on the first of the 4 study days. Then pulmonary bioavailability was determined with the charcoal-block method (2) and the subject was given a placebo inhaler to practice inhalation once every day at home until he or she arrived at the clinic the next week for a new determination of pulmonary bioavailability. This time, no instruction was given on how to use the inhaler. This procedure was then repeated a third and a fourth time before changing over to the other inhaler. The calculation of the values given was based on the nominal dose.

Table D–1 Lung Deposition (% of Nominal Dose) of Terbutaline Sulfate, Inhaled via Turbuhaler or pMDI, and Its Intra- and Intervariation

	Turbuhaler	pMDI	P value
Mean value, %	19.5	6.3	<.0001
Intravariation, CV %	32.9	64.7	.008
Intervariation, CV %	28.4	61.8	.03

CV, coefficient of variation.

Intraindividual Variability

For each type of inhaler and subject, a coefficient of variation, CV, was calculated from the four inhalations. The mean CV was 32.9% for Turbuhaler and 64.7% for the pMDI. The means of the calculated CVs for the pMDI and Turbuhaler were then compared. The CV ratio for Turbuhaler versus the pMDI was 50.0%, with confidence limits 32.4 and 79.9%, giving a P value of .008. Thus, the intraindividual variation in pulmonary bioavailability was significantly lower for Turbuhaler than for the pMDI.

Interindividual Variability

To obtain a value for the interindividual variability, the means for each subject and device were calculated. The variability in the individual means was then compared between devices. The CV was 28.4% for Turbuhaler and 61.8% for the pMDI; the difference reached statistical significance ($P = .03$). The mean lung deposition was also obtained in this analysis. The percentage of the nominal dose reaching the lungs was 19.5% for Turbuhaler and 6.3% for the pMDI. Deposition was about 3.1 times larger with Turbuhaler (95% confidence limits were 2.2 and 4.4; $P < .0001$).

In Vitro

The in vitro evaluation was done by analyzing 10 consecutive single doses from 10 inhalers derived from the same batches as the ones used in the in vivo study. Within-device variability, expressed as the CV, was 6.4% for the pMDI and 18.2% for Turbuhaler. The difference was significant. Also the between-device variability was larger for Turbuhaler than for the pMDI; the ratio of CV was 2.0 with confidence limits 1.0 and 4.1.

In the present study, which tried to mimic a patient situation at the clinic, the observed variation in dose reaching the lung was significantly lower for Turbuhaler than for the pMDI. The observed larger variation for the dry-powder inhaler in vitro was not reflected in the in vivo situation.

The observed difference between in vitro and in vivo results may be due to the differences in the basic concept for pMDIs and DPIs. For DPIs, the "actuation" of the dose, and the inhalation is a continuous and, owing to the design of DPIs, well coordinated process; the generated aerosol forms part of the normal inhaled volume of air. For pMDIs, actuation and inhalation are two separate processes. The speed of the actuated aerosol is not in harmony with the normal inhalation. This difference is probably of major importance for the obtained results.

The larger in vitro variation, both within and between devices, observed with Turbuhaler compared with the pMDI was not reflected in a larger variation in the in vivo measurement. In fact, the in vivo variation in pulmonary bioavailability was significantly smaller for Turbuhaler than for the pMDI both between and within devices.

B. Lung Deposition and Effect

The amount of drug reaching the effector organ, the lungs, differs between different inhalers and the development of new inhalation devices raises the question regarding comparative efficacy for administering drug via inhalation by different devices.

In a study with 10 asthmatic subjects, the degree of lung deposition and the change in lung function was measured after single inhalations of 0.5 mg of terbutaline sulfate both via a pMDI and via Turbuhaler. The degree of lung deposition was evaluated using the charcoal-block method (2) and changes in pulmonary function were estimated by measuring FEV_1 and sGaw (specific airway conductance). The degree of lung deposition was 9% for the pMDI and 22% for Turbuhaler. The changes in FEV_1 and sGaw levels were, however, similar for both study days. Thus, although the amount of drug reaching the lungs via Turbuhaler was twice that via the pMDI, this difference was not reflected in the elicited effects. Differences in the regional distribution of the inhaled drug could be the cause; a more peripheral distribution of the active drug when given via Turbuhaler could be the underlying reason for the observed no difference in effect. Another possibility is that the chosen dose was on the plateau of the dose-response curve. If so, a potential difference would not be observed. The study was redone with these two considerations in mind: A lower dose level was added and the full range of spirometric parameters was measured.

Also in the second study, the drug was given via a pMDI and Turbuhaler (3). Two dose levels, 0.25 and 0.5 mg terbutaline sulfate, were used. Pulmonary deposition was evaluated with the charcoal-block method and lung function (FEV_1, FVC, FEF_{25}, FEF_{50}, FEF_{75}, PEF, and sGaw) was evaluated up to 6 hr after inhalation. Pulmonary deposition was 8.1 and 8.3% of the nominal dose (0.25 and 0.5 mg, respectively) for the pMDI days and 19.0 and 22.0% of the nominal dose for Turbuhaler days. Thus, also in this second study, the degree of lung deposition was at least twice as high with Turbuhaler as with the pMDI. The increase in FEV_1 after 0.25 mg via pMDI was significantly smaller than the increase after all other treatments. The increase in FEV_1 after inhalation of 0.25 mg via Turbuhaler was similar to the increase after 0.5 mg via the pMDI. An increase in the Turbuhaler dose from 0.25 to 0.5 mg only slightly increased the response. Other lung function variables exhibited a similar response.

Thus, expanding the study with a lower dose level made it possible to detect the difference in effect between the two devices. When only one dose level was used, the study was inconclusive.

We concluded that (1) dose-response studies should be performed with at least two dose levels to be conclusive; (2) the dose of terbutaline deposited in the lungs is dependent on the inhalation device; (3) Turbuhaler delivers about twice the amount of drug to the lungs as a pMDI; and (4) the observed difference in deposition is also reflected in the pulmonary effects.

References

1. Beckman O, Bondesson E, Asking L, Källén A, Borgström L. Intra- and interindividual variations in pulmonary deposition via Turbuhaler and a pMDI. Drug Delivery to the Lungs V, London, 1995, and J Aer Med, 1996.
2. Borgström L, Nilsson M. A method for determination of the absolute pulmonary bioavailability of inhaled drugs: terbutaline. Pharm Res 1990; 7:1068–1070.
3. Borgström L, Derom E, Ståhl E, Wåhlin-Boll E, Pauwels R. The inhalation device influences lung deposition and bronchodilating effect of terbutaline. Am J Respir Crit Care Med 1996; 153:1636–1640.

11

Adverse Effects of Beta$_2$-Agonists

CARL D. BURGESS, RICHARD BEASLEY, JULIAN CRANE, and NEIL PEARCE

Wellington School of Medicine
Wellington, New Zealand

I. Introduction

Adverse events from a medicine usually result from the known pharmacological effects of that medicine. These effects are always dose related, which is unlike idiosyncratic adverse events that are not dose related and occur more rarely.

It is unusual for a drug or a class of drugs to be associated with either the deterioration in the condition that they are supposed to alleviate or to increase the mortality from that disease, but these are the two properties that have been attributed to beta$_2$-adrenoreceptor agonists (β_2-agonists). It is these two potentially severe adverse events that have resulted in the controversy on how, or indeed whether, these drugs should be used in the treatment of asthma. There is some urgency in the need to resolve these questions as patients and prescribers enter the age of the long-acting β_2-agonists which are used on a regular basis.

The most important questions that require answering are, first, whether these two adverse effects pertain to all, some, or none of the β-agonists, and whether there is any connection between these two potential adverse events.

Table 1 Distribution and Effects of β-Receptor Stimulation in Humans

	β_1-receptor	β_2-receptor
Bronchial smooth muscle	0^a	Relaxation
Myocardium		
heart rate	Increase[b]	Increase
contractility	Increase[b]	Increase
Vascular smooth muscle	0	Relaxation
Cyclic AMP[c] (plasma)	Increase	Increase[b]
Cell membrane $Na^+K^+ATPase$	0	Stimulation, decrease potassium (plasma)
Glucose (blood)	0	Increase
Skeletal muscle	0	Tremor/? weakness

[a]No effect.
[b]Dominant effect.
[c]Adenosine monophosphate.

To answer these questions requires an understanding of the pharmacology of β-agonists. In this chapter, we address these questions in an attempt to relate them to the action of the β-agonists.

II. Acute Pharmacological Changes

β_2-Receptors are widely distributed in the body (Table 1). Stimulation of these receptors may result in acute responses which could prove harmful to patients (1–5). These responses have been implicated as perhaps the underlying cause for the increased mortality associated with some β-agonists (see below). There is some evidence that regular treatment (at least 6-hourly administration) with these agents results in tolerance to the systemic responses of β-agonists (6,7), with the implication being that these responses can be ignored. However, neither of these studies was performed when patients were either hypoxemic or hypoxemic and hypercapnic; both of which may occur in severe asthma and may alter responses to β-agonists. Such factors could be important, as most asthma deaths occur outside the hospital where additional oxygen is unavailable.

III. Asthma Mortality and Inhaled β-Agonists

The case-control studies from New Zealand (8–10) relating to the epidemic of asthma deaths occurring in that country in the late 1970s revived a debate that originally evolved in the 1960s regarding the association of β-agonist use and asthma mortality. However, as long ago as the 1940s, doubt had been expressed about the use of sympathomimetics by inhalation in patients with asthma (11). Soon after the formal introduction of epinephrine (adrenaline) by inhalation, there were reports of unexpected deaths. The deaths were usually preceded by a period of increasing tolerance to the bronchodilator effect of the drug with resultant increased frequency of usage. The recorded deaths were usually caused by cardiovascular collapse (11). Although no formal study was performed, it was estimated that epinephrine increased the risk of death by a factor of five (11).

The 1950s and 1960s saw the introduction of a number of preparations of isoprenaline by inhalation. In six countries, a high-strength formulation (isoprenaline forte) was also available. In these countries, there was a sudden increase in asthma deaths in the 1960s. There was also a positive association between the sales of isoprenaline forte and asthma deaths (12,13). At the time, it was suggested that a case-control study should be performed to confirm the association, but before this could be achieved, warnings were made regarding the safety of the high-strength preparation, and it was removed from over-the-counter sales, sales duly decreased, and asthma mortality decreased (14). Although there were criticisms of the isoprenaline hypothesis, no alternative hypothesis was put forward for this sudden increase and decrease in asthma mortality after isoprenaline forte was no longer used. The underlying cause was thought to be due to cardiac arrhythmias, because the deaths were sudden (15). Although ventricular fibrillation was suspected, it was not evident in patients who were monitored. A clue to the mechanism of death was demonstrated in animal studies. Collins et al. (16) showed that dogs could tolerate massive doses of intravenous isoprenaline (500 μg/kg) when breathing room air, but much smaller doses (10 μg/kg) caused fatal inotropic failure when the dogs were hypoxic (PaO_2 = 40 mm Hg). In a further study, McDevitt et al. (17) showed that both the degree of hypoxemia and dose of isoprenaline were of importance in determining whether death occurred, with either alone unlikely to cause death. The deaths were always asystolic. Just prior to death, there was an increase in heart rate and blood pressure which was followed rapidly by bradycardia, idioventricular rhythm, and death. Similar effects in the same model have been demonstrated with salbutamol and orciprenaline (18). The effect of the β-agonists in this model can be prevented with propranolol pretreatment, confirming that this is a β-receptor phenomenon. Other workers have shown that isoprenaline administration can produce myocardial necrosis (19), and isoprenaline infusion has been associated with fatal myocardial toxicity when used in status asthmaticus (20).

A second epidemic of asthma deaths occurred in the late 1970s in New Zealand. It was not until 1989 that the epidemic was linked to the use of inhaled fenoterol (8–10). Three case-control studies were performed examining asthma mortality and β-agonist prescription between 1977 and 1987. The findings of an increased risk of death with a particular β-agonist aroused a great deal of controversy and criticism (21,22). However, the second and third case-control studies confirmed the first study and all three demonstrated an increased risk of death in those patients prescribed fenoterol. The more severe the asthma, the higher the relative risk of death (Table 2). At the time of the epidemic, most patients with asthma were treated with inhaled β-agonists; therefore the increased risk of death with fenoterol was not that compared with no β-agonist at all but rather to salbutamol (the market share was approximately 30% for fenoterol and 70% for salbutamol). One cause for concern was that fenoterol was prescribed to patients with more severe disease, which may have accounted for the findings in the case-control studies. However, there was no evidence that this was the case, and, furthermore, there was also no evidence that undertreatment with corticosteroids occurred in only the fenoterol group. The epidemiological studies led to a number of laboratory-based studies that investigated whether there were significant pharmacological differences between the commonly used β₂-agonists (see below). Meanwhile, in May 1989, the New Zealand Health Department removed the subsidy for fenoterol prescriptions and sent warnings to practitioners regarding the danger of this drug. Sales of fenoterol promptly plummeted, and mortality decreased dramatically (Fig. 1) and have since remained at similar levels as those found in other countries despite increased total sales of β₂-agonists.

Soon after the findings of the case-control studies, the manufacturers of fenoterol funded a study of asthma deaths in Saskatchewan. When analyzed in the same fashion as the New Zealand studies, similar results were found; namely, inhaled fenoterol was associated with a marked increase in the relative risk of death when compared with salbutamol (23). Once more there was no evidence of confounding by severity. A second report of the full cohort from Saskatchewan noted that the relative risk of death with fenoterol was 11.8 (24), which was far greater than that found in the New Zealand case-control studies. The Canadian investigators suggested that the association of increased asthma mortality was not a fenoterol phenomenon but was also associated with all β-agonists in general (more particularly salbutamol). These conclusions are, however, probably incorrect for a number of reasons: First, the conclusion (that the association was with all β-agonists) did not involve the primary hypothesis of the study; second, there were nonasthmatics in the control group; and last, because this conclusion was not apparent in the initial analyses, but was only found after complex multivariant analysis, it involves questionable assumptions (25–28). Furthermore, no other study has found an association between β-agonists as a class and asthma deaths (29).

The pharmacological studies can be divided into those that were performed in animals and those that were performed in humans.

Table 2 Studies of Prescribed β-Agonist Therapy and Asthma Deaths (23)[a]

	1st NZ study (8)[a]	2nd NZ study (9)[a]	3rd NZ study (10)[a,b]	Saskatchewan study (case-control)	Saskatchewan study (cohort)
Study period	1981–1983	1977–1981	1981–1987	1980–1987	1980–1987
Study base	All asthmatics	Patients with a hospital admission for asthma in previous year	Patients with a hospital admission for asthma in previous year	Patients with 10 different asthma prescriptions during 1978–1987	Patients with 10 different asthma prescriptions during 1978–1987
Study design	Case control	Nested case-control	Nested case-control	Nested case-control	Cohort
Matching for severity?	Yes (hospital admission controls)	Yes (hospital admission controls)	Yes (hospital admission controls)	No	No
Source of drug information	Family physician and routine hospital records	Routine hospital records	Routine hospital records	Routine prescription records	Routine prescription records
Main exposure information	Prescribed medication[c]	Prescribed medication[c]	Prescribed medication[c]	Dispensed medication	Dispensed medication
Additional information	None	None	None	Number of units/month	Number of units/month
Information on use?	No	No	No	No	No
Severity markers	Hospital admission, oral steroids, 3+ categories of drugs	Hospital admissions, oral steroids, 3+ categories of drugs	Hospital admissions, oral steroids, 3+ categories of drugs, peak flows, PaCO₂, psychotropic drugs	Hospital admissions, oral steroids	Hospital admissions, oral steroids

(continued)

Table 2 Continued

	1st NZ study (8)[a]	2nd NZ study (9)[a]	3rd NZ study (10)[a,b]	Saskatchewan study (case-control)	Saskatchewan study (cohort)
Odds ratio:					
fenoterol	1.6	2.0	2.1	5.3	11.8
salbutamol	0.7	0.7	0.6	1.0	1.1
both drugs	2.0	3.2	4.6	4.4	8.7
fenoterol only	1.6	1.9	2.0	3.7	8.1
salbutamol only[d]	1.0	1.0	1.0	1.0	1.0
neither	1.0	1.1	0.3	0.3	0.2

[a]Numbers in parentheses refer to reference numbers.
[b]Findings using control group A.
[c]Prescribed medication is synonymous with dispensed medication, since prescribed b-agonists were free during the study period.
[d]Reference category.

Source: Crane J, Pearce N, Burgess C, Beasley R. Thorax 1995; 50(suppl 1):S5–S10.

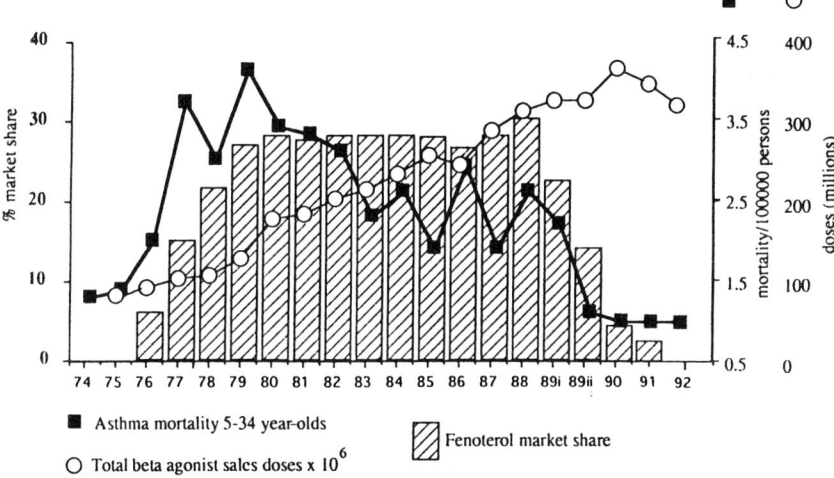

Figure 1 Trends in asthma mortality (per 100,000), fenoterol market share, and total β-agonist sales in New Zealand 1974–1982.

A. Animal Studies

Studies in animals have shown that both isoprenaline and fenoterol behave as full agonists at the β₂-receptor, whereas salbutamol and terbutaline act as partial agonists (30–32). Therefore, both fenoterol and isoprenaline will have the potential to cause greater acute effects than either salbutamol or terbutaline. In a recent study in sheep, Pack et al. (33) investigated the myocardial effects of isoprenaline, fenoterol, salbutamol, and saline when the animals breathed room air and also when they were breathing an hypoxic gas mixture. There were major differences in the pathological findings. At postmortem, myocardial lesions were found in all the sheep receiving β-agonists. Subendocardial hemorrhage was seen in all four of those sheep given fenoterol, whereas it only occurred in one of the four sheep given salbutamol or isoprenaline. The fenoterol-treated animals had the most severe myocardial damage. Fenoterol and isoprenaline were also shown to increase heart rate significantly more than salbutamol during both the period when the sheep breathed room air or the hypoxic gas mixture.

B. Human Studies

In Vitro Studies

In an in vitro study using human ventricular strips, fenoterol was shown to have far greater intrinsic activity than salbutamol (37). The increased inotropic effect with salbutamol was dependent on β_2-receptor stimulation only, whereas fenoterol stimulated both β_1- and β_2-receptors. In a further study of human atrial myocardium, salbutamol was shown to exert its positive inotropic effect through β_2-receptor stimulation only and acted as a partial agonist when compared with isoprenaline (35).

In Vivo Studies

There have been a number of studies in nonasthmatic and asthmatic individuals comparing the cardiovascular and hypokalemic effects of fenoterol, salbutamol, terbutaline, and isoprenaline (36–41). All studies demonstrate that fenoterol has greater cardiovascular and hypokalemic effects than salbutamol and greater intrinsic myocardial effects than terbutaline. Fenoterol's positive inotropic effect is equivalent to isoprenaline when supratherapeutic doses are inhaled (39).

In order to further define any pharmacological differences, two studies have been performed in humans investigating the systemic effects of salbutamol and fenoterol when very large doses of both were administered. The purpose of these studies was to assess whether there was any evidence for salbutamol behaving as a partial agonist when compared with fenoterol (42,43). In both studies, subjects were given incremental doses of the drugs; in one study in volunteers (42), the maximum response was reached, but in the other, patients received a fixed total dose (4000 μg) (43). In the first study (42), salbutamol acted as a partial agonist when compared with fenoterol for both cardiovascular and metabolic effects (Fig. 2, Table 3). In the second study, Lipworth et al. (43) showed almost identical results in patients with asthma, although they make the point that they had not reached the maximum effects. Nonetheless, it is clear that fenoterol is more potent in their model. Of interest was their finding that there was no difference between the two drugs in the degree of bronchodilatation attained by the patients.

A number of studies have been performed demonstrating that the cardiovascular effects of β-agonists are potentiated when the subjects breathe an hypoxic or hypoxic and hypercapnic gas mixture (see Fig. 2) (44–46). The findings of an increase in chronotropy or inotropy would suggest increased myocardial oxygen consumption which could be detrimental if an asthmatic was using large doses of β-agonists and was hypoxemic. The effects are likely to be a class effect, although the more potent β-agonists are more likely to have greater effects.

Therefore, the pharmacological evidence provides support for the epidemiological findings. There are indeed differences between the β-agonists which may explain the increased risk of asthma deaths with some of these agents. Both fenoterol and isoprenaline are full agonists on the cardiovascular

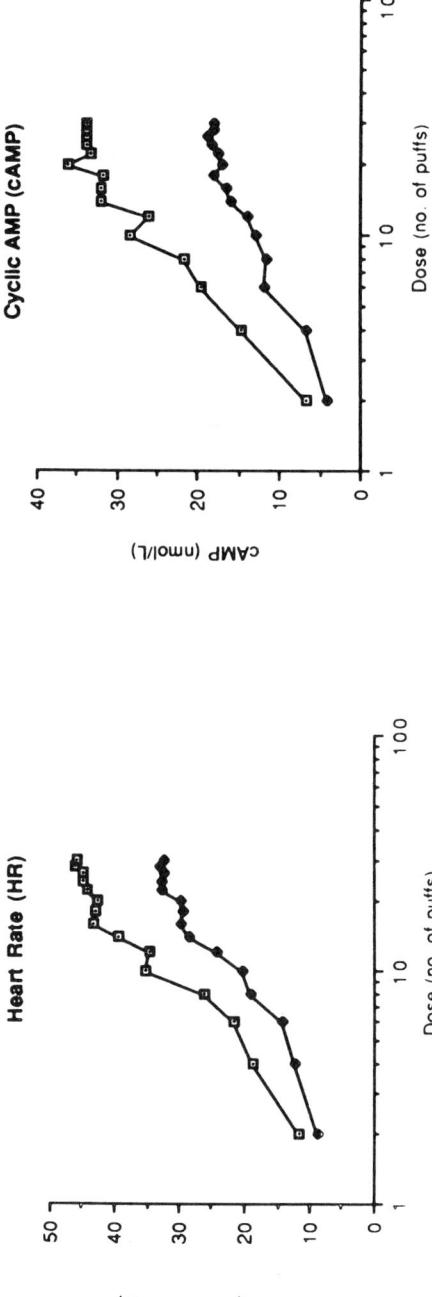

Figure 2 Cumulative log-dose response curves for heart rate and cyclic AMP following incremental doses of fenoterol (□) and salbutamol (◆). (From Burgess CD. An Overview of Experimental Methods. In: Beasley R, Pearce NE, eds. The Role of Beta Receptor Agonist Therapy in Asthma Mortality. CRC Press, Ann Arbor, MI: 1993:127–148.)

Table 3   The Maximum (Emax) Responses and Dose Required to Reach 50% of the Maximum Response to Fenoterol (ED_{50F}) of Fenoterol and Salbutamol

	Emax		ED_{50F} $(\mu g)^a$	
	Fenoterol	Salbutamol	Fenoterol	Salbutamol
QS_2I^c (msec)	-71.8^b	−57.5	767^b	1234
	(−42.8 to −94.5)	(−30.4 to −97.7)	(300 to 1200)	(800 to 2950)
Plasma potassium	−1.40	−1.03	1348	2365
(nM)	(−0.9 to −1.72)	(−0.47 to −1.50)	(550 to 2600)	(1400 to 3250)
cAMP (nM)	33.8	18.1	1085	2454
	(18.0 to 59.7)	(14.2 to 21.4)	(420 to 2160)	(900 to 4800)
Heart rate	44.9	32.5	1170	2312
(beats/min)	(14.7 to 70.3)	(10.1 to 52.0)	(370 to 2350)	(1600 to 4800)

Note: Potency ratios for QS_2I, plasma potassium, cAMP (cyclic adenosine monophosphate), and heart rate were 1.61, 1.75, 2.26, and 1.98, respectively.
[a]The mean dose (range) of salbutamol and fenoterol (μg) required to reach 50% of the maximum fenoterol effect.
[b]Values are means with ranges given in parentheses.
[c]QS_2I, total electromechanical systole, a measure of inotropy (the greater the negative result, the greater the degree of potential inotrophy–see Ref. 36).
Source: Burgess C. In: Beasley R, Pearce NE, eds. An Overview of Experimental Methods. The Role of Beta Receptor Agonist Therapy in Asthma Therapy. Ann Arbor, MI: 1993:127–148.

system when compared with salbutamol and terbutaline, and fenoterol may be less selective for the β_2-receptor than the other β_2-agonists.

IV. Chronic Adverse Effects: Increase in Asthma Severity

The advent of portable inhaled therapy allowed patients with asthma the opportunity of directing their own management. They were given the use of agents that were not only highly effective but were more rapid in onset. Not surprisingly, such preparations proved popular. Although initially recommended for as-needed use, over time prescribers have advised that they be used on a regular basis with additional doses on demand. It is the regular use of these agents that has led some investigators to question whether such practice may result in a deterioration in asthma with increasing symptoms (47). Like the reactivation of the mortality debate, the reporting of tolerance or tachyphylaxis is not new. In 1948, Benson and Perlman (11) reported that tachyphylaxis occurred with adrenaline (epinephrine), and soon after isoprenaline's introduction, there were reports of the development of refractory asthma with constant use of this agent (48,49).

However, the problem surfaced again following a study from Sears et al. (50). They demonstrated that there was an increase in the severity of asthma

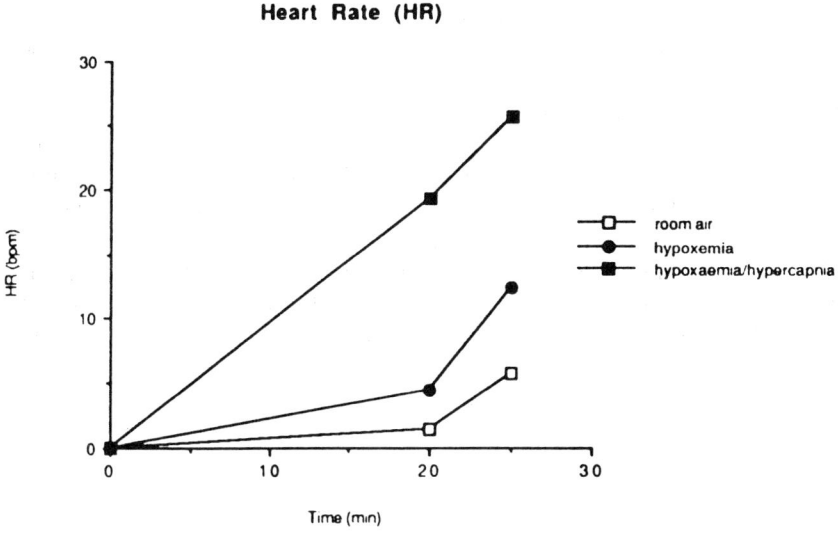

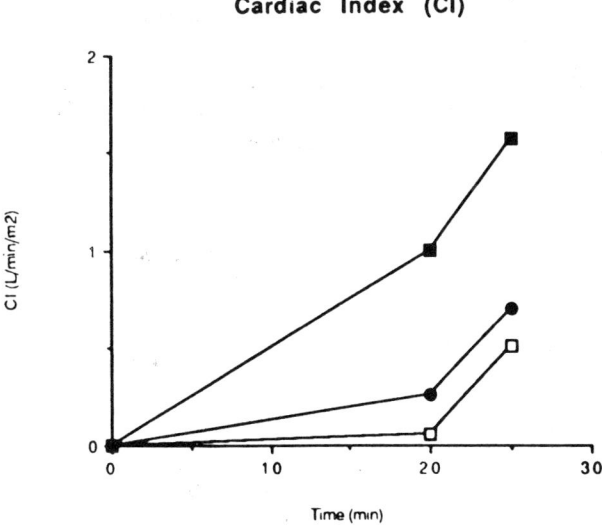

Figure 3 Effect of gas mixtures and isoprenaline on heart rate and cardiac index in nine healthy subjects. Isoprenaline (400 μg) was administered 20 min after the gas mixture. (From Bremner P, Burgess C, McHaffie D, Robinson B, Galletly D, Buckley D, Beasley R, Purdie G, Crane J. Clin Pharmacol Ther 1994; 56:302–308.) (From Ref. 46.)

when patients were given regular inhaled fenoterol rather than fenoterol on demand. They also noted a small, but significant, increase in bronchial hyper-responsiveness (BHR) with regular treatment. The investigators suggested that these findings are likely to occur with all β-agonists, and they recommended that these agents should only be used on demand, but the maximum on-demand dose has not been defined. Whether their findings with fenoterol can be extrapolated to other β-agonists is open to doubt. In an earlier study with fenoterol, it was shown that regular treatment with fenoterol led to a significant deterioration in lung function, whereas this did not occur when the patients were treated with terbutaline (51). Furthermore, using a similar design to that of Sears et al. (50), Chapman et al. (52) showed that asthma control

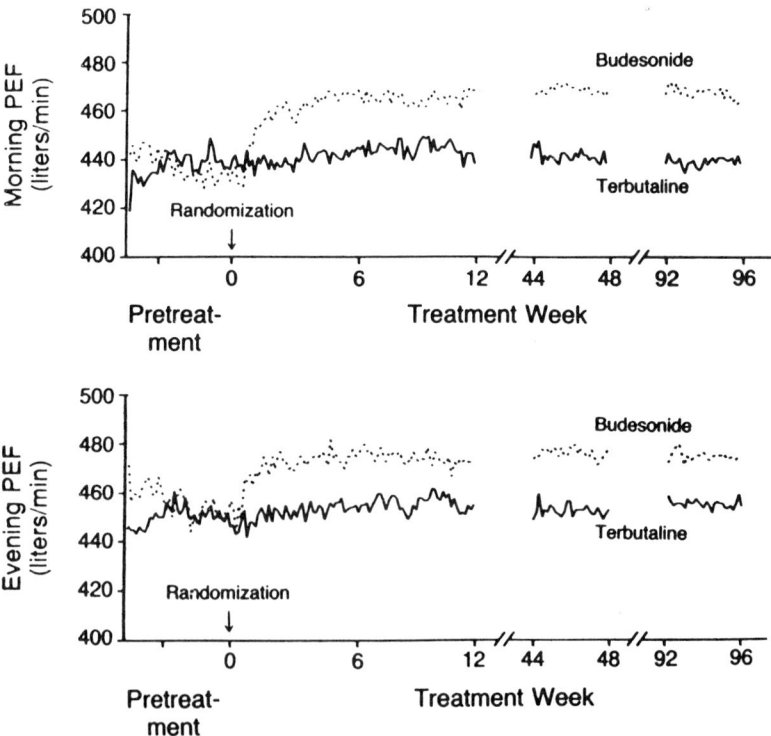

Figure 4   Effect of regular terbutaline or budesonide on morning and evening peak expiratory flow (PEF). (From Haahtela T, Jarvinen M, Kava T, Kiviranta K, Koskinen S, Lehtonen K, Nikanda K, Persson T, Reinikainen K, Selroos O, Sovijarvi A, Stenius-Aarniola B, Svan T, Tammivara R, Laitenen L. N Engl J Med 1991; 325:388–392.) (From Ref. 53.)

was superior when salbutamol was used regularly when compared with on-demand treatment. Finally, in a study performed over a 2-year period, regular inhaled terbutaline was not associated with deterioration in morning or evening peak flow (Fig. 4). However, this study did not include an on-demand comparative group (53). Despite BHR decreasing (Fig. 5), there was an excess of withdrawals from the β-agonist group when compared with a group treated with inhaled corticosteroids. However, at this time, the evidence suggesting that deterioration in lung function occurs with all β-agonists is lacking.

The underlying cause that has been proposed for deterioration in asthma control is that continuous bronchodilatation leads to decreased perception of bronchial symptoms, with consequent poorer compliance with anti-inflammatory medication and a lack of avoidance of exposure to allergens. This leads to increased BHR, with an increased decline in lung function (54). Therefore, an increased BHR could be used as a surrogate for a decrease in lung function. A number of studies have demonstrated increased BHR with β_2-agonists (50, 54–58). However, in some of these studies, BHR was measured after the β_2-agonist had been stopped (57), when one may predict that the airways would be hyperresponsive. Second, on some occasions, BHR has not increased and may in fact have decreased (53,59). And although BHR has been shown to increase during a study, the final result was no different to the pre–β_2-agonist

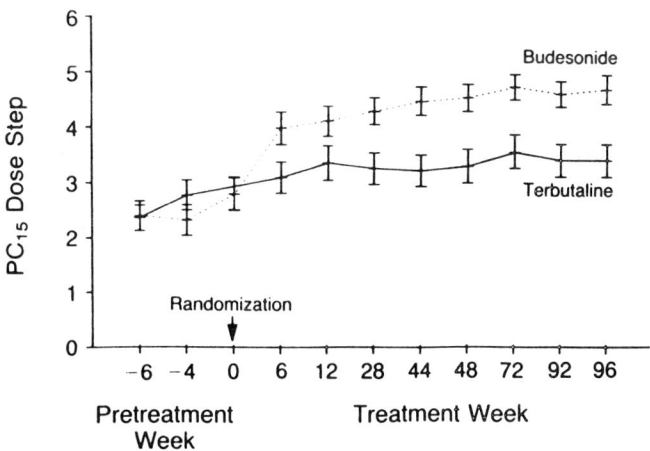

Figure 5 Effect of regular terbutaline or budesonide on the provocative concentrations of histamine (PC_{15}, mean ± SEM). (From Haahtela T, Jarvinen M, Kava T, Kiviranta K, Koskinen S, Lehtonen K, Nikanda K, Persson T, Reinikainen K, Selroos O, Sovijarvi A, Stenius-Aarniola B, Svan T, Tammivara R, Laitenen L. N Engl J Med 1991; 325:388–392.) (From Ref. 53.)

treatment measurement (60,61). Finally, none of these studies has shown satisfactorily that an increase in BHR is associated with a decrease in lung function. Therefore, the evidence that either salbutamol or terbutaline alter BHR consistently or lung function adversely is not convincing.

Long-acting agents such as salmeterol and formoterol will cause 24-hr β_2-receptor stimulation. Theoretically, this could lead to downregulation of the β_2-receptor with evidence of tolerance and perhaps a poor response to other bronchodilators when there is an exacerbation of asthma. This could, for example, lead to an increased number of additional admissions to intensive care units for ventilation. At present, there is no evidence that this is the case, but it may be too early to come to a conclusion regarding this latter point. Neither of the agents seems to induce tolerance to their bronchodilator effects (62,63). The initial decrease in BHR found with salmeterol decreases with time, but it was found to be lower than the pretreatment value (Fig. 6). At the same time as the BHR was rising, there was no evidence of any decrease in the

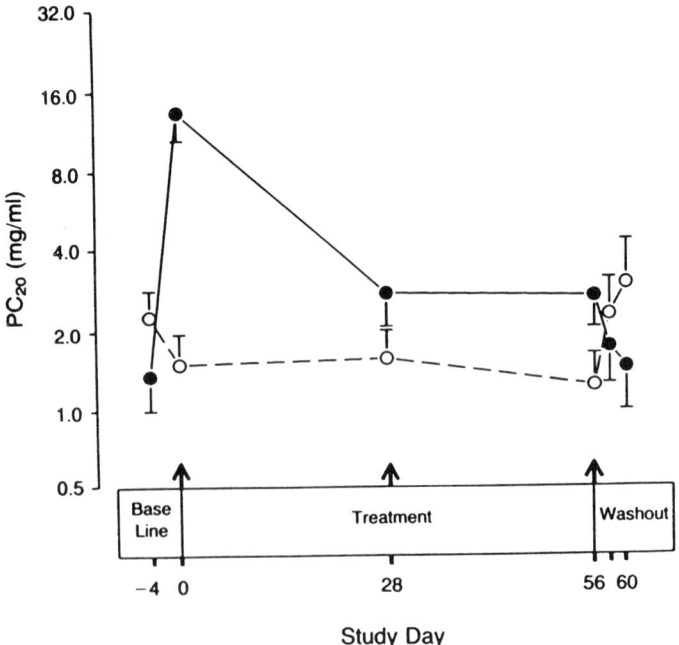

Figure 6   Mean ($\pm$ SE) airway responsiveness to methacholine (PC_{20}) one hour after inhalation (arrows) of salmeterol ($\bullet$) or placebo ($\bigcirc$). (From Ref. 61.)

bronchodilator effect with salmeterol or of any clinical deterioration in any of the patients (61) (see Fig. 7).

In a large safety study of 25,180 patients to assess an increased risk of death (16,787 patients on salmeterol; 8393 patients on salbutamol), 12 patients died in the salmeterol group compared with 2 in the salbutamol group (64). This difference was not significant. In other studies, salmeterol has been shown to be superior to salbutamol (65) with no increase in adverse effects, and it has proved to be superior to an increased dosage of beclomethasone dipropionate in patients with mild to moderate asthma (66). Of some concern, however, is that there has been a case report reporting near-fatal attacks in three patients soon after starting treatment with salmeterol (67), but other studies have not confirmed worsening asthma with this agent (61,65).

Therefore, once again, it is the potent full agonists (isoprenaline, epinephrine, and fenoterol) that seem to be at greater risk of causing worsening asthma than the partial agonists.

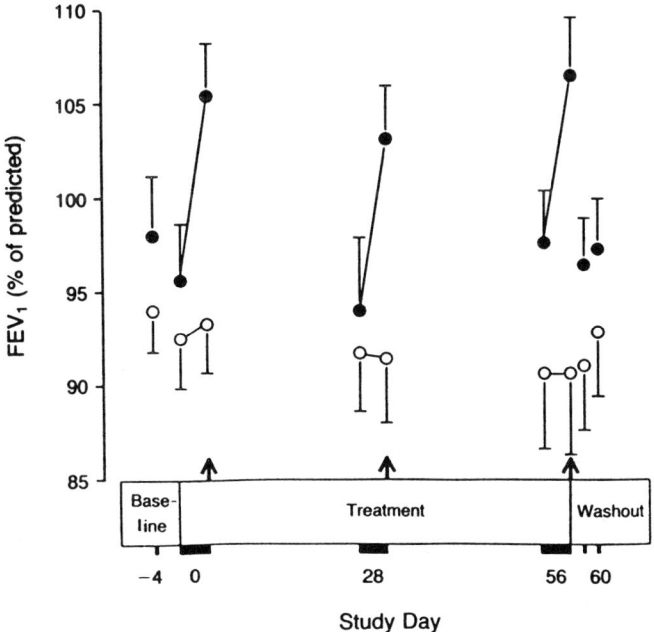

Figure 7 Mean (± SE) FEV₁ before and after inhalation (arrows) of salmeterol (●) or placebo (○). (From Ref. 61.)

V. Conclusions

The evidence that mortality, as an adverse effect, is related to agents such as fenoterol and isoprenaline is extremely convincing. In considering the adverse effect of increased morbidity, there is evidence that fenoterol increases asthma severity in mild asthmatics, but such evidence is not clearly available for either salbutamol or terbutaline. Further long-term studies will be required to be performed in those patients using the new long-acting β-agonists. The picture of increased morbidity and mortality with β-agonists is remarkably similar to antiarrhythmic drugs, where some are obviously more arrhythmogenic than others, and some may even increase the risk of death when compared with no treatment. In the case of β-agonists, it is the full, nonselective agonists which seem to have the greatest propensity for causing these adverse effects, and they should be avoided altogether.

Acknowledgment

We would like to thank Helen Bark for typing the manuscript.

References

1. Motomura S, Zerkowski HR, Daul A, Brodde O-E. On the physiologic role of β_2 adrenoceptors in the human heart: *In vitro* and *in vivo* studies. Am Heart J 1990; 119:608–619.
2. Struthers AD, Reid JL. The role of adrenomedullary catecholamines in potassium homeostasis. Clin Sci 1984; 66:377–382.
3. Strauss MH, Reeves RA, Smith DL, Leenen FHH. The role of cardiac beta-1 receptors in the haemodynamic response to a beta-2 agonist. Clin Pharmacol Ther 1986; 40:108–115.
4. Scheinin M, Koulu M, Laurikainen E, Allonen H. Hypokalaemia and other nonbronchial effects of inhaled fenoterol and salbutamol: a placebo controlled dose-response study in healthy volunteers. Br J Clin Pharmacol 1987; 24:645–653.
5. Kendall MJ, Haffner CA. The acute unwanted effects of beta-2 receptor agonist therapy. In: Beasley R, Pearce NE, eds. The Role of Beta Receptor Agonist Therapy in Asthma Mortality. Ann Arbor, MI: CRC Press, 1993:163–199.
6. Bengtsson B, Fagerstrom PO. Extrapulmonary effect of terbutaline during prolonged administration. Clin Pharmacol Ther 1982; 31:726–732.
7. Lipworth BJ, Struthers AD, McDevitt DG. Tachyphylaxis to systemic but not airway responses during prolonged therapy with high dose inhaled salbutamol in asthmatics. Am Rev Respir Dis 1989; 140:586–592.
8. Crane J, Pearce NE, Flatt A, Burgess C, Jackson R, Kwong T, Ball M, Beasley R. Prescribed fenoterol and death from asthma in New Zealand. 1981–83. Case-control study. Lancet 1989; 1:917–922.

9. Pearce N, Grainger J, Atkinson M, Crane J, Burgess C, Culling C, Windom H, Beasley R. Case-control study of prescribed fenoterol and death from asthma in New Zealand, 1977–81. Thorax 1990; 45:170–175.

10. Grainger J, Woodman K, Pearce N, Crane J, Burgess C, Keane A, Beasley R. Prescribed fenoterol and death from asthma in New Zealand, 1981–7: a further case-control study. Thorax 1991; 46:105–111.

11. Benson RL, Perlman F. Clinical effects of epinephrine by inhalation. J Allergy 1948; 19:129–140.

12. Speizer FE, Doll R. A century of asthma deaths in young people. Br Med J 1968; 3:245–246.

13. Speizer FE, Doll R, Heaf P. Observations on recent increase in mortality from asthma. Br Med J 1968; 1:335–339.

14. Asthma death. A question answered (editorial). Br Med J 1972; 2:443–444.

15. Fraser P, Speizer FE, Waters SDM, Doll R, Mann NM. The circumstances preceding death from asthma in young people in 1968 to 1969. Br J Dis Chest 1971; 65:71–84.

16. Collins JM, McDevitt DG, Shanks RG, Swanton JG. The cardiotoxicity of isoprenaline during hypoxia. Br J Pharmacol 1969; 36:35–45.

17. McDevitt D, Shanks R, Swanton J. Further observations on the cardiotoxicity of isoprenaline during hypoxia. Br J Pharmacol 1974; 50:335–344.

18. Shanks R. The role of hypoxemia in determining the cardiovascular response to beta receptor agonist drugs. In: Beasley R, Pearce NE, eds. The Role of Beta Receptor Agonist Therapy in Asthma Mortality. Ann Arbor, MI: CRC Press, 1993: 149–159.

19. Rona G, Chappel C, Balazs T, Gaudry R. An infarct-like myocardial lesion and other toxic manifestations produced by isoproterenol in the rat. Arch Pathol 1959; 67:43–55.

20. Kurland G, Williams J, Lewiston N. Fatal myocardial toxicity during continuous intravenous isoproterenol therapy of asthma. J Allergy Clin Immunol 1979; 63: 407–411.

21. O'Donnell TV, Holst P, Rea HH, Sears MR. Fenoterol and fatal asthma (letter). Lancet 1989; 1:1070–1071.

22. Poole C, Lanes SF, Walker AM. Fenoterol and fatal asthma (letter). Lancet 1990; 1:920.

23. Spitzer WO, Suissa S, Ernst P, Horwitz RI, Habbick B, Cockroft D, Boivin J-F, McNutt M, Buist AS, Rebuck AS. Beta agonists and the risk of asthma death in near-fatal asthma. N Engl J Med 1992; 326:501–506.

24. Suissa S, Ernst P, Boivin JF, Horwitz RI, Habbick B, Cockroft D, Blais L, McNutt M, Buist AS, Spitzer WO. A cohort analysis of excess mortality in asthma and the use of inhaled β agonists. Am J Respir Crit Care Med 1994; 149:604–610.

25. Horwitz RI, Spitzer WO, Buist S, Cockroft D, Ernst P, Habbick B, Hemmelgarn B, McNutt M, Rebuck A, Suissa S. Clinical complexity and epidemiologic uncertainty in case-control research: Fenoterol and asthma management. Chest 1991; 100:1586–1591.

26. Hensley MJ. Fenoterol and death from asthma (letter). Med J Aust 1992; 157:568.

27. Pearce N, Crane J, Burgess C, Beasley R. Re: The association between agonist use and death from asthma (letter). JAMA 1994; 271:822–823.

28. Pearce NE, Crane J, Burgess C, Beasley R, Jackson R. Fenoterol, beta agonists and asthma deaths (letter). N Engl J Med 1992; 327:355–356.
29. Mullin M, Mullin B, Carey M. The association between beta agonist use and death from asthma. JAMA 1993; 270:1842–1845.
30. Brittain RT, Deane CM, Jack D. Sympathomimetic bronchodilator drugs. Pharmacol Ther 1976; 2:423–462.
31. Raper C, Malta E. Salbutamol: agonistic and antagonistic activity at beta adrenoceptor sites. J Pharm Pharmacol 1973; 25:661–663.
32. Malta E, Raper C. Non-catechol phenylethanolamines: Agonistic and antagonistic actions on beta adrenoceptors in isolated tissues from the guinea pig. Clin Exp Pharmacol Physiol 1974; 1:259–268.
33. Pack RJ, Alley MR, Dallimore JA, Lapwood KR, Burgess C, Crane J. The myocardial effects of fenoterol, isoprenaline and salbutamol in normoxic and hypoxic sheep. Int J Exp Pathol 1994; 75:357–362.
34. Mügge A, Posselt D, Reimer U, Schmitz W, Scholz H. Effects of the beta-2 adrenoceptor agonists fenoterol and salbutamol on force of contraction in isolated human ventricular myocardium. Klin Wochenschr 1985; 63:26–31.
35. Hall HA, Kaumann AJ, Brown MJ. Selective β_1-adrenoceptor blockade enhances positive inotropic responses to endogenous catecholamines mediated through β_2-adrenoceptors in human atrial myocardium. Circ Res 1990; 66:1610–1623.
36. Crane J, Burgess C, Beasley R. Cardiovascular and hypokalaemic effects of inhaled salbutamol, fenoterol and isoprenaline. Thorax 1989; 44:136–140.
37. Flatt A, Crane J, Purdie G, Pearce N, Burgess C, Beasley R. The cardiovascular effects of beta adrenergic agonists administered by nebulisation. Postgrad Med J 1990; 66:98–101.
38. Burgess C, Windom H, Pearce N, Marshall S, Beasley R, Siebers R, Crane J. Lack of evidence for beta-2 receptor selectivity. A study of metaproterenol, fenoterol, isoproterenol and epinephrine in patients with asthma. Am Rev Respir Dis 1991; 143:444–446.
39. Gray BJ, Frame MH, Costello JF. A comparative double-blind study of the bronchodilator effects and side effects of inhaled fenoterol and terbutaline administered in equipotent doses. Br J Dis Chest 1982; 76:341–350.
40. Bremner P, Burgess C, Woodman K, Marshall S, Crane J, Pearce N, Beasley R. Nebulised fenoterol causes greater cardiovascular and hypokalaemic effects than equivalent bronchodilator doses of salbutamol in asthmatics. Respir Med 1992; 86:419–423.
41. Wong CS, Pavord ID, Williams J, Britton JR, Tattersfield AE. Bronchodilator, cardiovascular and hypokalaemic effects of fenoterol, salbutamol and terbutaline in asthma. Lancet 1990; 1:1396–1399.
42. Burgess C, Bremner P, Beasley R, Siebers R, Carne J, D'Souza W, Pearce N. A comparison of the maximum cardiovascular and metabolic effects of salbutamol and fenoterol (abstract). Am Rev Respir Dis 1992; 145:A67.
43. Lipworth BJ, Newnham DM, Clark RA, Dhillon BP, Winter JH, McDevitt DG. Comparison of the relative airways and systemic potencies of inhaled fenoterol and salbutamol in asthmatic patients. Thorax 1995; 50:54–61.

44. Leitch AG, Clancy LJ, Costello JF, Flenley DC. Effect of intravenous infusion of salbutamol on the ventilatory response to carbon dioxide and hypoxia, and on heart rate and plasma potassium in normal men. Br Med J 1976; 1:365–367.
45. Bremner P, Burgess C, Crane J, McHaffie D, Galletly D, Pearce N, Woodman K, Beasley R. Cardiovascular effects of fenoterol under conditions of hypoxaemia. Thorax 1992; 47:814–817.
46. Bremner P, Burgess C, McHaffie D, Robinson B, Galletly D, Buckley D, Beasley R, Purdie G, Crane J. The effect of hypercapnia and hypoxaemia on the cardiovascular responses to isoproterenol. Clin Pharmacol Ther 1994; 56:302–308.
47. Sears MR, Taylor DR. The β2 agonist controversy. Drug Safety 1994; 11:259–283.
48. Lowell FC, Curry JJ, Schiller JW. A clinical and experimental study of isuprel in spontaneous and induced asthma. N Engl J Med 1949; 240:45–51.
49. van Metre TE. adverse effects of inhalation of excessive amounts of nebulised amounts of isoproterenol in *status asthmaticus*. J Allergy 1969; 43:101–113.
50. Sears MR, Taylor DR, Print CG, Lake DC, Quingquing L, Flannery DM, Yates DM, Lucas MK, Herbison GP. Regular inhaled β-agonist treatment in bronchial asthma. Lancet 1990; 336:1391–1396.
51. Trembath PW, Greenacre JK, Anderson M, Dimmock S, Mansfield L, Wadsworth J, Green M. Comparison of four weeks treatment with fenoterol and terbutaline aerosol in adult asthmatics. A double-blind cross-over study. J Clin Immunol 1979; 63:395–400.
52. Chapman KR, Keston S, Szalai JP. Regular v as-needed inhaled salbutamol in asthma control. Lancet 1994; 343:1379–1382.
53. Haahtela T, Jarvinen M, Kava T, Kiviranta K, Koskinen S, Lehtonen K, Nikanda K, Persson T, Reinikainen K, Selroos O, Sovijarvi A, Stenius-Aarniola B, Svan T, Tammivara R, Laitenen L. Comparison of a β2 agonist, terbutaline, with an inhaled corticosteroid, budesonide, in newly detected asthma. N Engl J Med 1991; 325: 388–392.
54. van Schayck CP, Cloosterman SGM, Hofland ID, van Herwaarden CLA, van Weel C. How detrimental is chronic use of bronchodilators in asthma and chronic obstructive pulmonary disease? Am J Respir Crit Care Med 1995; 151:1317–1319.
55. Kerrebijn KF, van Essen-Zandvliet EDM, Neijens HJ. Effect of long term treatment with inhaled corticosteroids and beta agonists on the bronchial hyperresponsiveness in children with asthma. J Clin Immunol 1987; 79:653–659.
56. Kraan J, Koeter GH, van der Mark TH, Sluiter HJ, de Vries K. Changes in bronchial reactivity induced by four weeks of treatment with anti-asthmatic drugs in patients with allergic asthma: a comparison between budesonide and terbutaline. J Clin Immunol 1985; 76:628–636.
57. Vathenen AS, Higgins BG, Knox AJ, Britton JR, Tattersfield AE. Rebound increase in bronchial hyperresponsiveness after treatment with inhaled terbutaline. Lancet 1988; 1:554–558.
58. van Schayck CP, Graafsma SA, Visch MB, Dompeling E, van Weel C, van Herwaarden CLA. Increased bronchial responsiveness after inhaling salbutamol during one year is not caused by sub-sensitisation to salbutamol. J Clin Immunol 1990; 86:793–800.

59. Kerstjens HAM, Brand PLP, Hughes MD, Ribinson NJ, Postma DS, Sluiter HJ, Bleecker ER, Dekhuizen R, de Jong PM, Mengelers HJJ, Overbeek SE, Schoonbrood DFME. A comparison of bronchodilator therapy with or without inhaled corticosteroid therapy for obstructive airways disease. N Engl J Med 1992; 327: 1413–1419.
60. O'Connor BJ, Aikman SL, Barnes PJ. Tolerance to non-bronchodilator effect of inhaled β_2-agonists in asthma. N Engl J Med 1992; 327:1205–1208.
61. Cheung D, Timmers MC, Zwinderman AH, Bel EH, Dijkman JH, Sterk PJ. Long term effects of a long-acting β_2 adrenoceptor agonist, salmeterol, on airway hyperresponsiveness in patients with mild asthma. N Engl J Med 1992; 327:1198–1203.
62. Ullman A, hedner J, Svedmyr N. Inhaled salmeterol and salbutamol in asthmatic patients: An evaluation of asthma symptoms and the possible development of tachyphylaxis. Am Rev Respir Dis 1990; 142:571–575.
63. Arvidsson P, Larsson S, Lopfdahal C-G, Melander B, Wahlander L, Svedmyr N. Formoterol, a new long-acting bronchodilator for inhalation. Eur Respir J 1989; 2:325–330.
64. Castle W, Fuller R, Hall J, Palmer J. Serevent nationwide surveillance study: comparison of salmeterol with salbutamol in asthmatic patients who require regular bronchodilator treatment. Br Med J 1993; 306:1034–1037.
65. Juniper EF, Johnston PR, Borkhoff CM, Guyatt GH, Boulet L-P, Haukioja A. Quality of life in asthma clinical trials: Comparison of salmeterol and salbutamol. Am J Respir Crit Care Med 1995; 151:66–70.
66. Greening AP, Ind PW, Northfield M, Shaw G. Added salmeterol vs higher dose corticosteroid in asthma patients with symptoms on existing inhaled corticosteroid. Lancet 1994; 344:219–224.
67. Clark CE, Ferguson AD, Siddorn JA. Respiratory arrest in young asthmatics on salmeterol. Respir Med 1993; 87:227–228.

Discussion

KENNETH R. CHAPMAN

The Toronto Hospital and University of Toronto, Toronto, Ontario, Canada

A. Introduction

Given the widespread distribution of β_2-receptors in the body and the systemic absorption of inhaled β_2-agonists, one must be impressed not with the adverse effects of these agents but with their remarkable safety. Although there is continuing debate about possible worsening of asthma following the regular chronic administration of these drugs, there is little doubt that their hemodynamic and metabolic impact is minimal in almost all clinical situations.

B. Acute Pharmacological Changes

The cardiovascular consequences of β₂-agonist administration have been well described and seem qualitatively similar among the various bronchodilating agents in common clinical usage. Although the unintended increases in heart rate, stroke volume, and cardiac output are minimized by inhaling rather than swallowing or injecting these bronchodilators, even two MDI puffs (400 μg) of fenoterol produce easily measured cardiovascular changes. We have shown in a series of studies that normal volunteers exhibit cardiac output increases averaging 25–45% following acute administration of β₂-agonist in this fashion (1–3). However, the mechanism of these changes should be outlined clearly. Although β₂-receptors may be found within the myocardium, it is unlikely that stimulation of these receptors accounts for the major cardiovascular consequences of β₂-agonist inhalation. It is more likely that the cardiac output increase that follows β₂-agonist inhalation is a consequence of peripheral vasodilatation and afterload reduction. Thus, the increase in cardiac output is achieved with little or no increase in myocardial stress or myocardial oxygen demand. Indeed, β₂-agonists have been used successfully as therapeutic afterload-reducing agents in the treatment of congestive heart failure (4,5). Although Burgess and colleagues have argued that fenoterol is less β₂ selective and has more β₁-agonist properties than other available agents, the evidence for this is not consistent. The pretreatment with the β₁-selective blocker atenolol blunts but does not abolish the cardiac output increase that follows the administration of either fenoterol or terbutaline (3,6). Both agents continue to produce their cardiovascular effects primarily by β₂-receptor stimulation and afterload reduction.

C. Asthma Mortality and Inhaled β₂-Agonists

To clarify the putative relationship between β₂-agonists and asthma deaths, it would be more helpful to exclude references to isoproterenol, a nonselective agent. There is clearly an association between the frequent use of β₂-agonists and an increased risk from death from asthma (7,8). Although this is sometimes reported as a startling revelation of major importance, it would be more astonishing if there were no relationship between the use of quick-relief bronchodilators and deaths from asthma. Patients with more severe disease are more likely to self-administer medications that provide rapid relief. Thus the need for inhaled bronchodilator is a good marker of disease severity, and consensus guidelines for the management of asthma often offer the patient's use of β₂-agonist as a useful monitoring tool to guide prescribing. Given this intuitively obvious explanation of the association between β₂-agonist use and asthma mortality, epidemiologists have worked diligently to "control" for the confounding factor of disease severity. One must question, however, the ability of an epidemiological study to control for disease severity when assessment of asthma severity is a major problem in individual patient-physician encounters. Asthma specialists continue to hold symposia debating what measurements should be used to monitor asthma's management (9). Similar symposia continue to be held debating optimal endpoints for clinical research in asthma management (10–13). If we are unable to agree on the optimal endpoints for our clinical care and research trials, is it plausible that epidemiologists working with the blunt instruments of chart review and patient recall can quantify measures of severity with useful accuracy? Even if the optimal markers of disease severity were agreed on, physicians have been notoriously poor at estimating accurately the severity of the asthma suffered by their patients. Numerous surveys of primary practice have shown undertreatment of asthma with poor attention to follow-up care and the minimal use of objective measures such as pulmonary function testing (14). Patients at greatest risk of asthma death are often those with poorest perception of their own disease severity (15). Unfortunately, primary care physicians remain curiously reluctant to use spirometric monitoring of obstructive lung disease (16).

Burgess and colleagues have contended that fenoterol is more strongly associated with asthma deaths than salbutamol or other β_2-agonists. This has led us to explore the possibility that fenoterol imposes greater cardiovascular risk than other β_2-agonist bronchodilators because of full agonist activity at the receptor and lesser beta$_2$ selectivity. However, in the Saskatchewan database study, fenoterol and salbutamol were associated with equal risk of asthma death when compared on a microgram per microgram basis (7). If the frequent use of β_2-agonist is a marker of increased asthma severity and increased risk of death common to all agents in this class, how can one explain three case-control studies from New Zealand that report a greater risk for fenoterol than other β_2-agonists? It could be argued convincingly that fenoterol, a β_2-agonist available in a higher dose formulation than other β_2-agonists, was marketed selectively and successfully for use in severe disease. As discussed above, correcting for disease severity in epidemiological studies is not a simple task. However, a published survey of New Zealand physicians established that they were more likely to have prescribed fenoterol for severe disease than for mild disease. Such data could explain the increased association found in the case-control studies.

The data presented in Figure 1 in Section III by Burgess and colleagues would offer considerable reassurance to those fearful of fenoterol's reported hazards. Between 1979 and 1985, fenoterol's market share remained relatively constant at approximately 28%, whereas mortality plummeted by 54%. As reassuring as these data are, one is even more reassured when market share is translated into absolute amounts of fenoterol inhaled. As has been noted, asthma death rates in New Zealand fell despite uninterrupted increases in the sales of β₂-agonists. Although the market share of fenoterol began to decrease significantly in the late 1980s, more doses of this drug were being sold than ever before. In 1989, when New Zealand's asthma mortality was lower than it had been for more than a decade, 49,950,000 doses of fenoterol were used, an amount 41% higher than in 1979 at the height of the asthma death epidemic. A revised figure (Fig. D–1) has been prepared from the data presented in Figure 1 mentioned above.

If the two quantities of β₂-agonist use and asthma mortality were changing together, it would be tempting to assume the relationship was causal. However, the association between any two such variables may be influenced indirectly through a third factor. In the present example, asthma death rates and β₂-agonist prescriptions may both have risen because the prevalence and severity of asthma are increasing. There is ample evidence from many Western nations that support this assertion (17–19).

It is always helpful if epidemiological findings can be made sense of by biologically plausible mechanisms. The unintended cardiovascular effects of β₂-agonist would appear at first examination to provide such plausibility. However, it is curious that increases in asthma death rates are most evident among relatively young adults, which are those we would think of as being at least risk from myocardial stresses. In a careful review of asthmatics suffering near fatal

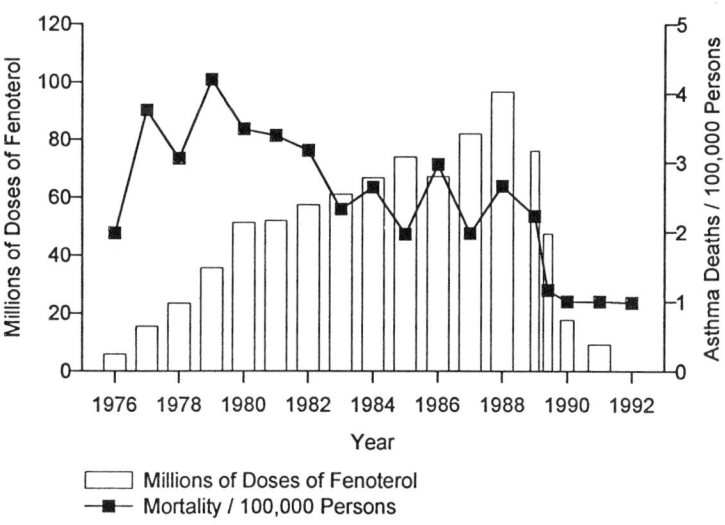

Figure D–1 Trends in asthma mortality (per 100,000) and total doses of fenoterol sold in New Zealand 1974–1982. Asthma deaths began to decrease before any decrease in total fenoterol sales. (Adapted from Fig. 1 in Section III.)

episodes, Molfino and colleagues described the presence of bradycardic dysrythmias that were the consequence of asphyxia and resolved despite the continued aggressive use of inhaled β_2-agonist bronchodilators (20).

D. The Larger Clinical Context

The β_2-agonist debate has been useful in shifting primary care physicians' prescribing practices away from the regular use of bronchodilators as a primary means of controlling disease. However, continued focus on putative adverse effects of β_2-agonists may become counterproductive if more important issues are overlooked. This is evident when discussing possible harmful effects of β_2-agonist administration to the hypoxemic myocardium. These concerns have no relevance in the day-to-day prescription of β_2-agonist for the occasional relief of asthmatic symptoms. It is important to note that the increased risk associated with β-agonist use is not linearly related to dose but is seen only at dosages exceeding eight puffs per day (21). Such concerns also have no immediate application to the treatment of status asthmaticus. No one has advocated that β_2-agonist bronchodilators be withheld from the patient with acute severe asthma, but everyone has appropriately advised that supplemental oxygen should be given. Debating the merits of a particular β_2-agonist selection for the moribund asthmatic is like discussing the merits of various antilock braking systems for the drunk driver about to hit a bridge abutment. Clearly, the more important intervention is prevention of such crises. If the current β_2-agonist debate convinces physicians that they will safeguard their patients by writing fewer β_2-agonist prescriptions or by switching the brand name they have written, it would do a great disservice to the care of asthmatic patients. Our resources would be better spent ensuring that asthmatic patients were offered education with their prescriptions so that they were able to recognize the warning signs of worsening asthma and understood the appropriate self-help responses. Vigorous public and professional educational initiatives in New Zealand seem more plausible explanations for the gratifying decrease in New Zealand's asthma rates than the greater or lesser availability of any single bronchodilator.

Our debate about the potential hazard of a class of drugs, or even one particular drug within that class, returns to an unfortunate paradigm of healthcare delivery. In many medical encounters, physicians and patients share a mistaken belief that optimum management of a medical problem depends primarily on prescription of the correct drug or combination of drugs. Most medical encounters are for common incurable processes such as asthma. In such a setting, the patient's intelligent participation and the medical regimen plus appropriate life style changes are required. When the disease is as variable as asthma, the patient's active participation becomes even more important. It would be unwise for physicians to seek a single perfect prescription that would provide optimal asthma management. It would be equally naive to seek out a single therapeutic agent to account for unwanted effects.

References

1. Chapman KR, Smith DL, Rebuck AS, Leenen FH. Hemodynamic effects of inhaled ipratropium bromide, alone and combined with an inhaled beta 2-agonist. Am Rev Respir Dis 1985; 132:845–847.
2. Chapman KR, Smith DL, Rebuck AS, Leenen FH. Hemodynamic effects of an inhaled beta-2 agonist. Clin Pharmacol Ther 1984; 35:762–767.
3. Chapman KR, Galko BM, Smith DL, Leenen FH. Effects of atenolol vs diltiazem on the haemodynamic effects of an inhaled beta 2-adrenoceptor agonist. Br J Clin Pharmacol 1989; 27:268–271.
4. Bourdillon PD, Dawson JR, Foale RA, Timmis AD, Poole-Wilson PA, Sutton GC. Salbutamol in treatment of heart failure. Br Heart J 1980; 43:206–210.
5. Sharma B, Goodwin JF. Beneficial effect of salbutamol on cardiac function in severe congestive cardiomyopathy. Effect on systolic and diastolic function of the left ventricle. Circulation 1978; 58:449–460.
6. Strauss MH, Reeves RA, Smith DL, Leenen FH. The role of cardiac beta-1 receptors in the hemodynamic response to a beta-2 agonist. Clin Pharmacol Ther 1986; 40:108–115.
7. Spitzer WO, Suissa S, Ernst P, Horwitz RI, Habbick B, Cockcroft D, et al. The use of β-agonists and the risk of death and near death from asthma. N Engl J Med 1992; 326:501–506.
8. Mullen M, Mullen B, Carey M. The association between beta-agonist use and death from asthma. A meta-analytic integration of case-control studies. JAMA 1993; 270:1842–1845.
9. Anonymous. Asthma—what are the important experiments? State of the art/conference summary. Am Rev Respir Dis 1988; 138:730–744.
10. Bailey WC, Wilson SR, Weiss KB, Windsor RA, Wolle JM. Measures for use in asthma clinical research. Am J Respir Crit Care Med 1994; 149(suppl):S1–S8.
11. Enright PL, Lebowitz MD, Cockroft DW. Physiologic measures: Pulmonary function tests. Am J Respir Crit Care Med 1994; 149(suppl):S9–S18.
12. O'Connor GT, Weiss ST. Clinical and symptom measures. Am J Respir Crit Care Med 1994; 149(suppl):S21–S28.
13. Richards JM Jr, Hemstreet MP. Measures of life quality, role performance, and functional status in asthma research. Am J Respir Crit Care Med 1994; 149(suppl): S31–S39.
14. Rea HH, Scragg R, Jackson R, Beaglehole R, Fenwock J, Sutherland DC. A case-control study of deaths from asthma. Thorax 1986; 41:833–839.
15. Burdon JG, Juniper EF, Killian KJ, Hargreave FE, Campbell EJ. The perception of breathlessness in asthma. Am Rev Respir Dis 1982; 126:825–828.
16. Kesten S, Chapman KR. Physician perceptions and management of COPD. Chest 1993; 104:254–258.

17. Shaw RA, Crane J, O'Donnell TV, Porteous LE, Coleman ED. Increasing asthma prevalence in a rural New Zealand adolescent population: 1975–89. Arch Dis Child 1990; 65:1319–1323.
18. Burr ML, Butland BK, King S, Vaughan-Williams E. Changes in asthma prevalence: two surveys 15 years apart. Arch Dis Child 1989; 64:1452–1456.
19. Weitzman M, Gortmaker SL, Sobol AM, Perrin JM. Recent trends in the prevalence and severity of childhood asthma. JAMA 1992; 268:2673–2677.
20. Molfino NA, Nannini LJ, Martelli AN, Slutsky AS. Respiratory arrest in near-fatal asthma. N Engl J Med 1991; 324:285–288.
21. Suissa S, Ernst P, Boivin J-F, Horwitz RI, Habbick B, Cockcroft D, et al. A cohort analysis of excess mortality in asthma and the use of inhaled β-agonists. Am J Respir Crit Care Med 1994; 149:604–610.

12

Clinical Studies of Beta-Agonists in Adults

A. E. TATTERSFIELD

University of Nottingham
Nottingham, England

I. Introduction

Whatever the attributes of a drug in the laboratory or in challenge studies in humans, the ultimate test is how it performs in clinical practice in the patients for whom it is intended. The crucial clinical question for beta-agonists as with all drugs relates to their efficacy and safety in a clinical setting and the balance between the two. The shorter-acting β-agonists such as salbutamol and terbutaline have been on the market for over 20 years and were introduced at a time when the need for longer-term clinical trials was not appreciated. These have been carried out more recently in response to some concerns about safety. The longer-acting β-agonists, salmeterol and formoterol, were developed in the 1980s and have undergone more extensive and sophisticated clinical trials at an earlier stage of development. Since there are important differences in the clinical effects of the longer- and shorter-acting β-agonists, the two types of β-agonists are considered separately.

The inhaled route provides therapeutic selectivity compared to the oral route and most of the important clinical studies in patients with asthma relate to the use of β-agonists given by inhalation. The role of oral β-agonists is discussed briefly at the end of the chapter.

II. Shorter-Acting β-Agonists

The shorter-acting β-agonists when given by inhalation as a single dose are very efficacious in relieving acute attacks of asthma whether mild or severe. Single doses are also very effective in preventing acute episodes of broncho-constriction if given prior to exposure to the constrictor challenge. They have been used in this way to prevent exercise-induced bronchoconstriction for many years. These points are well accepted and do not merit further discussion.

The question at issue is the efficacy and side effects of the shorter-acting β-agonists when given on a regular basis to patients with asthma. A large number of studies have addressed this question over the last few years. Before discussing the clinical outcome in these studies, it is relevant to review briefly the changes in bronchial reactivity that occur during and following regular treatment with β-agonists.

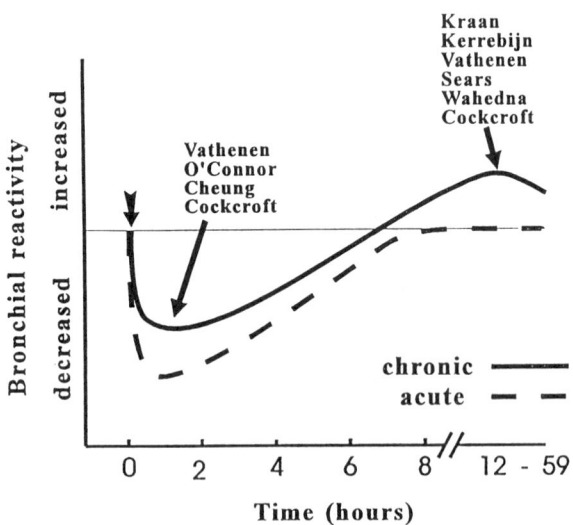

Figure 1   Schematic representation of change in reactivity following a single dose of a β-agonist (- - - -) and after regular treatment (——). A single dose protects against a bronchoconstrictor challenge (reduction in bronchial reactivity). With regular treatment, the protective effect of the β-agonist against the constrictor challenge is reduced and, once the bronchodilator effect has worn off, there is a rebound increase in bronchial reactivity. The names indicate the first authors of studies demonstrating these effects (see Tables 1–4).

A. Changes in Bronchial Responsiveness During and Following Regular β-Agonist Treatment

In addition to causing bronchodilatation, β-agonists protect against a wide range of nonspecific airway constrictor stimuli such as histamine, cold air challenge, and exercise (1,2). Several studies have measured bronchial reactivity, usually to histamine or methacholine, in asthmatic subjects during and following regular treatment with a β-agonist. Treatment on a regular basis has been associated with the two changes in bronchial reactivity demonstrated in Fig. 1: First, there is a reduction in the ability of β-agonists to protect against constrictor challenges, and second, there is a rebound increase in bronchial reactivity and sometimes a fall in lung function as the effect of the β-agonist wears off (Tables 1 and 2).

Gibson and colleagues first demonstrated the loss of protection against a constrictor challenge in asthmatic subjects following regular β-agonist treatment (3). In their study, the protective effect of inhaled salbutamol (200 μg) against an exercise challenge was reduced following oral salbutamol (16 mg daily) for 4–20 weeks, although the bronchodilator response to salbutamol was maintained. They found a similar but nonsignificant trend in subjects receiving regular inhaled salbutamol (800 μg daily) (4). Vathenen et al. showed that the protection afforded by inhaled terbutaline against histamine-induced bronchoconstriction was reduced after 2 weeks' regular treatment with inhaled terbutaline in a placebo-controlled study (5). Further studies have shown loss of protection by terbutaline against adenosine monophosphate (AMP) and methacholine (6) and by salbutamol against the early response to antigen (7), and a nonsignificant trend in the same direction has been seen in other studies (8).

Table 1 Studies Showing Loss of Protection by Shorter-Acting β-Agonists Against Constrictor Challenge

Reference	Drug and dose	Challenge
3	Oral salbutamol, 16 mg daily for 4–20 weeks	Exercise
5	Inhaled terbutaline, 750 μg tid for 2 weeks	Histamine
6	Terbutaline, 500 μg qid for 1 week	AMP
		Methacholine
7	Inhaled salbutamol, 200 μg qid for 2 weeks	Antigen
		Methacholine

AMP, adenosine monophosphate.

Table 2 Details of Studies in Which Change in Bronchial Reactivity Has Been Measured After Cessation of Treatment with Inhaled β-Agonists

Reference	No. of subjects	Treatment, dose, duration	Challenge	Time after last dose (hr)	Change in PD_{20} in doubling doses (DD)
Placebo-controlled studies					
5	8	Terbutaline, 750 μg tid for 2 wk	Histamine	23	-1.5
10	64	Fenoterol, 400 μg qid for 24 wk	Methacholine	>6	-0.6
8	11	Salbutamol, 200 μg tid Broxaterol, 400 μg tds Both for 3 wk	Histamine	12–59 12–59	-1.47 -0.95 Both at 59 hr
7	13	Salbutamol, 200 μg qid for 2 wk	Antigen Methacholine	>8	-0.91 No change
19	41	Terbutaline, 1 mg tds for 2–4 wk	Antigen Histamine	33 18	+0.58 -0.3

Nonplacebo-controlled studies

15[a]	8	Salbutamol, up to 500 μg qid for 4 wk	Histamine	12	NS inc in response to histamine after regular treatment in atopic subjects
4	8	Salbutamol, 200 μg qid for 4 wk	Histamine	>6	−0.25 (NS)
13	7	Terbutaline, 500 μg tid for 26 wk	Methacholine	12–16	−0.6 after 2 wk
12	17	Terbutaline, 500 μg qid for 4 wk	Histamine	12–16	−0.6 after 2 wk
74	15	Salbutamol, 400 μg qid for 1 yr	Histamine	8	−0.7
18	8	Fenoterol, 200 μg qid	Histamine	12	+1.0

Studies in which there have been a large number of dropouts or other treatment has been added have been excluded (e.g., Refs. 28 and 29).

NS, Nonsignificant.

[a]Change in bronchial reactivity not measured in doubling doses.

A rebound increase in bronchial reactivity to allergen (7,9) and to non-specific stimuli (5,6,8,10,12–14,74) has been seen in most but not all studies that have measured bronchial reactivity after the acute protective effect of the β-agonist has worn off (see Table 2). The increase in reactivity (usually measured as the fall in PD_{20} or PC_{20} (i.e., the provocative dose or concentration of an agonist such as histamine that causes a 20% fall in FEV_1) has been seen after fenoterol, terbutaline, and salbutamol use. It is not obviously related to duration of treatment and has been seen after treatment for only 1 week (6). It is not clear when the maximum increase in bronchial reactivity occurs, although it may be somewhere in excess of 16 hr following the last dose of treatment, since the greatest changes were seen in the study by Vathenen et al. (5) (1.5 doubling doses) and Wahedna et al. (8) (1.7 doubling doses) when measurements were made 23 and 59 hr after stopping regular terbutaline and salbutamol, respectively. In the study by Wahedna et al. (8), there was also a 10% reduction in FEV_1 12 hr after the last dose of terbutaline treatment compared with placebo. A fall in FEV_1 had also been observed following cessation of β-agonist treatment in three earlier studies (15–17), and the annual decline in FEV_1 was greater (72 ml) in patients taking 400 μg of regular salbutamol (or ipratropium bromide) than after intermittent bronchodilator use (20 ml) in a study by van Schayck et al. (11) in 223 patients with asthma or chronic obstructive airways disease (COAD).

Interpretation of the data on bronchial reactivity should be cautious, as the findings have not always been consistent. Nearly all studies have shown a loss of protection with the regular use of β-agonists, however, and in most this has been statistically significant (see Table 1). The majority of studies have shown a rebound increase in bronchial reactivity, although some have not (14, 18,19). We were unable to show any increase in the response to antigen following regular terbutaline, for example (19). Several studies have not shown a decrease in FEV_1 with regular β-agonists, although FEV_1 was often not a primary endpoint and relatively few studies have been placebo controlled. One problem with all studies is that the timing of measurements may not have been optimal, since the time course of the changes in bronchial reactivity has not been determined. Despite these caveats, there seems little doubt that regular treatment with β-agonists reduces the protective effect of the β-agonist against constrictor stimuli, and it seems very probable that regular treatment is associated with a small increase in bronchial reactivity and in some instances a fall in FEV_1. These effects are a manifestation of tolerance, which may affect β-receptors on mast cells to a greater extent than those on smooth muscle, since bronchodilator responsiveness is usually maintained with regular β-agonists in patients with asthma. The clinical significance of these findings is discussed later in relation to the findings in clinical studies discussed below.

B. Efficacy and Safety of Regular β-Agonist Treatment

Clinical Comparisons with Placebo

Several recent studies have compared the effects of regular β-agonists with placebo in patients with asthma and concentrating primarily on clinical outcomes rather than bronchial reactivity.

Sears et al. (10) carried out a 6-month crossover study in patients with moderate asthma and found that patients were somewhat worse on regular treatment with fenoterol (400 μg qid) compared with placebo, with both groups being allowed relief β-agonist as needed. FEV_1 and morning peak flow rates were lower, symptoms were greater, and time to relapse was shorter (20) in the patients taking regular fenoterol despite the fact that steroid dosage was slightly higher during the fenoterol period. The main endpoint was an overall within subject comparison of the two 6-month periods combining the different endpoints in a predetermined hierarchical assessment. Of the 57 patients showing a significant difference between periods, 40 were better on placebo compared with 17 on regular fenoterol. Similar conclusions were reached by van Schayck et al. (11) in their study in 223 patients with asthma or COAD in which the fall in FEV_1 over 12 months was greater with regular bronchodilator treatment compared with intermittent bronchodilator use, although there was no difference in exacerbations, symptoms, or quality of life. The difference in decline in FEV_1 was not seen after further follow-up though a reduction in the number of subjects makes interpretation difficult (21).

Some recent studies have not confirmed a deleterious effect with regular β-agonist treatment. In a large crossover study by Chapman et al. (22), 341 patients with asthma taking salbutamol as needed were randomized to salbutamol, 200 μg qid, and placebo for 2 weeks each. There was no difference in morning or evening peak flow rates between treatments, but asthma symptoms and asthma control assessed by the "Sears criteria" described above were slightly better with regular salbutamol treatment. The findings in a recent crossover study of 140 patients by Juniper et al. (23), designed primarily to assess quality of life, are broadly in agreement with those of Chapman et al. Patients with mild to moderate asthma were randomized to salmeterol, 50 μg bd, salbutamol, 200 μg qid, or placebo for 4 weeks each. The study showed very little difference between salbutamol and placebo, and although the trends were in favor of regular salbutamol, they were of borderline statistical significance and deemed by the investigators to be clinically unimportant. Finally, in an uncontrolled study by Heino (24), 54 patients with asthma changed from regular β-agonists to β-agonist "as needed". Peak flow and symptoms deteriorated from week 1 on regular β-agonist treatment to week 3 of as-needed treatment.

Whether the differences between the findings of Sears et al. (10) and those of Chapman et al. (22) and Juniper et al. (23) are due to differences in the β-agonist studied (fenoterol vs salbutamol), the duration of treatment (26 vs 2 and 4 weeks) or the much higher relative dose of fenoterol cannot be determined from the studies. In all cases, the differences between β-agonist treatment and placebo were small, and this is perhaps the main conclusion to be drawn.

One of the reasons why regular β-agonist treatment is not effective is seen in the more detailed time profile of airway function in the studies by Pearlman et al. (25) and D'Alonzo et al. (26). The studies are similar in design, being parallel group comparisons of the response to treatment with placebo, salmeterol, 42 μg bd, and salbutamol, 180 μg qid, for 3 months, and both had a large number of subjects (234 and 322, respectively) with relatively few withdrawals. FEV_1 was measured hourly for 12 hr during the day on the first and last day of regular treatment (Fig. 2). Patients on placebo showed little change in FEV_1 over the 12 hrs, whereas patients on salbutamol showed a large on/off effect, with good bronchodilatation initially after each dose but a fall to baseline before the end of the 6 hr. The area under the salbutamol time course curve was slightly lower after 3 months in one study (26), and although this was not significant, the reduction was greater and significant in the patients taking an inhaled steroid; a similar but nonsignificant difference between users and nonusers of inhaled steroids was seen in the study by Pearlman et al. (25). Morning PEF was slightly lower following salbutamol compared with placebo in both studies (by –6 and –13 L/min).

Comparison with Nedocromil and Inhaled Corticosteroids

When treatment with regular inhaled salbutamol, 180 μg qid, was compared with nedocromil sodium, 4 mg qid, over a 4-week period in a parallel group study of 212 patients with symptomatic asthma, symptoms and bronchial reactivity improved to a greater extent with nedocromil (27). There was no evidence of any improvement in the group given regular salbutamol.

Haahtela et al. (28) compared the response to budesonide, 600 μg bd, with inhaled terbutaline, 375 μg bd, over 2 years in 103 adults with newly detected asthma who had not previously taken an inhaled corticosteroid. Patients on budesonide fared better in terms of symptom control, morning peak flow rate, and supplemental β-agonist use, a finding confirmed in children (29). In the group treated with terbutaline, FEV_1, PEF, and bronchial reactivity to histamine were similar at the end of the 2 years to the values on entry. These measurements will overestimate the efficacy of terbutaline, however, since almost half the patients had either withdrawn or had had theophylline added to their treatment by the end of the study; a placebo limb is needed to estimate the true effect of β-agonists.

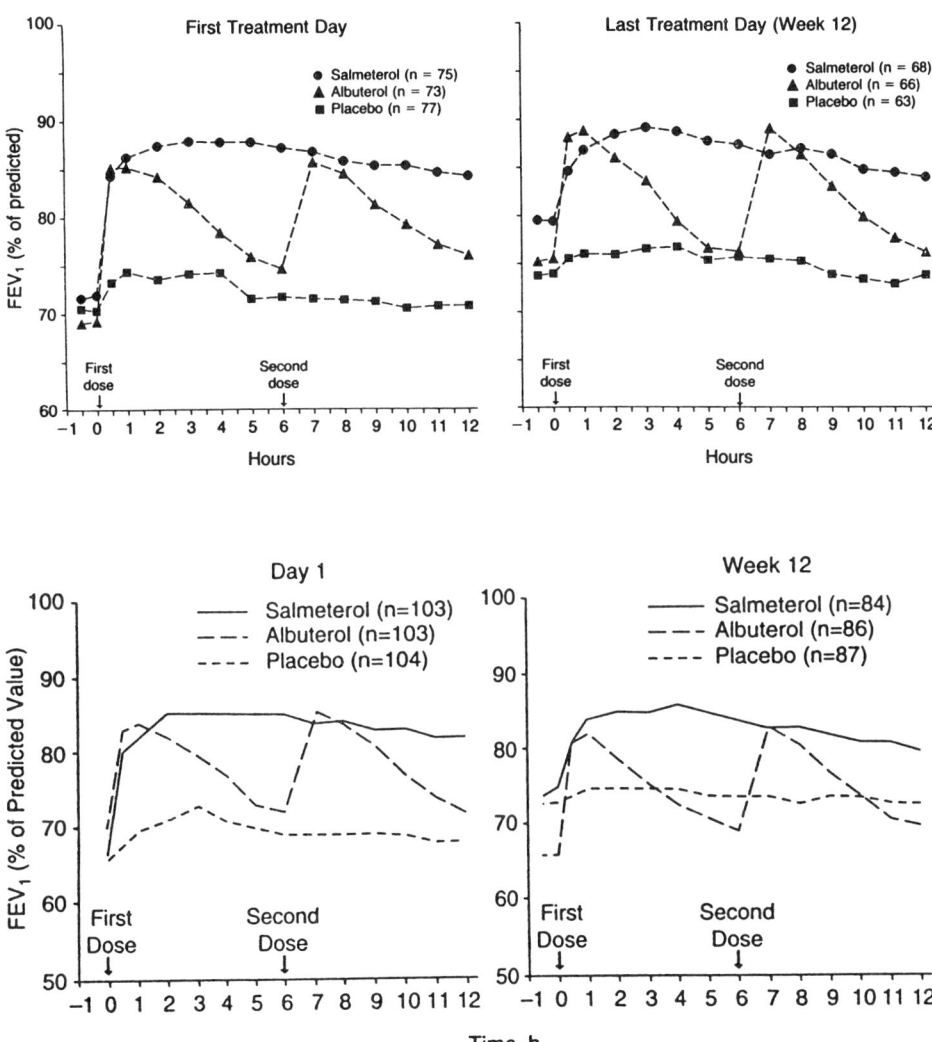

Figure 2 Graphs showing change in FEV1 over 12 hr in patients taking placebo, salmeterol, 42 μg bd, or salbutamol, 200 μg qid, for 3 months. The figures on the left show the changes on day 1 of treatment and the figure on the right those on the last day of treatment. The effect of salbutamol shows an on/off effect compared with salmeterol and in the D'Alonzo study dips below the placebo values at 6 hr. (Data from Refs. 25 and 26.)

Safety

Stimulation of β-receptors in organs other than the lung can cause adverse effects. The main problems reported by patients are tremor, headache, palpitations, and flushing. Metabolic studies show various changes with β-agonists of which hypokalemia is the most important, although this may not be maintained with regular treatment (30). The main concerns with β-agonists relate to their possible role in the epidemics of asthma deaths in the 1960s and more recently in New Zealand. These studies raise the question as to whether β-agonists may occasionally cause a dysrhythmia or whether patients may under certain circumstances develop tolerance to their effects and as a consequence take increasing doses to try to overcome the reduced efficacy. There is evidence that some patients taking very high doses of isoprenaline in the 1960s improved when the dose was reduced (31,32). The doses in the 1960s were very high compared with current doses; whether asthma control would be better if patients currently taking a β-agonist on a regular basis could be weaned to a lower dose or intermittent treatment is as yet uncertain. The arguments in this debate are complex and are discussed elsewhere (2,30). Serious adverse effects are clearly rare with the currently used shorter-acting β-agonists. They could nevertheless be important; for example, a fatal outcome in 1 in 8000 patients using a β-agonist would be very rare and undetectable in prospective trials; were this the case, however, it would account for half the asthma deaths in those under age 55 in the United Kingdom.

III. Longer-Acting β-Agonists

The longer-acting β-agonists, salmeterol and formoterol, have a different role in the management of asthma. Both are normally given on a regular daily basis and should not be used for relief of episodes of bronchoconstriction.

A. Efficacy

Salmeterol

A large number of clinical studies have compared regular treatment with salmeterol with placebo or regular short-acting β-agonists and, more recently, with inhaled corticosteroids. Other studies have compared different doses of salmeterol or have looked at its role in particular situations such as nocturnal asthma.

Comparison with Shorter-Acting β-Agonists and Placebo

The controlled prospective studies comparing salmeterol with placebo and/or a short-acting β-agonist for 4 weeks or more are shown in Table 3. The studies

Table 3 Controlled Studies of 4 Weeks' Duration or More in Which Salmeterol Has Been Compared with Placebo or Short-Acting β-Agonist

Reference	No. of patients (no. on salmeterol)	Duration (weeks)	bd Salmeterol dose (μg)	Control drug
33	692 (520)	4	12.5, 50, 100	Placebo
34	427 (282)	6	50	Placebo
38	199 (55)	12	100	Placebo
25	234 (78)	12	42	Placebo + Salbutamol, 180 μg qid
26	257 (84)	12	42	Placebo + Salbutamol, 180 μg qid
23	140 (46)	12	50	Placebo + Salbutamol, 200 μg qid
35	667 (334)	12	50	Salbutamol, 200 μg bd
36	388 (190)	12	50	Salbutamol, 400 μg qid
37	25180 (14113)	16	50	Salbutamol, 200 μg qid
64	23 (10)	8	50	Placebo
63	24 (12)	8	50	Placebo
40	9 (9)[a]	8	50	Placebo
65	20 (10)	6	50	Salbutamol, 400 μg bd

The last four studies are concerned specifically with bronchial reactivity (63–65) or bronchoalveolar lavage (40) and not with other clinical outcomes.
[a]Crossover study.

have lasted from 4 to 16 weeks, and the number of patients receiving salmeterol range from 10 to 14113 (25,26,33–39).

When compared with placebo, salmeterol has been shown to cause sustained bronchodilatation (25,26), a reduction in symptoms (25,26,33,34), and an improvement in asthma-specific quality of life (23). Most studies have not, however, demonstrated a reduction in exacerbations of asthma (25,26,33,34, 38). In a recent crossover study (abstract only), treatment with salmeterol, 50 μg bd, and placebo was given for 6 months each. Salmeterol treatment was associated with a reduction in inhaled steroid use, symptoms, and bronchodilator use and an increase in FEV_1 and PEF (39).

When salmeterol has been compared with regular shorter-acting β-agonists (invariably salbutamol to date), similar conclusions can be drawn. Bronchodilatation is usually greater and better maintained throughout the day (25, 26), symptoms are reduced (25,26,35,36), and quality of life is improved (23). It has again been difficult in most studies to demonstrate a reduction in exacerbations of asthma with salmeterol (25,26,34–36). The lack of effect on exacerbations may be because this is determined by the extent of airway inflammation, and this was not reduced after treatment with salmeterol as judged by measurement of inflammatory cell profiles in bronchoalveolar lavage (40). it could, however, be because many studies were not large enough and not designed primarily to measure the rate of exacerbations. Exacerbations are a particularly difficult endpoint in clinical trials and may be documented as a side effect or as a withdrawal (and sometimes as both in the same study). In a large postmarketing surveillance study of salmeterol (37) in which 25,180 patients were randomized to salbutamol or salmeterol, asthma exacerbations were lower in the salmeterol group (2.91 vs 3.79%); there was, however, no placebo group for comparison.

The studies by Pearlman et al. (25) and D'Alonzo et al. (26) demonstrate the difference in the effect of salmeterol and salbutamol on airway function most clearly (see Fig. 2). The sustained bronchodilatation with salmeterol over 12 daytime hours is evident and the response showed no decline over the 3 months of the study. It was associated with a reduction in both daytime and nighttime symptoms, as in other studies. The efficacy of salmeterol appeared to be similar whether or not patients were taking an inhaled corticosteroid, as in other studies.

Comparison with Inhaled Corticosteroids

There are no published data on the relative effects of the long-acting β-agonists compared with an inhaled corticosteroid in steroid naive patients. In a parallel group study, Greening and colleagues (41) studied the effect of adding salmeterol or increasing the dose of an inhaled steroid in patients with asthma who were symptomatic on beclomethasone diproprionate (BDP), 200 μg twice daily. Patients were randomized to receive either BDP, 500 μg bd, or BDP, 200 μg bd, plus salmeterol, 50 μg bd, for 6 months. Of the 290 patients who completed the study, there was a greater increase in morning and evening peak flow and a greater reduction in daytime and nighttime symptoms in the salmeterol group with no difference between groups in the number of exacerbations. There were a large number of withdrawals in this study (136), although the number was similar in each group. In a study with a similar design, Woolcock et al. (42) randomized patients with inadequately controlled asthma to receive BDP, 500 μg bd, combined with salmeterol, 50 μg bd or 100 μg bd, or BDP, 1000 μg bd, for 6 months. Asthma symptoms and peak flow (but not exacerbations) improved in patients in the two limbs containing salmeterol compared with the high-dose BDP group, with no difference between salmeterol, 50 and 100 μg bd, in terms of efficacy.

Comparison with Other Bronchodilators

Salmeterol, 50 μg bd, provided better symptom control and fewer side effects than a combination of theophylline, 300 mg, with ketotifen, 1 mg bd, in a multicenter 4-week crossover study (43). Salmeterol, 50 μg bd, also provided better asthma control (improved morning and evening peak flow and reduction in symptoms) than theophylline alone following individual dose titration of theophylline, with fewer adverse effects with salmeterol, although the latter was not statistically significant (44).

Nocturnal and Exercise-Induced Asthma

The long-acting β-agonists were expected to be of particular value in nocturnal asthma, and a reduction in nocturnal symptoms has been seen with salmeterol in most of the larger studies detailed in Table 3 (25,26,33–36). Sleep quality and overnight lung function were studied specifically in a crossover study of 20 patients given placebo or salmeterol, 50 or 100 μg bd, for 2 weeks each (45). Salmeterol improved evening and morning peak flow and caused some reduction in the overnight fall in peak flow. The 100-μg bd dose of salmeterol provided no added benefit over that seen with 50-μg bd dose. There was a significant improvement in sleep architecture with the 50-μg dose.

Salmeterol when given as a single dose causes a reduction in exercise-induced bronchoconstriction over 12 hr (46,47). The protective effect was attenuated, however, when salmeterol, 50 μg bd, was given for 4 weeks (48).

Formoterol

There are fewer long-term studies with formoterol (Table 4), but in those that have been published, the findings are similar to those of salmeterol in that formoterol has caused sustained bronchodilatation and a reduction in symptoms compared with salbutamol (49–52). In the study by Kesten et al. (50), the improvement in FEV_1 and PEF was maintained over 3 months. A large multicenter parallel group study published in abstract form only as yet found that

Table 4 Controlled Studies of 4 Weeks' Duration or More in Which Formoterol Has Been Compared with Short-Acting β-Agonist

Reference	No. of patients (no. on formoterol)	Duration (weeks)	bd Formoterol dose (μg)	Control drug
49	16[a]	4	24	Salbutamol, 400 μg bd
50	145 (73)	12	12	Salbutamol, 200 μg qid
52	18 (10)	52	12	Salbutamol, 200 μg bd
51	35 (19)	4	24[b]	Salbutamol, 400 μg bd

[a]Crossover study.
[b]Could take more as necessary.

24 μg formoterol for 6 months produced a significant reduction in symptoms and bronchodilator use with a mean increase in PEF of 28 L/min compared with placebo (53). There are no published studies comparing formoterol with inhaled steroids or other established treatments for asthma as yet.

Nocturnal and Exercise-Induced Asthma

Formoterol, like salmeterol, has reduced nocturnal symptoms in the longer-term clinical studies (49,50). When studied specifically in asthma, 12 μg formoterol at 2200 hr reduced the fall in FEV_1 compared with 200 μg salbutamol (54). When given as a single dose, formoterol inhibits exercise-induced bronchoconstriction over 8 hr at least (55).

B. Adverse Effects of Long-Acting β-Agonists

The adverse effects reported with the long-acting β-agonists are largely those expected of a β-agonist—mainly tremor, headache, cramps, and palpitations. The frequency of these side effects with salmeterol, 50 μg bd, or formoterol, 12 μg bd, has generally been low and similar to those seen with regular salbutamol, 200 μg qid.

Higher doses of salmeterol have been associated with an increased incidence of side effects with usually little further benefit. When salmeterol, 100 μg bd, has been compared with 50-μg bd dose, it caused a greater increase in peak flow rate (though not FEV_1) and a greater reduction in symptoms in one study (56), but no greater benefit than the 50-μg bd dose in three other studies (33,42,45). In the study in which salmeterol, 100 μg bd, was compared with placebo over 12 weeks (38), the benefit from salmeterol was no greater than that seen in studies of smaller doses. Adverse effects, particularly tremor and palpitations, have been higher with the 100-μg dose (56,33), and have included one death (45). There is little information on the effect of the dose of formoterol with regular treatment. Of the four formoterol studies discussed above, two gave 12 μg bd and two gave 24 μg bd. The small size of the studies makes it difficult to determine whether the 24-μg dose causes a worthwhile increase in efficacy and the extent to which this increases adverse effects.

C. Other Safety Issues

Although the clinical studies are generally reassuring, there are some safety issues that merit discussion.

Bronchoconstriction

Bronchoconstriction can occur following inhalation of salmeterol by metered-dose inhaler, and although this is not common, it can be severe (57,58). It may be more likely to occur in patients whose asthma is deteriorating or poorly controlled. Bronchoconstriction has not been described with formoterol, probably because the drug's bronchodilator effect occurs more rapidly and counteracts the bronchoconstriction.

Partial Agonism

Salmeterol is a partial agonist compared with salbutamol and could therefore act as a partial *antagonist* by occupying β-receptors which would then not be available for a fuller β-agonist such as terbutaline or salbutamol should either be needed during an acute attack of asthma. We found no evidence of an inhibitory effect of salmeterol on the subsequent response to inhaled salbutamol in patients with stable asthma (59). The response to salbutamol following salmeterol was reduced in another study (60), but baseline FEV_1 was higher after salmeterol and the maximum FEV_1 achieved was not reduced. These data are reassuring, although the interaction of salmeterol and salbutamol in acute asthma, the situation in which such a negative interaction is most likely to occur, has not been studied.

Systemic Activity

Salmeterol shows marked $β_2$-selectivity in vitro and when given in recommended doses cardiovascular effects are generally minimal. When given in higher doses in dose-response studies in humans, salmeterol causes a steep increase in heart rate and QTc interval and a marked fall in serum potassium (a $β_2$-mediated effect) (59,61,62). These studies show a dose equivalence for systemic effects of around 8; that is, 50 $μg$ salmeterol is equivalent to 400 $μg$ salbutamol. These data suggest that salmeterol has been marketed at a relatively high dose compared with salbutamol. Salmeterol may have a high initial uptake by the heart, since the cardiovascular effects occur fairly rapidly after inhalation of high doses (400 $μg$). The systemic effects are small at recommended doses, but the studies highlight the propensity of salmeterol to cause systemic effects if taken in higher than recommended doses. These studies were carried out in fit subjects and do not exclude greater systemic effects in an occasional patient with a vulnerable myocardium and other risk factors following lower doses of salmeterol. The postmarketing surveillance study of salmeterol which showed a nonsignificant increase in mortality in patients on salmeterol (37) does not reassure on this point.

Tachyphylaxis Including Loss of Protection Against Constrictor Challenges

The protective effect of salmeterol and formoterol against bronchoconstrictor challenge such as exercise and methacholine is reduced with their continued use (48,63), but this is probably true for all β-agonists. The main clinical relevance of this is that the protective effect of the drugs against exercise may be less than would be anticipated from single-dose studies. There is no evidence of a rebound bronchoconstrictor effect after regular treatment with salmeterol (63,65), which may be related to the more gradual offset of action of these drugs compared with the shorter-acting β-agonists. Three studies have shown reduced bronchodilator responsiveness—to salbutamol after regular treatment with salmeterol (60) and to formoterol after regular treatment with formoterol (66,67), but the effects have been small and, in one instance, the maximum response achieved was unchanged (60).

D. Oral β-Agonists

When studied acutely, β-agonists cause more systemic and adverse effects with less benefit when given orally rather than by inhalation (68). This adverse ratio of benefit to side effects is presumably maintained with regular treatment. There are few published clinical studies of efficacy and safety of regular treatment with oral β-agonists in adults. Oral salbutamol is associated with loss of the protective effect of salbutamol against exercise-induced bronchoconstriction (3).

Bambuterol, a terbutaline carbamate prodrug, was designed to reduce the systemic adverse effects associated with oral β-agonists (69). It is protected against first-pass metabolism following oral absorption and has high affinity for lung tissue. It has a long half-life (20 hr) and is given once daily. The 20-mg dose of bambuterol has been shown to cause significant bronchodilatation (69, 70) and a reduction in nocturnal asthma (69), although its effect on symptoms was small in these studies. Its effect was larger in a recent multicenter study (abstract only) and comparable to salmeterol, $50 \mu g$ bd, in its effect on morning and evening PEF and reduction in nocturnal wakening (72). Bambuterol appears to cause fewer adverse effects, mainly tremor, than other oral β-agonists (73).

IV. Conclusions

Clinical studies of regular treatment with short-acting inhaled β-agonists have shown them to be less efficacious than inhaled corticosteroids, nedocromil, and longer-acting β-agonists. When compared with placebo in patients with asthma of mild or moderate severity, asthma control has sometimes been marginally worse and sometimes marginally better with regular β-agonist treatment. The main conclusion from these studies is that differences from placebo are marginal; when benefit has been seen, it has been very small, and in some situations, adverse effects appear to dominate. The lack of benefit may relate to the on/off effect demonstrated in the studies by Pearlman et al. (25) and D'Alonzo et al. (26) and the increase in bronchial reactivity that occurs temporarily when the bronchodilating effect of the β-agonist wears off. An increase in bronchial reactivity of around one doubling dose is small and unimportant for most patients. This may be the last straw for an occasional patient, however, and could account very rarely for a severe or even fatal episode of asthma. On the basis of the clinical evidence, there is no indication to use the shorter-acting β-agonists in any way other than for relief of symptoms in patients with mild to moderate asthma.

There are, however, a group of patients with severe asthma who continue to take short-acting β-agonists on a regular basis whether by nebulizer or by inhaler despite, in some instances, medical advice to the contrary. Whether some of these patients have developed tolerance to β-agonists and are taking high doses to try to overcome their reduced efficacy is as yet uncertain. More information on the beneficial and adverse effects of the shorter-acting β-agonists in this situation is needed before firm recommendations can be made.

Asthma control is improved with long-acting β-agonists, and this is maintained at least over 3 months. The longer-acting β-agonists provide greater benefit than placebo, short-acting β-agonists, and theophylline, and in patients taking an inhaled steroid, adding salmeterol appears to provide greater benefit than doubling the dose of the inhaled steroid. The long-acting β-agonists differ from inhaled steroids in that there is no evidence of a reduction in airway inflammation and their protective effect against constrictor stimuli is attenuated over time (11), whereas it increases with an inhaled steroid. Control is presumably achieved, therefore, by suppressing the consequences of inflammation rather than reducing the underlying inflammatory response. The reason for the difference in asthma control between regular short-acting β-agonist treatment and the long-acting β-agonists may relate to the on/off effect seen with shorter-acting β-agonists and the rebound increase in bronchial reactivity. This is particularly likely to occur overnight when the pharmacological effect of the shorter-acting β-agonists is insufficiently long to cover the early morning fall in airway caliber.

The clinical data with long-acting β-agonists in general are reassuring, although there are still some concerns that by providing symptomatic relief rather than reducing the underlying inflammatory process long-acting β_2-agonists may not reduce the incidence of severe exacerbations. They may also discourage patient compliance with inhaled corticosteroids. Salmeterol has been marketed at a relatively high dose and, for an inhaled drug, has a relatively small therapeutic window before systemic effects are apparent. Ensuring that the long-acting β-agonists are only given twice daily is therefore very important for safety. Although further studies are needed, it is reasonable on present evidence to consider a long-acting β-agonist as an alternative to high doses of corticosteroids in patients who are not well controlled on lower doses of an inhaled steroid.

Notes Since Publication

Drazen JM, Israel E, Boushey HA, Chinchilli VM, Fahy JV, Fish JE, Lazarus SC, Lemanske RF, Martin RJ, Peters SP, Sorkness C, Szefler SJ, for the National Heart, Lung, and Blood Institute's Asthma Clinical Research Network. Comparison of regularly scheduled with as-needed use of albuterol in mild asthma. N Engl J Med 1996; 335:841–847.

Apter AJ, Reisine ST, Willard A, Clive J, Wells M, Metersky M, McNally D, ZuWallack RL. The effect of inhaled albuterol in moderate to severe asthma. J Allergy Clin Immunol 1996; 98:295–301.

References

1. Tattersfield AE. Effect of β-agonists and anticholinergic drugs on bronchial reactivity. Am Rev Respir Dis 1987; 136:S64–S68.
2. Wong CS, Tattersfield AE. The long term effects of β-receptor agonist therapy in relation to morbidity and mortality. In: Beasley R, Pearce NE, eds. The Role of β-Receptor Agonist Therapy in Asthma Mortality. Boca Raton, FL: CRC Press, 1993:201–224.
3. Gibson GJ, Greenacre JK, Konig P, Conolly ME, Pride NB. Use of exercise challenge to investigate possible tolerance to β-adrenoceptor stimulation in asthma. Br J Dis Chest 1978; 72:199–206.
4. Peel ET, Gibson GJ. Effects of long term inhaled salbutamol therapy on the provocation of asthma by histamine. Am Rev Respir Dis 1980; 121:973–978.
5. Vathenen AS, Knox AJ, Higgins BG, Britton JR, Tattersfield AE. Rebound increase in bronchial responsiveness after treatment with inhaled terbutaline. Lancet 1988; 1:554–558.
6. O'Connor BJ, Aikman SL, Barnes PJ. Tolerance to the nonbronchodilator effects of inhaled β2-agonists in asthma. N Engl J Med 1992; 327:1204–1208.
7. Cockcroft DW, McParland CP, Britto SA, Swystun VA, Rutherford BC. Regular inhaled salbutamol and airway responsiveness to allergen. Lancet 1993; 342:833–837.
8. Wahedna I, Wong CS, Wisniewski AFZ, Pavord ID, Tattersfield AE. Asthma control during and after cessation of regular β2-agonist treatment. Am Rev Respir Dis 1993; 148:707–712.
9. Cockcroft DW, O'Byrne PM, Swystun VA, Bhagat R. Regular use of inhaled albuterol and the allergen-induced late asthmatic response. J Allergy Clin Immunol 1995; 96:44–49.
10. Sears MR, Taylor DR, Print CG, Lake DC, Li Q, Flannery EM, Yates DM, Lucas MK, Herbison GP. Regular inhaled β-agonist treatment in bronchial asthma. Lancet 1990; 336:1391–1396.

11. van Schayck CP, Dompeling E, van Herwaarden CLA, Folgering H, Verbeek ALM, van der Hoogen HJM, van Weel C. Bronchodilator treatment in moderate asthma or chronic bronchitis: continuous or on demand: A randomised controlled study. Br Med J 1991; 303:1426–1431.

12. Kraan J, Koeter GH, van der Mark TH, Sluiter HJ, de Vries K. Changes in bronchial reactivity induced by 4 weeks of treatment with anti-asthmatic drugs in patients with allergic asthma: a comparison between budesonide and terbutaline. J Allergy Clin Immunol 1985; 76:628–636.

13. Kerrebijn KF, van Essen-Zandvliet EEM, Neijens HJ. Effect of long term treatment with inhaled corticosteroids and β-agonists on the bronchial responsiveness in children with asthma. J Allergy Clin Immunol 1987; 79:653–659.

14. Joad JP, Ahrens RC, Lindgren SC, Weinberger MM. Relative efficacy of maintenance therapy with theophylline, inhaled albuterol, and the combination for chronic asthma. J Allergy Clin Immunol 1987; 79:78–85.

15. Harvey JE, Tattersfield AE. Airway response to salbutamol: effect of regular salbutamol inhalations in normal, atopic, and asthmatic subjects. Thorax 1982; 37:280–287.

16. Van Arsdel PP, Schaffrin RM, Rosenblatt J, Sprenkle AC, Altman LC. Evaluation of oral fenoterol in chronic asthmatic patients. Chest 1978; 73:997–998.

17. Trembath PW, Greenacre JK, Anderson M, Dimmock S, Mansfield L, Wadsworth J, Green M. Comparison of four weeks' treatment with fenoterol and terbutaline aerosols in adult asthmatics. A double blind crossover study. J Allergy Clin Immunol 1979; 63:395.

18. Raes M, Mulder P, Kerrebijn KF. Long term effect of ipratropium bromide and fenoterol on the bronchial hyperresponsiveness to histamine in children with asthma. J Allergy Clin Immunol 1989; 84:874–879.

19. Wong CS, Wahedna I, Pavord ID, Tattersfield AE. Effect of regular terbutaline and budesonide on bronchial reactivity to allergen challenge. Am J Respir Crit Care Med 1994; 150:1268–1273.

20. Taylor DR, Sears MR, Herbison GP, Flannery EM, Pring CG, Lake DC, Yates DM, Lucas MK, Li Q. Regular inhaled β-agonist in asthma: effects on exacerbations and lung function. Thorax 1993; 48:134–138.

21. van Schayck CP, Dompeling E, van Herwaarden CLA. Continuous versus on demand use of bronchodilators in non-steroid asthma and chronic bronchitis: four-year follow-up randomised controlled study. Br J Gen Pract 1995;

22. Chapman KR, Kesten S, Szalai JP. Regular vs as-needed inhaled salbutamol in asthma control. Lancet 1994; 343:1379–1382.

23. Juniper EF, Johnston PR, Borkhoff CM, Guyatt GH, Boulet L-P, Haukioja A. Quality of life in asthma clinical trials: comparison of salmeterol and salbutamol. Am J Respir Crit Care Med 1995; 151:66–70.

24. Heino M. Regularly inhaled β-agonists with steroids are not harmful in stable asthma. J Allergy Clin Immunol 1994; 93:80–84.

25. Pearlman DS, Chervinski P, LaForce C, et al. A comparison of salmeterol with albuterol in the treatment of mild-to-moderate asthma. N Engl J Med 1992; 327:1420–1425.

26. D'Alonzo GE, Nathan RA, Henochowicz S, Morris RJ, Ratner P, Rennard SI. Salmeterol xinofoate as maintenance therapy compared with albuterol in patients with asthma. JAMA 1994; 271:1412–1416.

27. Wasserman SI, Furukawa CT, Henochowicz SI, Marcoux JP, Prenner BM, Findlay SR, Gross GN, Hudson LD, Myers DJ, Steinberg P. Asthma symptoms and airway hyperresponsiveness are lower during treatment with nedocromil sodium than during treatment with regular inhaled albuterol. J Allergy Clin Immunol 1995; 95:541–547.

28. Haahtela J, Järvinen M, Kava T, et al. Comparison of a β_2-agonist, terbutaline, with an inhaled corticosteroid, budesonide, in newly detected asthma. N Engl J Med 1991; 325:388–392.

29. van Essen-Zandvliet EE, Hughes MD, Waalkens HJ, Duiverman EJ, Pocock SJ, Kerrebijn KF, The Dutch Chronic Non-Specific Lung Disease Study Group. Effects of 22 months of treatment with inhaled corticosteroids and/or β_2-agonists on lung function, airway responsiveness, and symptoms in children with asthma. Am Rev Respir Dis 1992; 146:547–554.

30. Tattersfield AE, Britton JR. β-adrenoceptor agonists. In: Barnes PJ, Roger IW, Thomson NC, eds. Asthma: Basic Mechanisms and Clinical Management. London: Academic Press, 1992:527–554.

31. Van Metre TE. Adverse effects of inhalation of excessive amounts of nebulised isoproterenol in status asthmaticus. J Allergy 1969; 43:101–113.

32. Reisman RE. Asthma induced by adrenergic aerosols. J Allergy 1970; 46:162–177.

33. Dahl R, Earnshaw JS, Palmer JBD. Salmeterol: a four week study of a long acting β-adrenoceptor agonist for the treatment of reversible airways disease. Eur Respir J 1991; 4:1178–1184.

34. Jones KP. Salmeterol xinofoate in the treatment of mild to moderate asthma in primary care. Thorax 1994; 49:971–975.

35. Britton MG, Earnshaw JS, Palmer JBD. A twelve month comparison of salmeterol with salbutamol in asthmatic patients. Eur Respir J 1992; 5:1062–1067.

36. Lundback B, Rawlinson DW, Palmer JBD. Twelve month comparison of salmeterol and salbutamol as dry powder formulations in asthmatic patients. Thorax 1993; 48:148–153.

37. Castle W, Fuller R, Hall J, Palmer J. Serevent nationwide surveillance study: comparison of salmeterol with salbutamol in patients who require regular bronchodilator treatment. Br Med J 1992; 306:1034–1037.

38. Boyd G on behalf of a UK Study group. Salmeterol xinofoate in asthmatic patients under consideration for maintenance oral corticosteroid therapy. Eur Respir J 1995; 8:1494–1498.

39. Tattersfield AE, Wilding P, Thompson-Coon J, Clark M, Lewis S. Efficacy and safety of long term treatment with salmeterol in adults with asthma. Am J Respir Crit Care Med 1996; 153:A66.

40. Gardiner PV, Ward C, Booth H, Allison A, Hendrick DJ, Walters EH. Effect of eight weeks of treatment with salmeterol on bronchoalveolar lavage inflammatory indices in asthmatics. Am J Respir Crit Care Med 1994; 150:1006–1011.

41. Greening AP, Ind PW, Northfield M, Shaw G. Added salmeterol versus higher-dose corticosteroid in asthma patients with symptoms on existing inhaled corticosteroid. Lancet 1994; 344:219–224.

42. Woolcock A, Lundback B, Ringdal N, Jacques LA. Comparison of addition of salmeterol to inhaled steroids with doubling of the dose of inhaled steroids. Am Rev Respir Dis 1996; 153:1481–1488.

43. Muir JF, Bertin L, Georges D, French Multicentre Study Group. Salmeterol versus slow-release theophylline combined with ketotifen in nocturnal asthma: a multicentre trial. Eur Respir J 1992; 5:1197–1200.

44. Fjellbirkeland L, Gulsvik A, Palmer JBD. The efficacy and tolerability of inhaled salmeterol and individually dose-titrated, sustained-release theophylline in patients with reversible airways disease. Respir Med 1994; 88:599–607.

45. Fitzpatrick MF, Mackay T, Driver H, Douglas NJ. Salmeterol in nocturnal asthma: a double blind, placebo controlled trial of a long acting inhaled β_2-agonist. Br Med J 1990; 301:1365–1368.

46. Kemp JP, Dockhorn RJ, Busse WW, Bleecker ER, Van As A. Prolonged effect of inhaled salmeterol against exercise-induced bronchospasm. Am J Respir Crit Care Med 1994; 150:1612–1615.

47. Robertson W, Simkins J, O'Hickey SP, Freeman S, Cayton RM. Does single dose salmeterol affect exercise capacity in asthmatic men? Eur Respir J 1994; 7:1978–1984.

48. Ramage L, Lipworth BJ, Ingram CG, Cree IA, Dhillon DP. Reduced protection against exercise-induced bronchoconstriction after chronic dosing with salmeterol. Respir Med 1994; 88:363–368.

49. Wallin A, Melander B, Rosenhall L, Sandström T, Wåhlander L. Formoterol, a new long acting β_2-agonist for inhalation twice daily, compared with salbutamol in the treatment of asthma. Thorax 1990; 45:259–261.

50. Kesten S, Chapman KR, Broder I, Cartier A, Hyland RH, Knight A, Malo JL, Mazza JA, Moote DW, Small P, Tarlo S, Gontovnick L, Rebuck AS. A three-month comparison of twice daily inhaled formoterol versus four times daily inhaled albuterol in the management of stable asthma. Am Rev Respir Dis 1991; 144:622–625.

51. Midgren B, Melander B, Persson G. Formoterol, a new long acting β_2-agonist, inhaled twice daily, in stable asthmatic subjects. Chest 1992; 101:1019–1022.

52. Arvidsson P, Larsson S, Lofdahl C-G, Melander B, Svedmyr N, Wahlander L. Inhaled formoterol during one year in asthma: a comparison with salbutamol. Eur Respir J 1991; 4:1168–1173.

53. van der Molen T, Turner MO, Postma DS, Sears MR, for the Canadian and the Dutch D2522 investigators. An international multi-centre randomized controlled trial of formoterol in asthmatics requiring inhaled corticosteroid. Eur Respir J 1995; 8:2S.

54. Maesen FPV, Smeets JJ, Gubbelmans HLL, Zweers PGMA. Formoterol in the treatment of nocturnal asthma. Chest 1990; 98:866–870.

55. Patessio A, Podda A, Carone M, Trombetta N, Donner CF. Protective effect and duration of action of formoterol aerosol on exercise-induced asthma. Eur Respir J 1991; 4:296–330.

56. Palmer JBD, Stuart AM, Shepherd GL, Viskum K. Inhaled salmeterol in the treatment of patients with moderate to severe reversible obstructive airway disease—a 3-month comparison of the efficacy and safety of twice-daily salmeterol (100 μg) with salmeterol (50 μg). Respir Med 1992; 86:409–417.

57. Wilkinson JRW, Roberts JA, Bradding P, Holgate ST, Howarth PH. Paradoxical bronchoconstriction in asthmatic patients after salmeterol by metered dose inhaler. Br Med J 1992; 305:931–932.

58. Anon. Change to US Serevent labelling. SCRIP 1994 (1995) 25.

59. Smyth ET, Pavord ID, Wong CS, Wisniewski AF, Williams J, Tattersfield AE. Interaction and dose equivalence of salbutamol and salmeterol in patients with asthma. Br Med J 1993; 306:543–545.

60. Grove A, Lipworth BJ. Bronchodilator subsensitivity to salbutamol after twice daily salmeterol in asthmatic patients. Lancet 1995; 346:201–206.

61. Bennett JA, Smyth ET, Pavord ID, Wilding PJ, Tattersfield AE. Systemic effects of salbutamol and salmeterol in patients with asthma. Thorax 1994; 49:771–774.

62. Bennett JA, Tattersfield AE. Dose equivalence of systemic effects from non cumulative doses of salmeterol and salbutamol in healthy subjects. Thorax 1995; 50:A77.

63. Cheung D, Timmers MK, Zwinderman AH, Bel EH, Dijkman JH, Sterk PJ. Long term effects of a long acting β_2-adrenoceptor agonist, salmeterol, on airway hyperresponsiveness in patients with mild asthma. N Engl J Med 1992; 327:1198–1203.

64. Booth H, Fishwick K, Harkawat R, Devereux G, Hendrick DJ, Walters EH. Changes in methacholine-induced bronchoconstriction with the long acting β_2-agonist salmeterol in mild to moderate asthmatic patients. Thorax 1993; 48:1121–1124.

65. Beach JR, Young CL, Harkawat R, Gardiner PV, Avery AJ, Coward GA, Walters EH, Hendrick DJ. Effect on airway responsiveness of six weeks treatment with salmeterol. Pulmon Pharmacol 1993; 6:155–157.

66. Newnham DM, Grove A, McDevitt DG, Lipworth BJ. Subsensitivity of bronchodilator and systemic β_2-adrenoceptor responses after regular twice daily treatment with eformoterol dry powder in asthmatic patients. Thorax 1995; 50:497–504.

67. Newnham DM, McDevitt DG, Lipworth BJ. Bronchodilator subsensitivity after chronic dosing with eformoterol in patients with asthma. Am J Med 1994; 97:29–37.

68. Larsson S, Svedmyr N. Bronchodilating effects and side effects of β_2-adrenoceptor stimulants by different modes of administration (tablets, metered aerosol and combinations thereof). Am Rev Respir Dis 1977; 116:861–869.

69. Vilsvik JS, Langaker O, Persson G, Ringdal N, Schaanning J, Kvelstad G, Svensson K, Holthe S, Soliman S. Bambuterol: a new long acting bronchodilating prodrug. Ann Allergy 1991; 66:315–319.

70. Persson G, Baas A, Knight A, Larsen B, Olsson H. One month treatment with the once daily oral β_2-agonist bambuterol in asthmatic patients. Eur Respir J 1995; 8:34–39.

71. Petrie GR, Chookang JY, Hassan WU, Morrison JF, O'Reilly JF, Pearson SB, Shneerson JM, Tang OT, Ning ACWS, Turbitt ML. Bambuterol: effective in nocturnal asthma. Respir Med 1993; 87:581–585.

72. Wallaert B and the French Bambuterol Study Group, Ostinelli J, Arnould B. Long acting β_2-agonists: a comaprison of oral bambuterol and inhaled salmeterol in asthmatic patients with nocturnal symptoms. Eur Respir J 1995; 8:1S.

73. Fugleholm AM, Ibsen TB, Laxmyr L, Svendsen UG. Therapeutic equivalence between bambuterol, 10 mg once daily, and terbutaline controlled release, 5 mg twice daily, in mild to moderate asthma. Eur Respir J 1993; 6:1474–1478.

74. van Schayck CP, Graafsma SJ, Visch MB, Dompeling E, van Weel, van Herwaarden CLA. Increased bronchial hyperresponsiveness after inhaling salbutamol during 1 year is not caused by subsensitization to salbutamol. J Allergy Clin Immunol 1990; 86:793–800.

Discussion

MALCOLM R. SEARS

McMaster University, Hamilton, Ontario, Canada

A. Introduction

Professor Tattersfield has reviewed many studies addressing the efficacy and safety of short- and long-acting beta-agonist medications in the management of asthma. Although there is no doubt as to their efficacy as bronchodilators, concerns have been identified with respect to rebound hyperresponsiveness, decreased control of asthma with regular use, tachyphylaxis to bronchoprotective effects, interactions with corticosteroids, and their possible role in increasing morbidity and mortality of asthma. The short- and long-acting β-agonists differ in some respects, and so they are discussed separately.

B. Short-Acting β-Agonists

Rebound Airway Hyperresponsiveness

Dr. Robin Taylor and I also reviewed the literature regarding the effects of short-acting β-agonists on airway responsiveness, and we have published similar reviews agreeing that overall there is an increase in airway responsiveness during and following use of β-agonists, although studies vary in the magnitude of effect (1,2). Among studies that do not show increased airway responsiveness, there is often a substantial dropout rate among those treated with a regular β-agonist which minimizes the likelihood of detecting the adverse effect.

Asthma Control

The debate over the deleterious effects of regular short-acting β-agonist use on the control of asthma that we reported (3,4) has been fueled by other studies which have either not shown an adverse effect (5) or have reported benefit from regular treatment (6). The duration of the studies, and the potency of the β-agonist used, are likely to be significant factors influencing different outcomes of such studies (7). Although detectable adverse effects are generally small, in population terms these small shifts in severity may translate into a substantial increase in the prevalence of more severe disease, increasing the population susceptible to life-threatening episodes (2).

Studies of withdrawal of β-agonists have been few to date, which is in part due to difficulties in designing and conducting well-controlled studies, but early results have been presented from the United Kingdom, United States, and Japan showing benefit from lower or as-needed doses (8–12). The study of Heino (13) is flawed on several counts, being nonrandomized, uncontrolled, of minimal duration, in patients with little if any room for improvement, and with no data on actual β-agonist usage (14). Heino showed simply that the withdrawal of low-dose twice-daily β-agonist for 2 weeks did not improve stable asthma in subjects using moderate doses of inhaled corticosteroid. The methodological problems inherent in the study make any further interpretation dubious. A recent larger longer trial in Germany, also unblinded but otherwise more substantive, showed a beneficial effect of withdrawing either salbutamol or fenoterol in the majority of subjects (12). The experience of many clinicians who have reduced utilization of inhaled β-agonist has confirmed reports of several decades ago that withdrawal of potent bronchodilators resulted in improvement rather than in deterioration of asthma (15, 16).

Interaction with Corticosteroids

As noted, in one study of regular salbutamol, the area under the bronchodilator dose-response curve decreased with regular use in subjects also taking inhaled corticosteroids (17). Other laboratory and clinical trial data add weight to the possibility of an interaction between high doses of β-agonists and corticosteroids. In our study of regular fenoterol versus as-needed β-agonist, the deleterious effect of fenoterol was not negated by any dose of inhaled corticosteroid (3); on the contrary, in the subgroup of eight patients using the most inhaled corticosteroid (over 1500 μg daily), seven deteriorated during regular fenoterol therapy, a higher proportion than among subjects not using any or lower doses of inhaled corticosteroid. Adcock et al. have demonstrated in vitro that high concentrations of β-agonist inhibit corticosteroid receptor function (18).

Comparison with Corticosteroid Therapy

In order to justify use of β-agonists as first-line treatment, studies are needed to show not only benefit compared with placebo but also greater benefit than alternative treatments. On the contrary, studies in adults and in children show that moderate doses of inhaled corticosteroid are substantially superior to regular inhaled β-agonist in reducing symptoms, improving lung function, and reducing airway hyperresponsiveness (19,20), inflammation (21), and mortality (22). Furthermore, delayed introduction of inhaled corticosteroid appears to produce less beneficial effect than if these drugs are used early as first-line treatment (23,24). This may reflect either progression of disease which has not been beneficially modified by β-agonist or deterioration of asthma as a direct result of several years of β-agonist monotherapy.

Effect of Short-Acting β-Agonists on Allergen Response

Cockcroft and colleagues have shown increases in both early-phase and late-phase responses toa llergen after treatment with regular salbutamol for only 1 or 2 weeks (25,26). This finding is consistent with previous reports of increased response to AMP (27) and provides at least one explanation of the adverse effect of β-agonists on asthma control in atopic subjects.

Conclusions Regarding Short-Acting β-Agonists

Few studies support the regular use of short-acting β-agonists as first-line or maintenance treatment for asthma, and several show significant deleterious effects from such regimens. Many of the criteria suggested by Bradford-Hill (28) for proposing a causal relationship between an intervention and an outcome (strength, consistency, temporality, a dose-response relationship, plausibility, experimental evidence, and coherence) are met in the studies of increasing asthma morbidity and mortality associated with higher-potency β-agonists (2). Potency of β-agonist is highly likely to influence adverse effects, most noticeably seen in the epidemics of asthma mortality observed coincident with the introduction of high-dose isoprenaline and fenoterol (2). A recent report shows a clear dose-response effect of regular β-agonist on airway responsiveness, with no change being found after salbutamol aerosol, 200 μg, three times daily for 1 month, whereas salbutamol, 2.5 mg, by nebulizer three times daily for 8 days increased airway responsiveness by almost fivefold, with PD_{20} falling from 1.95 to 0.43 mg (29). Withdrawal of frequent use of short-acting β-agonists is feasible in many subjects with benefit in control of asthma (8–12).

C. Long-Acting β-Agonists

Clinical Control of Asthma

Again there is no doubt as to the efficacy of these drugs in reducing symptoms of asthma and increasing lung function in the short and medium term. Their use is clearly more beneficial than the regular or frequent use of short-acting agents. To date, there has been no evidence of any increase in morbidity or mortality similar to that seen with the introduction of more potent short-acting β-agonists. Studies of formoterol and salmeterol have now continued for 6 months or more, with sustained bronchodilator effect and no loss of control or rebound increase in airway responsiveness. Questions regarding their safety relate primarily to concerns that their efficacy as bronchodilators may mask on-going airway inflammation that is characteristic of asthma, and to the concern that there may be an increased risk of mortality from the use of salmeterol.

Comparison with Inhaled Corticosteroids

Despite early claims, several biopsy and bronchoalveolar lavage studies show that long-acting β-agonists do not provide anti-inflammatory activity as judged by inflammatory cell counts and cytokine assays in contrast with corticosteroids (21,30–32). Clinical studies comparing the addition of salmeterol to an increased dose of inhaled corticosteroid have used relatively low corticosteroid doses (even when doubled), and their effect may well have been suboptimal (33,34). Such studies need to be repeated using noninvasive markers of inflammation to judge efficacy, such as differential cell counts in induced sputum.

Tachyphylaxis to Bronchoprotection

Several investigators have shown tachyphylaxis of bronchoprotection to methacholine or exercise with the regular use of long-acting β-agonists. Although single-dose studies show protection for up to 12 hr, bronchoprotective effects against AMP, exercise, or methacholine challenge diminish markedly within weeks (35,36). Cockcroft and colleagues have demonstrated tachyphylaxis to methacholine challenge by the third dose of regular treatment, with progressive tachyphylaxis to the seventh dose (37); this effect was not diminished by the concomitant use of inhaled corticosteroids (38). Hence, although the bronchodilitation effect persists, there is a substantial and early loss of the bronchoprotective effect, sharply reducing this justification for the regular use of long-acting β-agonists.

Increase Risk of Breakthrough Bronchoconstriction

Of even greater concern is the possibility that use of long-acting β-agonists could enhance airway responsiveness. Sterk and colleagues showed an increase in steepness of the dose-response curve to methacholine after salbutamol use (39). We have found similar results with salmeterol, and of particular note, we have shown that those with the lowest baseline FEV_1, who are in greatest need of bronchodilatation, show the greatest steepening of the dose-response curve (40). This raises the possibility that if breakthrough bronchoconstriction should occur despite the use of salmeterol, the rapidity of deterioration in asthma could be greater, a possibility suggested by some case reports (41). In our study, bronchoprotection against methacholine was greatest following a single dose of salbutamol, only slightly less following a salbutamol dose after 4 days of twice-daily treatment but substantially less following salmeterol after 4 days of twice-daily treatment, being less than 50% of the protection given by a single dose of salbutamol.

Asthma Mortality

The only study to address asthma mortality in salmeterol-treated patients reported a relative risk of 3 for asthma death compared with subjects treated with regular salbutamol, but this figure was not significant when examined without regard to age of patients (42). The age-related risks of death from asthma were not calculated by the investigators doing the study (43), but our examination of data subsequently provided by the investigators giving the age at death (44) suggested that younger people may have been more at risk (45). To determine whether there is an excess risk of mortality in any particular age group, four items of data are required—the age of each study subject, the age at death of all cases, the age distribution of all asthmatics in the community, and the age at death of asthmatics not in the study. Of these, community prevalence is more difficult but not impossible to obtain; all other data are known. In the UK study, there was a uniform risk of death across all age groups using salmeterol, which is quite different from the pattern seen in the community where greatest asthma prevalence is found in young people and most deaths occur in the elderly. Hence, there may be an increased risk of death among younger subjects using salmeterol.

Conclusions Regarding Long-Acting β-Agonists

Long-acting β-agonists represent an improvement in symptom-controlling therapy as compared with the frequent use of short-acting β-agonists. However, their lack of beneficial effect on airway inflammation, their potential for masking of progressive disease by providing longer symptom relief, and the uncertainty regarding interpretation of the postmarketing surveillance study raise concerns which should lead to detailed ongoing evaluation of the safety of β-agonists in the management of asthma.

References

1. Taylor DR, Sears MR. Bronchodilators and bronchial hyperresponsiveness. Thorax 1994; 49:190.
2. Sears MR, Taylor DR. The β$_2$-agonist controversy. Observations, explanations and relationship to asthma epidemiology. Drug Safety 1994; 11:259–283.
3. Sears MR, Taylor DR, Print CG, et al. Regular inhaled β-agonist treatment in bronchial asthma. Lancet 1990; 336:1391–1396.
4. Taylor DR, Sears MR, Herbison GP, et al. Regular inhaled β-agonist in asthma: effect on exacerbations and lung function. Thorax 1993; 48:134–138.

5. Ikeda K, Nakashima A, Tsukino M. Concomitant regular use of inhaled β₂-agonist additionally to sufficient doses of inhaled steroid did not attenuate morning baseline peak flow rate (PEFR) in asthma. Eur Respir J 1993; 6:602s.

6. Chapman KR, Kesten S, Szalai JP. Regular vs as-needed inhaled salbutamol in asthma control. Lancet 1994; 343:1379–1382.

7. Sears MR, Taylor DR. Regular beta-agonist therapy—the quality of the evidence. Eur Respir J 1992; 5:896–898.

8. Peters MJ, Yates DH, Chung KF, Barnes PJ. Beneficial effect of β₂-agonist dose reduction in asthma. Aust NZ J Med 1994; 24:460.

9. Yates DH, Peters MJ, Keatings V, Worsdell M, Barnes PJ. A comparison of the efficacy of a reduced dose albuterol with standard dosage for symptom relief in asthma. Am J Respir Crit Care Med 1994; 149:A205.

10. Gleason MC, Kamada AK, Nelson HS, Szefler SJ. "As needed" (prn) administration of inhaled beta-adrenergic agonists (iBAA): clinical experimence in pediatric patients. J Allergy Clin Immunol 1993; 91:165.

11. Katayama S, Sugitani A, Shibayama S, Yasuda K. Study of peak expiratory flow changes after cessation of regular fenoterol inhalation. Eur Respir J 1994; 7:261s.

12. Richter B, Buselic K, Heisters J, Richter A, Berger M. Continuous vs on demand inhaled β-agonist therapy on the basis of regular inhaled corticosteroids: a randomised controlled study. Eur Respir J 1995; 8(suppl 19):159s.

13. Heino M. Regularly inhaled β-agonists with steroids are not harmful in stable asthma. J Allergy Clin Immunol 1994; 93:80–84.

14. Sears MR, Taylor DR. Regularly inhaled β-agonists in stable asthma. J Allergy Clin Immunol 1995; 96:137.

15. Reisman RE. Asthma induced by adrenergic aerosols. J Allergy 1970; 40:162–177.

16. Eisenstadt WS, Nicholas SS. The adverse effect of adrenergic aerosols in bronchial asthma. Ann Allergy 1969; 27:283–288.

17. D'Alonzo GE, Nathan RA, Henochowicz S, Morris RJ, Ratner P, Rennard SI. Salmeterol xinofoate as maintenance therapy compared with albuterol in patients with asthma. JAMA 1994; 271:1412–1416.

18. Adcock IM, Peters MJ, Crown CR, Barnes PJ. Interactions between steroids and β-agonists in vitro. Eur Respir J 1994; 7:421s.

19. Haahtela T, Jarvinen M, Kava T, et al. Comparison of a β-agonist, terbutaline, with an inhaled corticosteroid, budesonide, in newly detected asthma. N Engl J Med 1991; 325:388–392.

20. Van Esses-Zandvliet EE, Hughes MD, Waalkens HJ, et al. Effects of 22 months of treatment with inhaled corticosteroids and/or beta-2-agonists on lung function, airway responsiveness, and symptoms in children with asthma. An Rev Respir Dis 1992; 146:547–554.

21. Laitinen LA, Laitinen A, Haahtela T. A comparative study of the effects of an inhaled corticosteroid, budesonide, and a β₂-agonist, terbutaline, on airway inflammation in newly diagnosed asthma: a randomised, double-blind parallel-group trial. J Allergy Clin Immunol 1992; 90:32–43.

22. Ernst P, Spitzer W, Suissa S, et al. Risk of fatal and near fatal asthma in relation to inhaled corticosteroid use. JAMA 1992; 268:3462–3464.

23. Pedersen S, Agertoft L. Effect of long term budesonide treatment on growth, weight and lung function in children with asthma. Am Rev Respir Dis 1993; 147: A265.

24. Haahtela T, Jarvinen M, Kava T, et al. Effects of reducing or discontinuing inhaled budesonide in patients with mild asthma. N Engl J Med 1994; 331:700–705.

25. Cockcroft DW, McPaarland CP, Britto SA, Swystun VA, Rutherford BC. Regular inhaled salbutamol and airway responsiveness to allergen. Lancet 1993; 342:833–837.

26. Cockcroft DW, O'Byrne PM, Swystun VA, Bhagat R. Regular use of inhaled albuterol and the allergen-induced late response. J Allergy Clin Immunol 1995; 96: 44–49.

27. O'Connor BJ, Aikman SL, Barnes PJ. Tolerance to the nonbronchodilator effects of inhaled β_2-agonists in asthma. N Engl J Med 1992; 327:1204–1208.

28. Bradford Hill A. The environment and disease: association or causation? Proc R Soc Med 1965; 58:295–300.

29. Krasnowska M, Malolepszy J, Liebhart E, Passowicz E, Fal AM. The influence of regular salbutamol inhalations on bronchial hyperreactivity in patients with bronchial asthma. Eur Respir J 1995; 8:260s.

30. Boulet L-P, Turcotte H, Dube J, Gagnon M, Lavioloeet M, Boutet M. Influence of salmeterol on chronic and acute antigen-induced airway inflammation. Am J Respir Crit Care Med 1994; 149:A804.

31. Gardiner PV, Ward C, Booth H, Allison A, Hendrick DJ, Walters EH. Effect of eight weeks of treatment with salmeterol on bronchoalveolar lavage inflammatory indices in asthmatics. Am J Respir Crit Care Med 1994; 150:1006–1011.

32. Booth H, Richmond I, Ward C, Gardiner PV, Harkawat R, Walters EH. Effect of high dose fluticasone propionate on airway inflammation in asthma. Am J Respir Crit Care Med 1995; 152:44–52.

33. Greening AP, Ind PW, Northfield M, Shaw G. Added salmeterol versus higher-dose corticosteroid on asthma patients with symptoms on existing inhaled corticosteroid. Lancet 1994; 344:219–224.

34. Woolcock A, Lundback B, Ringdal OLN, Jacques LA. Comparison of the effect of addition of salmeterol with doubling the inhaled steroid dose in asthmatic patients. Am J Respir Crit Care Med 1994; 149:A280.

35. Cheung D, Timmers MC, Zwinderman AH, Bel EH, Dikjman JH, Sterk PJ. Long-term effects of a long-acting β_2-adrenoceptor agonist, salmeterol, on airway hyper-responsiveness in patients with mild asthma. N Engl J Med 1992; 327:1198–1203.

36. Ramage L, Lipworth BJ, Ingram CG, Cree IA, Dhillon DP. Reduced bronchoprotection against exercise induced bronchoconstriction after chronic dosing with salmeterol. Respir Med 1994; 88:363–368.

37. Bhagat R, Kalra S, Swystun VA, Cockcroft DW. Rapid onset of tolerance to the bronchoprotective effect of salmeterol. Chest 1995; 108:1235–1239.

38. Kalra S, Swystun VA, Bhagat R, Cockcroft DW. Inhaled corticosteroids do not prevent the development of tolerance to the bronchoprotective effect of salmeterol. Chest 1996; 109:953–956.

39. Bel EH, Zwinderman AH, Timmers MC, Dijkman JH, Sterk PJ. The protective effect of a beta2 agonist against excessive airway narrowing in asthma and chronic obstructive lung disease. Thorax 1991; 46:9–14.

40. Wong AG, O'Shaughnessy AD, Walker CM, Sears MR. Effects of long-acting and short-acting B-agonists on methacholine dose response curves in asthmatics. Eur Respir J 1997. In press.

41. Clark CE, Ferguson AD, Siddorn JA. Respiratory arrests in young asthmatics on salmeterol. Respir Med 1993; 878;227–228.

42. Castle W, Fuller R, Hall J, Palmer J. Serevent nationwide surveillance study: comparison of salmeterol with salbutamol in asthmatic patients who require regular bronchodilator treatment. Br Med J 1993; 306:1034–1037.

43. Sears MR, Taylor DR. Bronchodilator treatment in asthma. Increase in deaths during salmeterol treatment unexplained. Br Med J 1993; 306:1610–1611.

44. Fuller RW, Castle WM, Hall JR, Palmer JBD. Bronchodilator treatment in asthma. Authors' reply. Br Med J 1993; 306:1611.

45. Sears MR, Taylor DR. Bronchodilator treatment in asthma. Br Med J 1993; 307:446.

Discussion

KENNETH R. CHAPMAN

The Toronto Hospital and University of Toronto, Toronto, Ontario, Canada

A. Studies of Bronchial Hyperreactivity

For many years, a slight decrease in bronchodilator effect has been a known consequence of chronic β_2-agonist bronchodilator use (1). Such tolerance or tachyphylaxis has been attributed to downregulation of the β_2-receptor and has been regarded of little clinical consequence. More recently, investigation with both short-acting and long-acting β_2-agonists has shown mild tolerance or tachyphylaxis to their bronchoprotective effects. Terbutaline given regularly for a period of 1 week was shown to be protective against the bronchoconstriction produced by inhaled cyclic AMP and inhaled methacholine (2). Salmeterol given for 2 months affords less protection against inhaled methacholine (3). However, the latter study reassures that these shifts in bronchoprotection are nonprogressive. That is, the loss of protection resulting from regular use of a β_2-agonist appears to occur in the first week or two of use and does not subsequently worsen.

Of greater concern are reports that the regular use of inhaled β_2-agonists can lead to increased nonspecific bronchial hyperreactivity and increased allergic hyperresponsiveness in subjects with mild asthma. For example, Vathenen has shown that following regular terbutaline use by a group of patients with mild asthma, methacholine PC_{20} drops slightly in the few days following withdrawal of the β_2-agonist (4). Similarly, Kraan and colleagues found significant shifts in methacholine PC_{20} in a group of mild asthmatics taking regular terbutaline for 2 weeks (5). Of note in the latter study, continued use of terbutaline for a further 2 weeks failed to lead to further decline in methacholine PC_{20}. Indeed, there was a return toward baseline, such that the methacholine PC_{20} following 4 weeks of regular terbutaline use was not significantly different from that measured at baseline. Thus, small changes in methacholine PC_{20} do not appear to be progressive over time. Even these minor acute changes do not appear consistently in all studies.

Allergen challenge in patients with mild allergic asthma appears to offer a more realistic laboratory model of naturally occurring asthma. Using allergen challenge, Cockcroft has shown that the regular use of an inhaled β_2-agonist is accompanied by measurable and statistically significant decreases in the provocative concentrations of allergen (6). Curiously, the same study did not show significant shifts in nonspecific bronchial responsiveness as assessed by methacholine challenge. Longer-term studies have not been undertaken to determine whether these changes are progressive or self-limited. Of greater concern is the validity of generalizing results from these studies to the larger population of asthmatics who use β_2-agonists. Of necessity, studies of nonspecific and specific bronchial hyperreactivity are undertaken in subjects with very mild asthma, which are subjects who would not normally use inhaled β_2-agonists on a regular or even frequent basis.

B. Clinical Trials

When published in 1990, the study by Sears and colleagues appeared to bridge the gap between small-scale laboratory studies of β_2-agonists' adverse effects and epidemiological studies associating β_2-agonists with increased morbidity (7). In their careful study, Sears and colleagues recruited a large number of subjects with mild to moderate asthma and asked them to take inhaled fenoterol by two schedules, regular and as needed, in a 1-year crossover trial. Their reporting of results seem to indicate dramatic disadvantages for the regular use of β_2-agonists by patients with asthma. A closer examination of their published data points out some limitations to the study and other possible conclusions. First, a relatively large number of patients initially randomized were lost to follow-up (24%). Second, the study was reported in unconventional terms without presentation of group means for most pulmonary function data. When later reported, these changes in lung function would prove to be relatively small. The variable most responsible for differences between regimens, the morning peak flow rate, differed approximately 10 L/min between treatment regimens (8). Finally, most subjects recruited suffered from relatively mild asthma and would have been unlikely to use regular β_2-agonists under usual clinical circumstances. Just as for laboratory trials of bronchial hyperresponsiveness, it is unclear that findings in these subjects can be extrapolated to patients with more severe disease.

It may also be worth stepping back from the 1-year fenoterol crossover trial and thinking of it as a series of "n-of-1" trials (9). Using this approach, the investigators found that approximately two of three of their patients did not benefit from the regular use of inhaled β_2-agonist. However, the remaining patients either had as good asthma control when taking β_2-agonists regularly as compared with "as needed" or they in fact had better asthma control. Twenty-seven percent, or almost one-third, of the patients had better asthma control taking β_2-agonist in a scheduled fashion. Such findings do not lead to a simple unitary conclusion. It would be unreasonable to state flatly that the regular use of inhaled β_2-agonists is unwarranted for all asthmatics. With further reflection, it seems likely that the population of patients recruited by Sears represents a reasonable cross section typical of primary practice where the majority of patients have mild disease, few have moderate disease, and exceedingly few have severe disease. If the need for β_2-agonists is correlated with disease severity, it would not be surprising to find a majority of patients preferring a β_2-agonist on an intermittent as-needed basis and a minority of patients preferring one on a regular basis.

Our group has reported an abbreviated crossover trial comparing regular inhaled salbutamol with as-needed salbutamol in 341 asthmatic patients (10). In contrast to the findings of Sears and colleagues, the majority of our patients had better symptom control using their β_2-agonist on a scheduled basis. Moreover, we could detect no adverse effect in terms of worsening morning or evening peak expiratory flow rate during the regular β_2-agonist treatment period. Although our study used inhaled salbutamol rather than inhaled fenoterol, we suspect that the difference between studies is not so much the choice of β_2-agonist as in the selection of patients. Patients with more severe disease were recruited for our study leading to the intuitively obvious and plausible finding that a regular β_2-agonist was more likely to be of symptomatic benefit.

C. β_2-Agonists vs. the Alternatives

Discussing the adverse effects of β_2-agonists without discussing the alternatives is unwise. If patients with symptomatic asthma are to be denied effective β_2-agonists, the remaining options are to suffer symptomatic disease without treatment or to receive alternative treatment. The contemporary approach is to offer inhaled corticosteroids or other inhaled anti-inflammatories in a preventive fashion.

Various national and international consensus guidelines currently advocate the early and sometimes aggressive use of inhaled corticosteroids to control disease (11,12). However, it would be prudent to note that our use of inhaled corticosteroids in this fashion is relatively recent and untested by appropriate clinical trials. Although the reasons for advocating anti-inflammatory therapy are plausible, they remain largely hypothetical. Goals such as inducing long-term remission and preventing airway remodeling are laudable but may apply to a minority of the asthmatic population at large (13). Such reservations would be of little concern if inhaled corticosteroid use were completely benign. However, this may not be the case.

There is increasing evidence that patients are receiving more inhaled corticosteroids than is absolutely essential for control of disease. For example, recently published studies of inhaled corticosteroid withdrawal in stable asthmatic patients have shown that as many as two-thirds may be taking more glucocorticoid than is necessary (14,15). Moreover, the dose response to inhaled corticosteroids remains a matter of some controversy. There is considerable evidence that the dose response to inhaled corticosteroids is not linear. Hummel and colleagues, for example, reported that the oral steroid-sparing properties of beclomethasone were no different between daily dosages of 400 and 1500 μg (16). Nonetheless, many international consensus guidelines advocate the use of inhaled corticosteroid dosage in excess of 1000 μg of beclomethasone per day (or equivalent) in the hope of extinguishing bronchodilator need.

With the earlier and more widespread use of inhaled corticosteroids in higher dosage, reports have begun to appear to systemic side effects. Easy bruising and dermal thinning are widely reported consequences of inhaled corticosteroid use (17). More worrisome, reports have begun to link the use of inhaled corticosteroids to decreases in bone density. For example, Packe and colleagues have recently reported that asthmatics using inhaled corticosteroids had significant decreases in bone density as compared with asthmatics who used bronchodilator alone (18). In their study, bone density was not different between asthmatics currently using inhaled corticosteroids and asthmatics currently using oral corticosteroids. These findings have been questioned; many of the patients currently taking inhaled corticosteroids had previously used oral corticosteroids. However, more recent studies have demonstrated decreases in bone density among asthmatics who have not used oral corticosteroids on a regular basis. Our group, for example, has recently reported significant decreases in bone density among asthmatics using moderate amounts of inhaled corticosteroid for 3–4 years in the absence of previous oral corticosteroid consumption (19). These decreases in bone density were correlated with the dose and duration of inhaled corticosteroids. This latter finding not only underscores the relationship between inhaled corticosteroid use and adverse connective tissue effects, but suggests that the effect may not be self-limited but rather may be progressive with continued use. Such findings should give pause to those who advocate the aggressive use of inhaled corticosteroids so as to extinguish all bronchodilator need. A more appropriate approach might be a thoughtful balancing of bronchodilator need and preventive therapy bearing in mind the risks of each pharmacological agent.

Against this background, the studies of Greening et al. and Woolcock et al. provide valuable information about the optimal balance of long-acting β_2-agonist bronchodilators and inhaled corticosteroids (20,21). Further study will be needed to determine the long-term consequences of the available therapeutic approaches. In a disease which lasts a lifetime, a study of even 6–12 months is relatively brief.

References

1. McFadden ER, Jr. Clinical use of beta-adrenergic agonists. J Allergy Clin Immunol 1985; 76:352–356.
2. O'Connor BJ, Aikman SL, Barnes PJ. Tolerance to the nonbronchodilator effects of inhaled β_2-agonists in asthma. N Engl J Med 1992; 327:1204–1208.
3. Cheung D, Timmers MC, Zwinderman AH, Bel EH, Dijkman JH, Sterk PJ. Long-term effects of a long-acting β_2-adrenoceptor agonist, salmeterol, on airway hyperresponsiveness in patients with mild asthma. N Engl J Med 1992; 327:1198–1203.
4. Vathenen AS, Knox AJ, Higgins BG, Britton JR, Tattersfield AE. Rebound increase in bronchial responsiveness after treatment with inhaled terbutaline. Lancet 1988; 1:554–558.
5. Kraan J, Koeter GH, v.d.Mark TW, Sluiter HJ, de Vries K. Changes in bronchial hyperreactivity induced by 4 weeks of treatment with antiasthmatic drugs in patients with allergic asthma: a comparison between budesonide and terbutaline. J Allergy Clin Immunol 1985; 76:628–636.
6. Cockcroft DW, McParland CP, Britto SA, Swystun VA, Rutherford BC. Regular inhaled salbutamol and airway responsiveness to allergen. Lancet 1993; 342:833–837.
7. Sears MR, Taylor DR, Print CG, Lake DC, Li QQ, Flannery EM, et al. Regular inhaled beta-agonist treatment in bronchial asthma. Lancet 1990; 336:1391–1396.
8. Sears MR. Should we be using β-agonists for treatment of chronic asthma? In: Costello JF, Mann RD, eds. Beta Agonists in the Treatment of Asthma. The proceedings of a symposium held at the Royal Society of Medicine, London, February 1992. New York: Parthenon, 1992:79–88.
9. Guyatt GH, Keller JL, Jaeschke R, Rosenbloom D, Adachi JD, Newhouse MT. The n-of-1 randomized controlled trial: clinical usefulness. Our three-year experience. Ann Intern Med 1990; 112:293–299.
10. Chapman KR, Kesten S, Szalai JP. Regular vs as-needed inhaled salbutamol in asthma control. Lancet 1994; 343:1379–1382.
11. Lenfant C, Sheffer AL, Bousquet J, Busse WW, Clark TJH, Dahl R, et al. International consensus report on diagnosis and management of asthma. Bethesda, MD: U.S. Department of Health and Human Services, Publication #92-3091. 1992.

12. British Thoracic Society, British Paediatric Association, Research Unit of the Royal College of Physicians of London, King's Fund Centre, National Asthma Campaign, Royal College of General Practitioners in Asthma Group, et al. Guidelines on the management of asthma. Thorax 1993; 48:S1–S24.

13. Bousquet J, Vignola AM, Chanez P, Campbell AM, Bonsignore G, Michel F-B. Airways remodelling in asthma: no doubt, no more. Int Arch Allergy Immunol 1995; 107:211–214.

14. Haahtela T, Järvinen M, Kava T, Kiviranta K, Koshinen S, Lehtonen K, et al. Effects of reducing or discontinuing inhaled budesonide in patients with mild asthma. N Engl J Med 1994; 331:700–705.

15. Agertoft L, Pedersen S. Importance of the inhalation device on the effect of budesonide. Arch Dis Child 1993; 69:130–133.

16. Hummel S, Lehtonen L. Comparison of oral-steroid sparing by high-dose and low-dose inhaled steroid in maintenance treatment of severe asthma. Lancet 1992; 340: 1483–1487.

17. Hanania NA, Chapman KR, Kesten S. Adverse effects of inhaled corticoids. Am J Med 1995; 98:196–208.

18. Packe GE, Douglas JG, McDonald AF, Robins SP, Reid DM. Bone density in asthmatic patients taking high dose inhaled beclomethasone dipropionate and intermittent system corticosteroids. Thorax 1992; 47:414–417.

19. Hanania NA, Chapman KR, Sturtridge WC, Szalai JP, Kesten S. Dose-related decrease in bone density among asthmatic patients treated with inhaled corticosteroids. J Allergy Clin Immunol 1995; 96:571–579.

20. Greening AP, Ind PW, Northfield M, Shaw G. Added salmeterol versus higher-dose corticosteroid in asthma patients with symptoms on existing inhaled corticosteroid. Lancet 1994; 344:219–224.

21. Woolcock A, Lundback B, Ringdal OLN, Jacques LA. Comparison of the effect of addition of salmeterol with doubling the inhaled steroid dose in asthmatic patients (abstr). Am J Respir Crit Care Med 1993; 149:A280.

13

Clinical Studies of Beta$_2$-Adrenergic Agonists in Children

F. ESTELLE R. SIMONS

University of Manitoba
Winnipeg, Manitoba, Canada

I. Introduction

In infants and children, as in adults, β_2-adrenergic agonists are the most effective bronchodilators available (1). Increasingly, the use of short acting β_2-adrenergic agonists is limited to the prevention of exercise-induced bronchospasm and the relief of breakthrough symptoms of wheeze, cough, and shortness of breath and acute asthma episodes (2). The basic pharmacology of β_2-adrenergic agonists is age independent (3,4) and is not reviewed here.

The clinical pharmacology of β_2-adrenergic agonists has been reasonably well studied in infants and children with asthma. Functional β_2-adrenoreceptors are present in the airways of young mammals (5). Short-acting β_2-adrenergic agonists have a bronchodilator and bronchoprotective effect in infants and young children (6–19). The degree of bronchodilation and bronchoprotection achieved is age related throughout infancy and early childhood.

Interpretation of the data on the effect of age and response to β_2-adrenergic agonists is complicated by the fact that the primary pathology of asthma may differ in infants and in young children compared with adults. In the very young, airway narrowing may be more due to fixed obstruction as a result of airway wall edema and excess mucus than to smooth muscle shortening. Edema is less likely to respond to β_2-adrenergic agonist treatment than smooth muscle spasm does. Also, the precise dose of β_2-adrenergic agonists administered by inhalation to very young patients may be difficult to control, especially if the medication is given by wet nebulization. Variables such as nose versus mouth breathing, inspiratory flow rate, airway geometry, nebulizer type, dilution volume, driving gas flow rate, and aerosol droplet size affect the site of deposition in the airway. The acidity, osmolarity, and preservative content of the solution being aerosolized may affect the bronchodilator response.

In a recent study in which children ages 3–9 years were trained to use a spirometer reliably and to complete dose-response curves, a significant age effect on bronchodilator response to nebulized salbutamol (albuterol) was

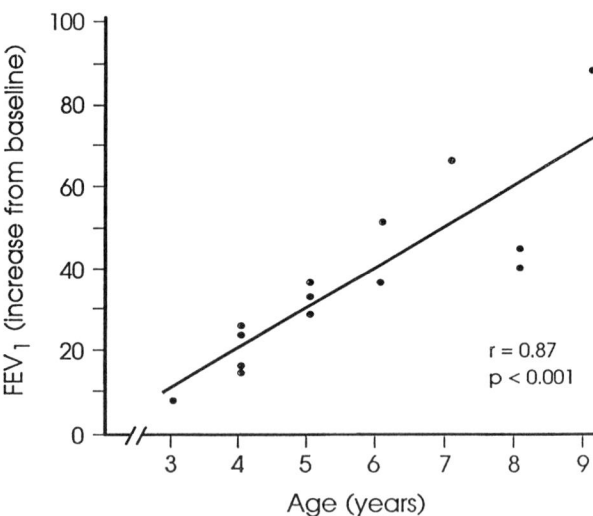

Figure 1 Asthmatic children aged 3–9 years with an FEV_1 <80% predicted were trained to produce an FEV_1 with a standard deviation of <200 ml. They completed a dose-response curve by inhaling nebulized salbutamol every 15 min up to a cumulative total of five doses (6.84 mg). FEV_1, FVC, and $FEF_{25-75\%}$ were measured in all subjects; SaO_2 and heart rate in some. The percentage increase in FEV_1 after the last salbutamol dose regressed with age as shown. Each point of data represents one child. A significant effect of age on the bronchodilator response (FEV_1, FVC) was detected, with older children responding better than younger ones, in whom the response plateaued after the maximum dose. (From Ref. 6.)

detected in the FEV_1 and the FVC. Despite receiving a lower microgram per kilogram dose, the older children had a greater improvement than the younger ones, in whom the response plateaued after the maximum dose of 6.84 mg (6) (Fig. 1).

The bronchoprotective effect of β_2-adrenergic agonists has been studied in infants as well as in children with chronic asthma (10–16). Even in infants less than 12 months of age, salbutamol has been shown to have a protective effect on the response to nebulized water, carbachol, methacholine (16) (Fig. 2), and histamine. Exercise-induced bronchospasm is the most practical and widely used model for the study of the onset and duration of the bronchoprotective effect of β_2-adrenergic agonists in young subjects (17–19). Using the exercise model, β_2-adrenergic agonists have also been studied in nonasthmatic children, in whom they do not enhance the submaximal running economy or peak oxygen consumption (20).

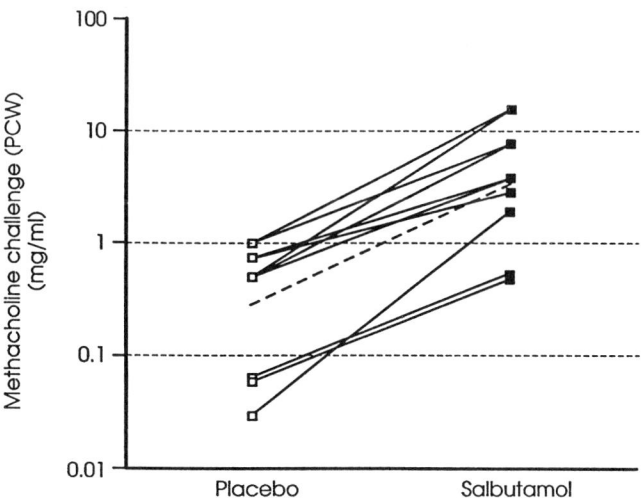

Figure 2 In a double-blind, crossover study, nine asthmatic children aged 2–5 years had a methacholine challenge test after placebo or salbutamol administered via metered-dose inhaler (MDI) and a Babyhaler (Glaxo Wellcome, U.K.). The provocative concentration causing wheezing (PCW) increased from a geometrical mean of 0.28 mg/ml after placebo to 3.59 mg/ml after albuterol ($P < .0001$), a protective effect of 3.87 ± 1.2 doubling doses. The dashed line indicates geometrical mean. Salbutamol reduces bronchial hyperreactivity in young wheezy children. (From Ref. 16.)

II. Chronic Asthma

A. Short-Acting β₂-Adrenergic Agonists

Studies of the comparative efficacy of inhaled short-acting β₂-adrenergic agonists in children with chronic asthma have been performed over a broad age range using many different medications and inhalation devices (21–27). The best-studied medications are salbutamol and terbutaline. All inhaled β₂-adrenergic agonists tested are effective bronchodilators for the relief of episodic wheezing, coughing, and shortness of breath in children with asthma regardless of the device used to administer them: metered-dose inhaler with or without valved aerosol spacer or various sized holding chamber, used with or without a face mask; and a variety of dry-powder inhalers, including the Turbuhaler (Astra Draco, Lund, Sweden), Rotahaler, Diskhaler (Glaxo Wellcome, U.K.), or Autohaler (3M Riker, USA).

In school-age children, superiority of one β₂-adrenergic agonist over another or of one inhalation device over another cannot be readily demonstrated. In younger children, the administration of β₂-adrenergic agonists via some inhalation devices is more effective than via others. For example, although approximately 50% of 4- and 5-year-olds can use the Turbuhaler satisfactorily after a single instruction (26) (Fig. 3), young patients may find other dry-powder inhalers such as the Diskhaler and Rotahaler more difficult to use, as they may not have a sufficiently high inspiratory flow rate to permit the powder to exit these devices.

Metered-dose inhalers provide an efficient means of medication delivery, but they require hand coordination with inspiration. In very young children, they must be used in conjunction with a spacer and a face mask. In infants and children under age 2 years, who have a small tidal volume, low-volume spacers (<350 ml) can be cleared more readily than high-volume spacers. In older children, the latter are more efficient, although rather more cumbersome. Evaluation of β₂-adrenergic agonists administered by metered-dose inhalers using nonchlorofluorocarbon propellants is underway in children (28).

The administration of β₂-adrenergic agonists by wet nebulization, air compressor, and face mask, although effective, is now seldom recommended for home use, as it is relatively inefficient, cumbersome, costly, and time consuming (29). A power source is required, and considerable training of caregivers is needed. In young asymptomatic infants, the administration of salbutamol by this route has caused paradoxical deterioration in lung function, and hypoxemia (30). The dose of the drug may be affected by the air entrainment which occurs when inspiratory flow exceeds nebulizer flow. When given a nebulizer solution concentration, infants who do not entrain will inspire a more concentrated aerosol than older children (31). Also,

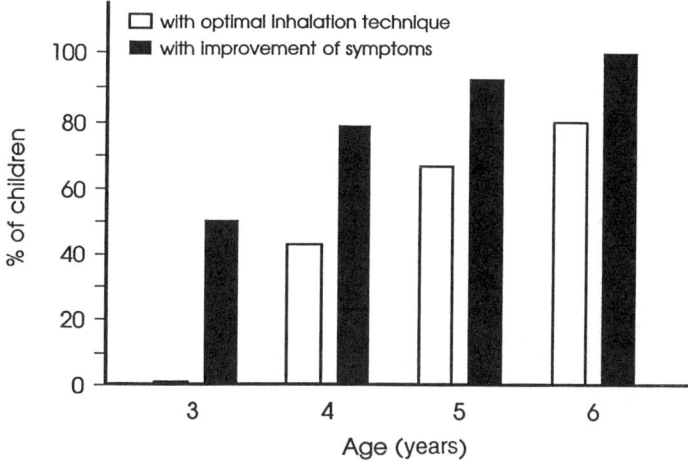

Figure 3 Fifty-nine unselected children with asthma aged 3–6 years old were given a single instruction in how to use the terbutaline Turbuhaler. No 3-year-olds, 43% of 4-year-olds, 67% of 5-year-olds, and 80% of 6-year-olds used the Turbuhaler correctly. Asthma symptoms improved in 50% of 3-year-olds and 79, 92, and 100% of 4-, 5-, and 6-year-olds, respectively. The Turbuhaler can be used satisfactorily in children as young as 4 years of age. (From Ref. 26.)

during home use, nebulizers have proved unhygienic, and may transmit *Pseudomonas* species and other potentially pathogenic aerobic, gram-negative bacteria (32).

B. Long-Acting β₂-Adrenergic Agonists

The long-acting β_2-adrenergic agonists salmeterol and formoterol have been reasonably well-studied in adolescents but not in infants or young children with regard to onset and duration of action (33–45). They provide excellent bronchodilation for 12–24 hr in older children and adolescents with chronic asthma (33–40). Significant bronchodilator action is present as early as 5, 10, or 15 min after a 25- or 50-μg salmeterol dose compared with placebo; however, the 25-μg dose of salmeterol produces significantly less bronchodilation than salbutamol, 200 μg, 5, 10, and 15 min after inhalation, and the 50-μg salmeterol dose produces significantly less bronchodilation than salbutamol 5 and 10 min after inhalation with no significant difference being noted at 15 min (34) (Fig. 4A).

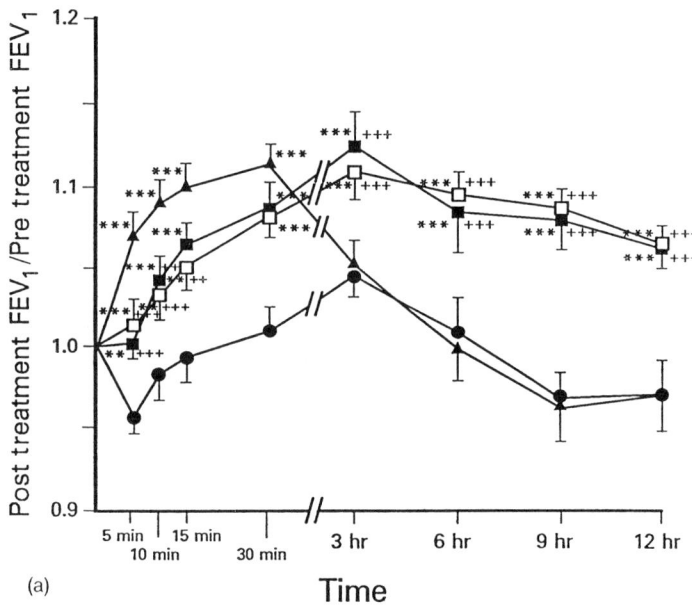

(a)

Time

Figure 4 In a double-blind, crossover study in 20 children, the bronchodilator and bronchoprotective effects of doses of salmeterol, 25 or 50 μg, salbutamol, 200 μg, and placebo were compared. (a) Mean baseline FEV_1 did not change significantly after placebo, but increased significantly from 5 to 30 min after salbutamol and from 5 min to 12 hr after salmeterol, 25 or 50 μg, compared with placebo. After both doses of salmeterol, FEV_1 was significantly lower than after salbutamol at 5 and 10 min but did not differ at 30 min, and it was significantly greater than after salbutamol from 3 to 12 hr. At 15 min, the effect of salmeterol, 50 μg, and salbutamol did not differ significantly. (b) After placebo, PC_{20} methacholine did not change. After salbutamol, PC_{20} increased significantly only at 30 min. After salmeterol, 25 or 50 μg, PC_{20} increased significantly from 30 min to 12 hr. Salmeterol, 25 and 50 μg, provided significantly greater broncho-protection than salbutamol from 3 to 12 hr and from 30 min to 12 hr, respectively, and over the latter time period, salmeterol, 50 μg, provided significantly better broncho-protection than salmeterol, 25 μg. The amount of change in PC_{20} accounted for by change in FEV_1 varied from 14 to 28%, indicating that protection against bronchocon-striction is not entirely dependent on bronchodilation. (From Ref. 34.)

A single dose of salmeterol, 25–50 μg (34) (Fig. 4B), or formoterol, 12 μg, also provides excellent protection against methacholine-induced broncho-spasm for 12–24 hr (34–37) and protection against exercise-induced broncho-spasm (EIB) for at least 8 hr (38–41). Like the short-acting β₂-adrenergic agonists, the long-acting medications shift the stimulus response curve to exercise in a beneficial direction. Unlike the short-acting medications,

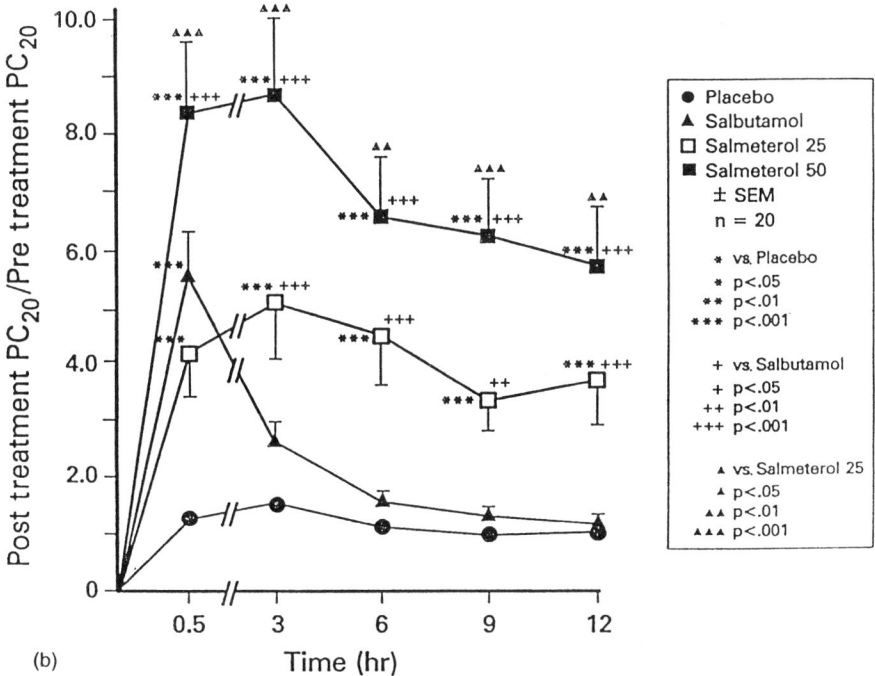

(b)

which do not entirely eliminate airflow obstruction, the long-acting β_2-adrenergic agonists may almost completely abolish the postexercise decrease in peak expiratory flow or FEV_1 throughout the dosing interval, thus potentially providing protection against exercise-induced asthma throughout the school day (41) (Fig. 5). In young subjects, there is preliminary evidence that the bronchoprotective effect of the long-acting β_2-adrenergic agonists may diminish during chronic use (41) (Fig. 6).

In multicenter studies of up to 1 year duration, salmeterol, 25 μg or 50 μg, twice daily regularly, in contrast to salbutamol, 200 μg, twice daily regularly, has decreased the need for "rescue" bronchodilator treatment and improved nocturnal asthma symptoms and morning peak expiratory flows measured before dosing of either β_2-adrenergic agonist (42–44). Salmeterol, 100 μg, twice daily has been found to be effective and well-tolerated in adolescents with severe chronic asthma in residential treatment (45). Additional long-term studies of regular administration of salmeterol in children have now been completed (see Discussion).

Guidelines prepared at the 1995 International Pediatric Consensus Conference on the Management of Asthma contain the recommendation that long-

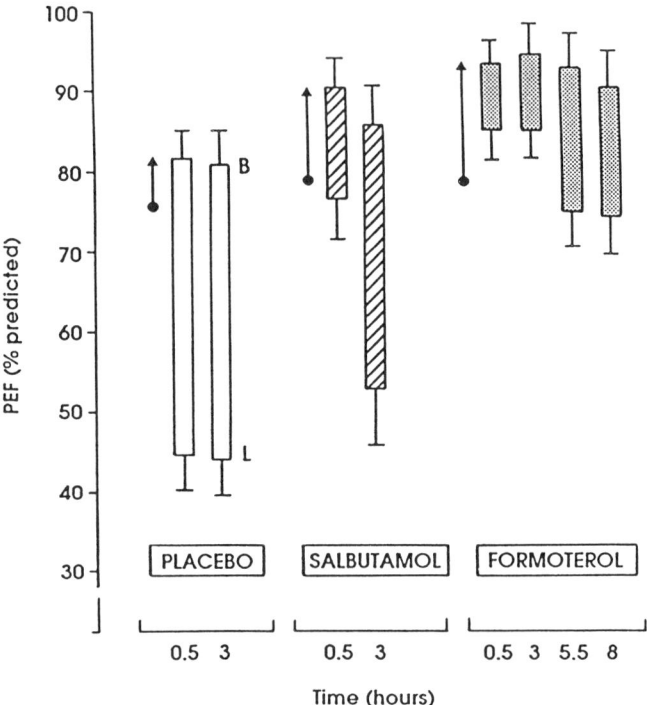

Figure 5 In a double-blind, crossover, placebo-controlled study in 12 children with exercise-induced asthma (greater than 25% fall from baseline FEV_1 on a pretrial standardized treadmill test), formoterol, 12 μg, blocked exercise-induced asthma significantly for 8 hr in contrast to salbutamol, 200 μg, which blocked it for 0.5 hr. The mean duration of a 50% reduction in exercise-induced asthma was 6.5 hr for formoterol and 1.5 hr for salbutamol. Placebo had no significant effect. The arrows indicate change in baseline after medications. B, pre-exercise baseline value. L, the lowest recorded value after exercise. (From Ref. 39.)

acting β_2-adrenergic agonists should be used only in conjunction with regular inhaled glucocorticoid treatment in children and should, in fact, be reserved for use in children requiring high-dose glucocorticoid treatment (2).

C. Oral β_2-Adrenergic Agonists

Salbutamol, terbutaline, metaproterenol, and other β_2-adrenergic agonists are available in oral formulations, including syrups, tablets, and granules. These formulations are still used in infants and young children despite their relatively

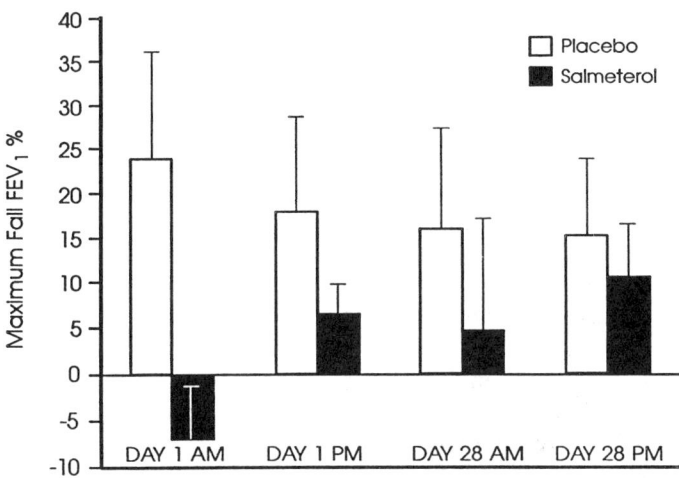

Figure 6 In a double-blind, crossover, placebo-controlled study in 14 adolescents, mean age 13 years, salmeterol, 50 µg, was administered once daily by a Nebulizer Chronolog which recorded the date, hour, and minute of the dose. It did not protect significantly (p = 0.1) against exercise-induced bronchospasm 9 hr after dosing on day 28 of treatment, compared to placebo, as it did 1 and 9 hours after dosing on day 1 of treatment (p = 0.0001, p = 0.0002) and 1 hour after dosing on day 28 of treatment (p = 0.0002) (from Ref. 41).

slow onset of action and less favorable benefit/risk ratio when compared with the same medication administered by inhalation. The efficacy and safety of oral β₂-adrenergic agonists has generally been studied during regular administration three or four times daily rather than during intermittent use for relief of breakthrough asthma symptoms (46–49). There is little to justify their use except that they are palatable and easy to administer. They are therefore prescribed for infants and children who dislike or refuse inhaled medications or whose parents are unable or unwilling to learn how to administer inhaled medications.

Therapeutic options with regard to other classes of oral bronchodilators are limited. Oral β₂-adrenergic agonists are as effective as methylxanthines, and if an oral bronchodilator is required, many physicians prefer to prescribe β₂-adrenergic agonists because of their relatively favorable safety profile and the absence of a need to monitor serum concentrations (50).

D. Concerns Regarding the Regular Use of β₂-Adrenergic Agonists in Children

The 1995 International Guidelines contained the recommendation that short-acting β₂-adrenergic agonists should be used in children only to prevent exercise-induced asthma and as rescue medications on an "as needed" or "on demand" or "rescue" basis to relieve intermittent "breakthrough" symptoms of wheezing, coughing, and shortness of breath. Regular daily use is not recommended. The use of inhaled β_2-adrenergic agonists on a rescue basis more than three times weekly at any level of treatment is deemed to be a signal that treatment of chronic inflammation in the airways needs to be started or increased (2).

There are several long-term, well-designed, well-controlled studies of regular β_2-adrenergic agonist use in children (51–54). In one double-blind study of 6 months duration in 19 children, budesonide, 200 μg, three times daily regularly was associated with significantly decreased bronchial hyperreactivity in 7 of 12 patients. In contrast, the seven children receiving terbutaline, 500 μg, three times daily regularly had a slight increase in bronchial hyperreactivity. The increase plateaued at 2–3 months and was not associated with a significant loss of bronchodilator effect. One of the seven children receiving terbutaline alone experienced an increase in asthma symptoms (51).

In another study of 8 weeks' duration, 12 children with mild asthma received budesonide, 200 μg, twice daily and terbutaline, 500 μg, four times daily regularly, and 15 children received placebo and terbutaline regularly. PC_{20} improved by 2.1 doubling doses in those inhaling both budesonide and terbutaline and by 1.3 doubling doses in those inhaling terbutaline and placebo. FEV_1 and diurnal variation of peak expiratory flow did not change in either group. The children treated with both budesonide and terbutaline also showed improvement in morning and nocturnal peak expiratory flows and decreased peak flow reversibility; they wheezed less but did not have decreased cough or shortness of breath (52).

In a larger double-blind, multicenter study, 116 children with asthma received either budesonide, 0.2 mg, plus salbutamol, 0.2 mg, three times daily or placebo plus salbutamol, 0.2 mg, three times daily. After a median follow-up time of 22 months, 45% of the children receiving the β_2-agonist alone had withdrawn from randomized treatment, mainly because of asthma symptoms, compared with withdrawal of only three children receiving concurrent treatment with budesonide and salbutamol. This study has been interpreted as providing evidence that regular treatment with β_2-adrenergic agonists such as salbutamol does not increase asthma symptoms, worsen pulmonary function, or increase bronchial hyperresponsiveness, but this interpretation is probably not valid because of the high drop-out rate in children being treated regularly with the β_2-agonist alone (53) (Fig. 7).

In another study, treatment with salbutamol, 200 μg, four times daily regularly for 6 months did not result in any loss of bronchodilator effect, but significant downregulation of β_2-receptors on peripheral mononuclear cells

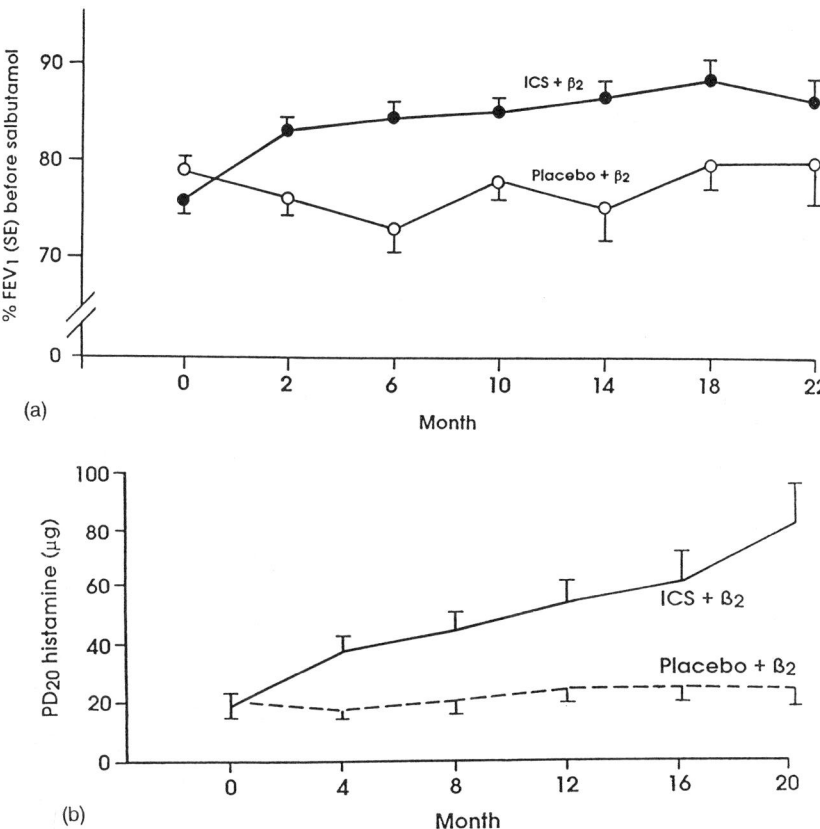

Figure 7 In a randomized double-blind, multicenter study, 116 children with asthma were treated with either budesonide, 0.2 mg, plus salbutamol, 0.2 mg, three times daily (ICS plus β_2) or salbutamol, 0.2 mg, plus placebo three times daily (placebo plus β_2) via metered-dose inhaler. (a) FEV_1 expressed as a percentage of predicted value for age, sex, and height showed an absolute increase of 7% after 2 months of treatment with ICS plus β_2 compared with a decrease of 4% after 2 months of treatment with placebo plus β_2, and this 11% difference was maintained after a median follow-up period of 22 months ($P < .0001$). (b) Mean airway responsiveness expressed as the provocative dose of histamine required to give a 20% fall in FEV_1 increased from baseline to 4 months by 0.98 doubling doses in the children receiving ICS plus β_2 compared with a decrease of 0.42 doubling doses in children receiving placebo plus β_2, a difference of 1.4 doubling doses ($P < .0001$). This difference had not plateaued after the median follow-up period of 22 months, by which time 26 patients (45%) of those receiving placebo plus β_2 had withdrawn from randomized treatment, mainly because of asthma symptoms, compared with 3 withdrawals in the group receiving ICS plus β_2 ($P < .00010$). Long-term regular treatment with a β_2-adrenergic agonist is undesirable. (From Ref. 53.)

occurred as early as the third to seventh day of treatment (54). Bronchoprotection was not tested.

E. Concerns Regarding Overuse of β_2-Adrenergic Agonists in Children

Short-acting inhaled β_2-adrenergic agonists are the most useful medications available for rescue treatment of asthma symptoms because of their rapid onset of action and lack of troublesome adverse effects. The lack of compliance with physician recommendations for β_2-adrenergic agonists use includes overuse as well as underuse, as documented by administering the medication using a Nebulizer Chronolog (Medtrac Technologies, Lakewood, CO) or other electronic device for timing inhalations (55). In children, as in adults, the frequency of β_2-adrenergic agonist inhalations serves as an indicator of asthma severity and the need for additional anti-inflammatory treatment.

In asthmatics of all ages, there are concerns that overuse of β_2-adrenergic agonists may contribute to increased mortality. In children, deaths from asthma are, fortunately, quite rare. Mortality is decreasing in preschoolers, and it has remained stable in children aged 5–15 years despite the increased prevalence of the disease and the widespread underuse of anti-inflammatory medications (56).

In most recent asthma mortality studies, although children age 5 years and older have been included, age-stratified data are not readily available (57–61). The mean age of the patients in these studies ranges from 12 to 32 years (62) (Fig. 8). There is some suggestion that the association between β_2-adrenergic agonist use and death increases as the mean age of the sample increases. Nevertheless, based on evidence obtained primarily in young adults and extrapolated to the pediatric age group, the use of more than one cannister of β_2-adrenergic agonist (200 doses) per month or equivalent by a child is generally considered to be a strong indicator that asthma is not optimally controlled, and that he or she may be at increased risk for morbidity and mortality. Further studies of this issue are needed in young children.

III. Acute Asthma

A. Use of β_2-Adrenergic Agonists in the Treatment of Acute Asthma

During the past two decades, bronchodilator treatment for children presenting to healthcare facilities with acute asthma episodes has changed dramatically. Injected epinephrine and intravenously administered aminophylline, the "gold standards" for more than half a century, have been replaced by the admini-

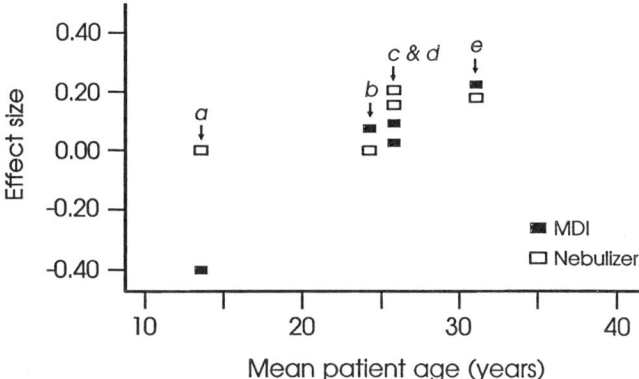

Figure 8 In case-controlled studies examining the use of β_2-adrenergic agonists among patients with asthma who died and among those who did not die, the association between β_2-adrenergic agonist use and death appears to be more likely in adults than in adolescents or children. The tendency for the β_2-adrenergic agonist–death relationship to increase as a function of sample age is significant for delivery via metered-dose inhaler (MDI) ($r = 0.954$, $z = 2.338$, $P = .00969$), although not for nebulizer delivery ($r = 0.692$, $z = 0.626$, $P = .2658$) or for oral delivery (not shown). (a, Ref. 57b, Ref. 59; c, Ref. 60; d, Ref. 58; e, Ref. 61.) (From Ref. 62.)

stration of the nebulized β_2-adrenergic agonists salbutamol or terbutaline (63–70). Various dosage regimens have been studied: for example, salbutamol low-dose, 0.05 mg/kg; standard dose, 0.15 mg/kg; and high dose, 0.3–0.5 mg/kg. A fixed-dose of salbutamol, 2.5 mg/2.5 ml, is as effective as a dose calculated on a milligram/kilogram basis. Various dose frequencies have also been studied, ranging from intermittent (every 3hr) to semicontinuous (every 20 min) to continuous nebulization, which, as might be expected, produces the most rapid improvement. Nebulized β_2-adrenergic agonists act locally in the airways; there is little correlation between serum β_2-adrenergic agonist concentrations and the increase in FEV_1 (64,65,69).

Optimally, volume fill in the nebulizer should be 4 ml in order to avoid the potential problem of a progressive increase in osmolality and resulting paradoxical bronchoconstriction which may occur during inhalation. The face mask should fit tightly, as if it is even 1 cm away from the face, medication delivery to the airways decreases by 50% or more. Mouth breathing rather than nasal breathing should be encouraged.

During severe acute asthma attacks, supplemental oxygen should be administered during β_2-adrenergic agonist treatment and oxygen saturation should be monitored (71–73). β_2-Adrenergic agonists may cause a transient decrease in arterial oxygen tension, due to ventilation/perfusion mismatching (74). Children with prolonged falls in SaO_2 should have a chest radiograph to facilitate identification and treatment of any pulmonary consolidation that may be present (75).

Recently, several groups of investigators have confirmed that during acute asthma episodes, the administration of salbutamol via metered-dose inhaler, face mask, and spacer is as effective or perhaps even more effective than intermittent nebulization via compressor and face mask (76–78). This method of administration is being used more frequently in hospitals, because it is cost effective with regard to the time required to administer medication to children by nurses or respiratory therapists (77) (Fig. 9). During acute asthma episodes, although peak inspiratory flow is reduced, most school-age children can still generate the required peak inspiratory flow needed to achieve bronchodilation from terbutaline administered via the Turbuhaler (79).

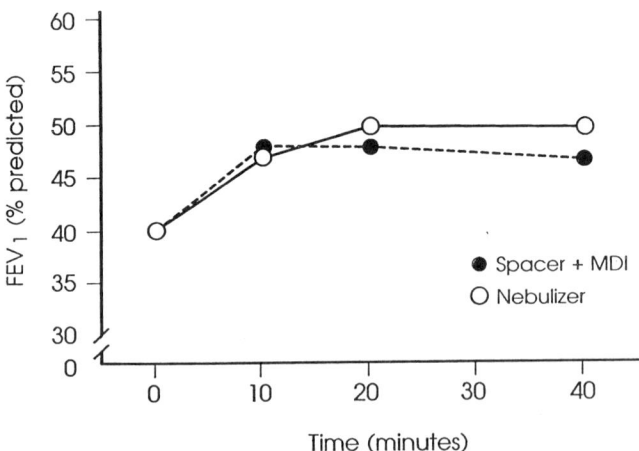

Figure 9 In a double-blind, 40-min study, 33 children in the emergency department (aged 6–14 years, FEV_1, 20–70% predicted) were given aerosolized salbutamol or placebo by MDI-spacer followed by salbutamol or placebo given by nebulizer with oxygen. The ratio of salbutamol doses administered by MDI-spacer/nebulizer was 1:5. No difference in the rate of improvement of clinical score, respiratory rate, SaO_2, or FEV_1 was noted between the two groups. Heart rate increased in the nebulizer group and decreased in the MDI-spacer group ($P < .05$). Spacers and nebulizers are equally effective in delivering β_2-agonists to children with acute asthma. (From Ref. 77.)

B. β₂-Adrenergic Agonists in Bronchiolitis

Discussion of the use of β₂-adrenergic agonists in acute asthma would be incomplete without mention of their use in bronchiolitis, as in infants with wheezing, coughing, or shortness of breath, it may be difficult to distinguish between acute asthma and bronchiolitis. Most of the early studies of β₂-adrenergic agonists in bronchiolitis were performed in small numbers of infants recovering in the hospital from severe bronchiolitis (80,81). Attempts to demonstrate efficacy, often unsuccessful, were generally made after sedation of the infants for pulmonary function tests such as the measurement of maximum flow at functional residual capacity (81). Although "negative" studies of β₂-adrenergic agonists in bronchiolitis continue to be published

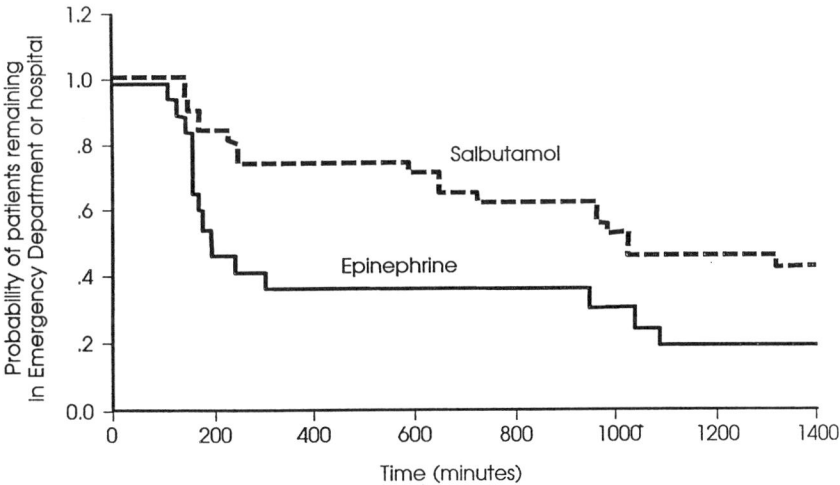

Figure 10   In a double-blind, parallel-group study, the efficacy of nebulized epinephrine was compared with that of nebulized salbutamol in the treatment of 42 infants with acute bronchiolitis. The mean ages of the groups were 0.4 ± 0.2 and 0.5 ± 0.2 years, respectively. The doses administered were epinephrine: 3 ml of 1/1000 solution and salbutamol: 0.3 ml of a 5 mg/mL solution combined with 2.7 ml of 0.9% saline. Both medications were administered by nebulizer with continuous-flow oxygen at 5–6 L/min. Mean percentage of oxygen saturation at 60 min was significantly higher in the epinephrine group. Thirty-three percent of the infants receiving epinephrine were admitted to the hospital compared with 81% of those receiving salbutamol ($P < .003$). The survival curve in the figure illustrates that epinephrine-treated infants spent a significantly shorter time in the emergency department at the hospital than salbutamol-treated infants did ($P < .02$). (From Ref. 89.)

(82,83), there is increasing evidence that salbutamol is effective in the treatment of this disorder, as documented using symptom scores, SaO_2, and respirosonography or other novel, noninvasive, objective methods of assessing lung function (84–87).

Nebulized epinephrine may be even more effective than nebulized salbutamol in bronchiolitis (88,89) in contrast to acute asthma in which injected epinephrine is less effective than nebulized salbutamol (63). In a recent study, faster discharge from the emergency department, a decreased hospital admission rate, increased oxygen saturation, and decreased heart rate were shown in infants receiving epinephrine compared with those receiving salbutamol. With the exception of pallor, adverse effects were not significantly more frequent in babies receiving epinephrine (89) (Fig. 10). Nebulized metaproterenol is also effective in the treatment of acute bronchiolitis (90).

A trial of β_2-adrenergic agonist treatment is generally given to all infants with bronchiolitis ill enough to require medical attention; however, the debate about the use of β_2-adrenergic agonists in this disorder will probably continue for some time.

IV. Additional Safety Issues Regarding β_2-Adrenergic Agonists in Children

A. Safety of Usual Doses

Despite the ubiquitous use of β_2-adrenergic agonists in children around the world, remarkably few adverse effects are attributed to these medications. Where reported, adverse effects are expected pharmacological actions that occur when the β_2-adrenergic agonists are absorbed into the systemic circulation. As the medications are nearly always given by inhalation, and as plasma concentrations are negligible, adverse effects are infrequent even in hospitalized children receiving semicontinuous or continuous nebulization (64,65,69,91–94). Cardiotoxicity does not occur with the β_2-selective agents, although transient elevation of creatinine kinase (MB) (CK-MB) may be noted (93). Transient hyperglycemia has also been reported (94). The commonest adverse effect is tremor caused by direct stimulation of the β_2-adrenergic receptors in skeletal muscle (95).

Although salbutamol does not penetrate the central nervous system to any significant extent, hallucinations have been reported after salbutamol inhalation from a metered-dose inhaler. They have been attributed to the chlorofluorocarbon propellant, which can produce hallucinations when administered alone (96).

An increased prevalence of dental caries has been reported in adults inhaling β_2-adrenergic agonists regularly, which has been attributed to decreased saliva secretion (97). This has not been confirmed in children. The regular administration of oral or even inhaled β_2-agonists impairs growth hormone secretion (98), but the clinical relevance of this observation is unknown. In any event, regular long-term β_2-agonist treatment is no longer recommended.

B. Intentional Overdose

After ingestion of doses averaging 10 times the therapeutic oral salbutamol dose, tachycardia, widened pulse pressure, agitation, irritability, nausea, and vomiting have been reported. Laboratory test abnormalities include hyperglycemia, delayed hypoglycemia, hypokalemia, hypomagnesemia, hypocarbia, increased white blood cell count, and ketonuria (99–104). The threshold salbutamol dose for development of three or more signs of toxicity is 1 mg/kg (99). After overdose, plasma salbutamol concentrations usually correlate with tachycardia and hypokalemia (100). Symptoms are usually transient. Although some patients require intravenous potassium treatment in the emergency department, hospitalization is almost never required and fatalities are virtually unknown (99–104).

V. Conclusions

In children with chronic asthma, β_2-adrenergic agonists used intermittently play an important role in the prevention of exercise-induced asthma and as rescue medications in the treatment of breakthrough acute asthma symptoms. They should be administered via the inhaled route wherever possible. Although β_2-adrenergic agonists are useful bronchodilators in infants, additional studies of their effect on the developing lung are needed. Regular administration of short-acting β_2-adrenergic agonists should be avoided. The role of the long-acting β_2-adrenergic agonists salmeterol and formoterol is being defined. At present, these medications are reserved for use in children with frequent breakthrough symptoms despite regular inhaled glucocorticoid use.

In acute asthma, β_2-adrenergic agonists are the most effective bronchodilators available. Although traditionally they have been administered by wet nebulization, there is a trend to administering them by metered-dose inhaler and a spacer device.

β_2-adrenergic agonists are relatively safe medications in the usual pharmacological sense. The main concerns are potential loss of their bronchoprotective effects during long-term regular use and their potential contribution to asthma morbidity and mortality if overused by young patients in lieu of adequate anti-inflammatory treatment.

Acknowledgment

We gratefully acknowledge the assistance of Lori McNiven.

References

1. Nelson HS. β-Adrenergic bronchodilators. N Engl J Med 1995; 333:499–506.
2. Warner JO, et al. Third international pediatric consensus on the management of childhood asthma. In press.
3. Barnes PJ. Beta-adrenergic receptors and their regulation. Am J Respir Crit Care Med 1995; 152:838–860.
4. Hochhaus G, Mollmann H. Pharmacokinetic/pharmacodynamic characteristics of the β-2-agonists terbutaline, salbutamol and fenoterol. Int J Clin Pharmacol Ther Toxicol 1992; 30:342–362.
5. Birnkrant DJ, Mader SL, Van Lunteren E, Davis PB. Chronic hypoxia increases β-adrenergic receptor density in the lungs of young and old rats. Mech Ageing Dev 1991; 60:135–142.
6. Turner DJ, Landau LI, LeSouëf PN. The effect of age on bronchodilator responsiveness. Pediatr Pulmonol 1993; 15:98–104.
7. Kraemer R, Frey U, Sommer CW, Russi E. Short-term effect of albuterol, delivered via a new auxiliary device, in wheezy infants. Am Rev Respir Dis 1991; 144: 347–351.
8. Waalkens HJ, Merkus PJFM, van Essen-Zandvliet EEM, Brand PLP, Gerritsen J, Duiverman EJ, Kerrebijn KF, Knol K, Quanjer PH, and the Dutch CNSLD Study Group. Assessment of bronchodilator response in children with asthma. Eur Respir J 1993; 6:645–651.
9. O'Callaghan C, Milner AD, Swarbrick A. Nebulised salbutamol does have a protective effect on airways in children under 1 year old. Arch Dis Child 1988; 63: 479–483.
10. Merkus PJFM, Eelkman Rooda HM, van Essen-Zandvliet EEM, Duiverman EJ, Quanjer PH, Kerrebijn KF. Assessment of bronchodilatation after spontaneous recovery from a histamine challenge in asthmatic children. Thorax 1992; 47:355–359.
11. Henderson AJW, Young S, Stick SM, Landau LI, LeSouëf PN. Effect of salbutamol on histamine induced bronchoconstriction in healthy infants. Thorax 1993; 48: 317–323.
12. Orlowski L, Zychowicz C, Migdal M, Gutkowski P. Effect of salbutamol on specific airway resistance in infants with a history of wheezing. Pediatr Pulmonol 1991; 10: 191–194.
13. Tepper RS. Airway reactivity in infants: a positive response to methacholine and metaproterenol. J Appl Physiol 1987; 62:1155–1159.
14. Wilts M, Hop WCJ, van der Heyden GHC, Kerrebijn KF, de Jongste JC. Measurement of bronchial responsiveness in young children: comparison of transcutaneous oxygen tension and functional residual capacity during induced bronchoconstriction and -dilatation. Pediatr Pulmonol 1992; 12:181–185.

15. Bibi H, Montgomery M, Pasterkamp H, Chernick V. Relationship between response to inhaled salbutamol and methacholine bronchial provocation in children with suspected asthma. Pediatr Pulmonol 1991; 10:244–248.
16. Avital A, Godfrey S, Schachter J, Springer C. Protective effect of albuterol delivered via a spacer device (Babyhaler) against methacholine induced bronchoconstriction in young wheezy children. Pediatr Pulmonol 1994; 17:281–284.
17. Shapiro GG, Kemp JP, DeJong R, et al. Effects of albuterol and procaterol on exercise-induced asthma. Ann Allergy 1990; 64:273–6.
18. Svenonius E, Arborelius M, Wiberg R, Stahl E, Svensson M. A comparison of terbutaline inhaled by Turbuhaler and by a chlorofluorocarbon inhaler in children with exercise-induced asthma. Allergy 1994; 49:408–412.
19. Lopes dos Santos JM, Costa H, Stahl E, Wiren JE. Bricanyl Turbuhaler and Ventolin Rotahaler in exercise-induced asthma in children. Allergy 1991; 46:203–205.
20. Unnithan VB, Thomson KJ, Aitchison TC, Paton JY. β2-agonists and running economy in prepubertal boys. Pediatr Pulmonol 1994; 17:378–382.
21. Connor WT, Dolovich MB, Frame RA, Newhouse MT. Reliable salbutamol administration in 6- to 36-month-old children by means of a metered dose inhaler and Aerochamber with mask. Pediatr Pulmonol 1989; 6:263–267.
22. Laberge S, Spier S, Drblik SP, Turgeon JP. Comparison of inhaled terbutaline administered by either the Turbuhaler dry powder inhaler or a metered-dose inhaler with spacer in preschool children with asthma. J Pediatr 1994; 124:815–817.
23. Völkl KP, Kroll VM, Wiesemann HG, Schneider B. Clinical efficacy of two β2-sympathicomimetics in different inhalers in children with asthma. Arzneim-Forsch/Drug Res 1991; 41:533–536.
24. Cunningham SJ, Crain EF. Reduction of morbidity in asthmatic children given a spacer device. Chest 1994; 106:753–757.
25. Green CP, Price JF. Bronchodilator effect of salbutamol via the Volumatic in children. Respir Med 1991; 85:325–326.
26. Goren A, Noviski N, Avital A, Maayan C, Stahl E, Godfrey S, Springer C. Assessment of the ability of young children to use a powder inhaler device (Turbuhaler). Pediatr Pulmonol 1994; 18:77–80.
27. Kesten S, Elias M, Cartier A, Chapman KR. Patient handling of a multidose dry powder inhalation device for albuterol. Chest 1994; 105:1077–1081.
28. Custovic A, Taggart SCO, Stuart A, Robinson A, Woodcock A. GR106642X: a new non-ozone depleting inhaler propellant in childhood asthma. Am J Respir Crit Care Med 1995; 151:A364.
29. Anonymous. The nebuliser epidemic. Lancet 1984; 2:789–790.
30. O'Callaghan C, Milner AD, Swarbrick A. Paradoxical deterioration in lung function after nebulised salbutamol in wheezy infants. Lancet 1986; 2:1424–1425.
31. Collis GG, Cole CH, LeSouëf PN. Dilution of nebulised aerosols by air entrainment in children. Lancet 1990; 336:341–343.
32. Wexler MR, Rhame FS, Blumenthal MN, Cameron SB, Juni BA, Fish LA. Transmission of gram-negative bacilli to asthmatic children via home nebulizers. Ann Allergy 1991; 66:267–271.
33. Foucard T, Lönnerholm G. A study with cumulative doses of formoterol and salbutamol in children with asthma. Eur Respir J 1991; 4:1174–1177.

34. Simons FER, Soni NR, Watson WTA, Becker AB. Bronchodilator and broncho-protective effects of salmeterol in young patients with asthma. J Allergy Clin Immunol 1992; 90:840–846.

35. Verberne AAPH, Hop WCJ, Bos AB, Kerrebijn KF. Effect of a single dose of inhaled salmeterol on baseline airway caliber and methacholine-induced airway obstruction in asthmatic children. J Allergy Clin Immunol 1993; 91:127–134.

36. Becker AB, Simons FER. Formoterol, a new long-acting selective β_2-adrenergic receptor agonist: double-blind comparison with salbutamol and placebo in children with asthma. J Allergy Clin Immunol 1989; 84:891–895.

37. Von Berg A, Berdel D. Efficacy of formoterol metered aerosol in children. Lung 1990; 168(suppl):90–98.

38. Green CP, Price JF. Prevention of exercise induced asthma by inhaled salmeterol xinafoate. Arch Dis Child 1992; 67:1014–1017.

39. Henriksen JM, Agertoft L, Pedersen S. Protective effect and duration of action of inhaled formoterol and salbutamol on exercise-induced asthma in children. J Allergy Clin Immunol 1992; 89:1176–1182.

40. Boner AL, Spezia A, Piovesan P, Chiocca E, Maiocchi G. Inhaled formoterol in the prevention of exercise-induced bronchoconstriction in asthmatic children. Am J Respir Crit Care Med 1994; 149:935–939.

41. Simons FER, Gerstner T, Cheang M. Tolerance to the bronchoprotective effect of salmeterol in adolescents with exercise-induced asthma. Pediatrics. In press.

42. Boner A. Salmeterol: long-term studies in children. Eur Respir J 1993; 15(suppl): 318s.

43. Verberne A, Lenney W, Kerrebijn KF, et al. A 3-way crossover study comparing twice daily dosing of salmeterol, 25 μg and 50 μg with placebo in children with mild to moderate reversible airways disease. Am Rev Respir Dis 1991; 143:A20.

44. Russell G, Williams DAJ, Weller P, Price JF. Salmeterol xinafoate in children on high dose inhaled steroids. Ann Allergy Asthma Immunol 1995; 75:423–428.

45. Hewer SL, Hobbs J, French D, Lenney W. Pilgrim's progress: the effect of salmeterol in older children with chronic severe asthma. Respir Med 1995; 89:435–440.

46. Fuglsang G, Hertz B, Holm E-B. No protection by oral terbutaline against exercise-induced asthma in children: a dose-response study. Eur Respir J 1993; 6:527–530.

47. Fuglsang G, Hertz B, Holm EB, Borgström L. Absolute bioavailability of terbutaline from a CR-granulate in asthmatic children. Biopharm Drug Disp 1990; 11: 85–90.

48. Mulligan S, Devane J, Martin M. Pharmacokinetic characteristics of a novel controlled-release sprinkle formulation of salbutamol. Eur J Drug Metab Pharmacokinet 1991; Special Issue No. 3:312–314.

49. LeBourgeois M, de Blic J, Chauvin J-P, Scheinmann P, Paupe J. Treatment of asthma with tulobuterol or albuterol in school-age children. Clin Ther 1990; 12: 513–519.

50. Rachelefsky GS, Katz RM, Mickey MR, Siegel SC. Metaproterenol and theophylline in asthmatic children. Ann Allergy 1980; 45:207–212.

51. Kerrebijn KF, van Essen-Zandvliet EEM, Neijens HJ. Effect of long-term treatment with inhaled corticosteroids and beta-agonists on the bronchial responsiveness in children with asthma. J Allergy Clin Immunol 1987; 79:653–659.
52. Waalkens HJ, Gerritsen J, Koëter GH, Krouwels FH, van Aalderen WMC, Knol K. Budesonide and terbutaline or terbutaline alone in children with mild asthma: effects on brochial hyperresponsiveness and diurnal variation in peak flow. Thorax 1991; 46:499–503.
53. Van Essen-Zandvliet EE, Hughes MD, Waalkens HJ, Duiverman EJ, Pocock SJ, Kerrebijn KF, The Dutch Chronic Non-Specific Lung Disease Study Group. Effects of 22 months of treatment with inhaled corticosteroids and/or beta-2-agonists on lung function, airway responsiveness, and symptoms in children with asthma. Am Rev Respir Dis 1992; 146:547–554.
54. Schuster A, Kozlik R, Reinhardt D. Influence of short- and long-term inhalation of salbutamol on lung function and β_2-adrenoceptors of mononuclear blood cells in asthmatic children. Eur J Pediatr 1991; 150:209–213.
55. Milgrom H, Bender B, Ackerson L, Bowry P, Smith B, Rand C. Children's compliance with inhaled asthma medications. J Allergy Clin Immunol 1995; 95:217.
56. Warner JO. Review of prescribed treatment for children with asthma in 1990. Br Med J 1995; 311:663–666.
57. Miller BD, Strunk RC. Circumstances surrounding the deaths of children due to asthma: A case-control study. Am J Dis Child 1989; 143:1294–1299.
58. Grainger J, Woodman K, Pearce N, Crane J, Burgess C, Keane A, Beasley R. Prescribed fenoterol and death from asthma in New Zealand, 1981–7: a further case-control study. Thorax 1991; 46:105–111.
59. Pearce N, Grainger J, Atkinson M, Crane J, Burgess C, Culling C, Windom H, Beasley R. Case-control study of prescribed fenoterol and death from asthma in New Zealand, 1977–81. Thorax 1990; 45:170–175.
60. Crane J, Pearce N, Flatt A, Burgess C, Jackson R, Kwong T, Ball M, Beasley R. Prescribed fenoterol and death from asthma in New Zealand, 1981–1983: case control study. Lancet 1989; 1:917–922.
61. Spitzer WO, Suissa S, Ernst P, Horwitz RI, Habbick B, Cockcroft D, Boivin J-F, McNutt M, Buist AS, Rebuck AS. The use of β-agonists and the risk of death and near death from asthma. N Engl J Med 1992; 326:501–506.
62. Mullen B. Asthma mortality and β_2-agonists: results of a meta-analysis of studies examining β_2-agonists. In: Stevens R, ed. International Respiratory Forum. Current Perspectives in β_2-agonist Therapy. Birkshire, UK: Colwood House, 1994:6–12.
63. Becker AB, Nelson NA, Simons FER. Inhaled salbutamol (albuterol) vs injected epinephrine in the treatment of acute asthma in children. J Pediatr 1983; 102:465–469.
64. Schuh S, Parkin P, Rajan A, Canny G, Healy R, Rieder M, Tan YK, Levison H, Soldin SJ. High- versus low-dose, frequently administered, nebulized albuterol in children with severe, acute asthma. Pediatrics 1989; 83:513–518.
65. Schuh S, Reider MJ, Canny G, Pender E, Forbes T, Tan YK, Bailey D, Levison H. Nebulized albuterol in acute childhood asthma: comparison of two doses. Pediatrics 1990; 86:509–513.

66. Bentur L, Canny GJ, Shields MD, Kerem E, Schuh S, Reisman JJ, Fakhoury K, Pedder L, Levison H. Controlled trial of nebulized albuterol in children younger than 2 years of age with acute asthma. Pediatrics 1992; 89:133–137.
67. Oberklaid F, Mellis CM, LeSouëf PN, Geelhoed GC, Maccarrone AL. A comparison of a bodyweight dose versus a fixed dose of nebulised salbutamol in acute asthma in children. Med J Aust 1993; 158:751–753.
68. Papo MC, Frank J, Thompson AE. A prospective, randomized study of continuous versus intermittent nebulized albuterol for severe status asthmaticus in children. Crit Care Med 1993; 21:1479–1486.
69. Moler FW, Johnson CE, Van Laanen C, Palmisano JM, Nasr SZ, Akingbola O. Continuous versus intermittent nebulized terbutaline: plasma levels and effects. Am J Respir Crit Care Med 1995; 151:602–606.
70. Lowenthal D, Kattan M. Facemasks versus mouthpieces for aerosol treatment of asthmatic children. Pediatr Pulmonol 1992; 14:192–196.
71. Seidenberg J, Mir Y, von der Hardt H. Hypoxaemia after nebulised salbutamol in wheezy infants: the importance of aerosol acidity. Arch Dis Child 1991; 66:672–675.
72. Holmgren D, Sixt R. Effects of salbutamol inhalations on transcutaneous blood gases in children during the acute asthmatic attack: from acute deterioration to recovery. Acta Paediatr 1994; 83:515–519.
73. Prendiville A, Rose A, Maxwell DL, Silverman M. Hypoxaemia in wheezy infants after bronchodilator treatment. Arch Dis Child 1987; 62:997–1000.
74. Yiallouros PK, Milner AD. Effective pulmonary blood flow in children with acute asthma attack requiring hospitalization. Pediatr Pulmonol 1994; 17:370–377.
75. Connett G, Lenney W. Prolonged hypoxaemia after nebulised salbutamol. Thorax 1993; 48:574–575.
76. Rubin BK, Nakanishi AK, Smith E, Lamb B, Albers GM. Albuterol administered by metered dose inhaler with a holding chamber is more effective than nebulization in treating acute asthma in children. Am J Respir Crit Care Med 1995; 151:A364.
77. Kerem E, Levison H, Schuh S, O'Brodovich H, Reisman J, Bentur L, Canny GJ. Efficacy of albuterol administered by nebulizer versus spacer device in children with acute asthma. J Pediatr 1993; 123:313–317.
78. Chou KJ, Cunningham SJ, Crain EF. Metered-dose inhalers with spacers vs nebulizers for pediatric asthma. Arch Pediatr Adolesc Med 1995; 149:201–205.
79. Drblik SP, Lapierre G, McManus B, Payer P, Thivierge R, Verdy I, Gaudreault P. Peak inspiratory flow (PIF) measured with and without the Turbuhaler (Tb) dry powder inhaler (DPI) in 6-16 year olds during an acute asthmatic episode. Am J Respir Crit Care Med 1995; 151:A365.
80. Stokes GM, Milner AD, Hodges IGC, et al. Nebulized therapy in acute severe bronchiolitis in infancy. Arch Dis Child 1983; 58:279–283.
81. Hughes DM, Lesouëf PN, Landau LI. Effect of salbutamol on respiratory mechanics in bronchiolitis. Pediatr Res 1987; 22:83–86.
82. Ho L, Collis G, Landau LI, Le Souef PN. Effect of salbutamol on oxygen saturation in bronchiolitis. Arch Dis Child 1991; 66:1061–1064.
83. Wang EEL, Milner R, Allen U, Maj H. Bronchodilators for treatment of mild bronchiolitis: a factorial randomised trial. Arch Dis Child 1992; 67:289–293.

84. Schuh S, Canny G, Reisman JJ, Kerem E, Bentur L, Petric M, Levison H. Nebulized albuterol in acute bronchiolitis. J Pediatr 1990; 117:633–637.

85. Schuh S, Johnson D, Canny G, Reisman J, Shields M, Kovesi T, Kerem E, Bentur L, Levison H, Jaffe D. Efficacy of adding nebulized ipratropium bromide to nebulized albuterol therapy in acute bronchiolitis. Pediatrics 1992; 90:920–923.

86. Tal A, Sanchez I, Pasterkamp H. Respirosonography in infants with acute bronchiolitis. Am J Dis Child 1991; 145:1405–1410.

87. Klassen TP, Rowe PC, Sutcliffe T, Ropp LJ, McDowell IW, Li MM. Randomized trial of salbutamol in acute bronchiolitis. J Pediatr 1991; 118:807–811.

88. Kristjánsson S, Lodrup Carlsen KC, Wennergren G, Strannegard I-L, Carlsen K-H. Nebulised racemic adrenaline in the treatment of acute bronchioilitis in infants and toddlers. Arch Dis Child 1993; 69:650–654.

89. Menon K, Sutcliffe T, Klassen TP. A randomized trial comparing the efficacy of epinephrine with salbutamol in the treatment of acute bronchiolitis. J Pediatr 1995; 126:1004–1007.

90. Alario AJ, Lewander WJ, Dennehy P, Seifer R, Mansell AL. The efficacy of nebulized metaproterenol in wheezing infants and young children. Am J Dis Child 1992; 146:412–418.

91. Kelly HW, McWilliams BC, Katz R, Murphy S. Safety of frequent high dose nebulized terbutaline in children with acute severe asthma. Ann Allergy 1990; 64:229–233.

92. Penna AC, Dawson KP, Manglick P, Tam J. Systemic absorption of salbutamol following nebulizer delivery in acute asthma. Acta Paediatr 1993; 82:963–966.

93. Katz RW, Kelly HW, Crowley MR, Grad R, McWilliams BC, Murphy SJ. Safety of continuous nebulized albuterol for bronchospasm in infants and children. Pediatrics 1993; 92:666–669.

94. Dawson KP, Penna AC, Manglick P. Acute asthma, salbutamol and hyperglycemia. Acta Paediatr 1995; 84:305–307.

95. Mazer B, Figueroa-Rosario W, Bender B. The effect of albuterol aerosol on fine-motor performance in children with chronic asthma. J Allergy Clin Immunol 1990; 86:243–248.

96. Schnapf BM, Santeiro ML. Beta-agonist inhaler causing hallucinations. Pediatr Emerg Care 1994; 10:87–88.

97. Ryberg M, Möller C, Ericson T. Saliva composition and caries development in asthmatic patients treated with β_2-adrenoceptor agonists: a 4-year follow-up study. Scand J Dent Res 1991; 99:212–218.

98. Ghigo E, Valetto MR, Gaggero L, Visca A, Valente F, Bellone J, Castello D, Camanni F. Therapeutical doses of salbutamol inhibit the somatotropic responsiveness to growth hormone-releasing hormone in asthmatic children. J Endocrinol Invest 1993; 16:271–275.

99. Wiley JR, Spiller HA, Krenzelok EP, Borys DJ. Unintentional albuterol ingestion in children. Pediatr Emerg Care 1994; 10:193–196.

100. Lewis LD, Essex E, Volans GN, Cochrane GM. A study of self poisoning with oral salbutamol—laboratory and clinical features. Hum Exp Toxicol 1993; 12: 397–401.

101. Leikin JB, Linowiecki KA, Soglin DF, Paloucek F. Hypokalemia after pediatric albuterol overdose: a case series. Am J Emerg Med 1994; 12:64–66.
102. Spiller HA, Ramoska EA, Henretig FM, Joffe M. A two-year retrospective study of accidental pediatric albuterol ingestions. Pediatr Emerg Care 1993; 9:338–340.
103. King WD, Holloway M, Palmisano PA. Albuterol overdose: a case report and differential diagnosis. Pediatr Emerg Care 1992; 8:268–271.
104. Wasserman D, Amitai Y. Hypoglycemia following albuterol overdose in a child. Am J Emerg Med 1992; 10:556–557.

Discussion

ANDREA VON BERG

Marienhospital Wesel, Wesel, Germany

A. Introduction

The position of short-acting β_2-agonists in the treatment of childhood asthma has been defined, whereas the place of the new long-acting β_2-agonists formoterol and salmeterol still remained a point in question, since too few data of long-term outcome were available until recently. Meanwhile results from long-term studies with both formoterol and salmeterol have been reported.

B. Long-Term Studies with Formoterol

Two studies investigated the efficacy and safety of formoterol monotherapy over a period of 3 months. An open study with regular 12 µg bd formoterol in 14 children aged 5–14 years with mild to moderate asthma showed a marked improvement in lung-function which was maintained throughout treatment. Additional 12 µg formoterol given 8 hr after the morning dose produced further bronchodilatation that diminished slightly although not significantly at the end of the treatment period, which might be interpreted as an indication for tolerance (Fig. D–1) (1).

A second parallel group study compared double-blind and double-dummy 12 µg bd formoterol versus 200 µg td salbutamol in 24 children aged 6–14 years with mild to moderate asthma. Lung function and histamine challenges were performed before treatment, on the first and 90th day of treatment 2 and 8 hr after the morning dose (formoterol), respectively, 2 hr after the morning and 4 hr after the midday dose (salbutamol) and 24 hr after the last dose (Fig. D–2a). In addition, bronchodilation tests with 12 µg formoterol and 200 µg salbutamol were performed on days 30 and 60, respectively (2). Compared with pretreatment, prechallenge lung function improved significantly at all time points during treatment with salbutamol except on day 90 4 hr postdose, but with formoterol only on day 1 2 hr postdose. Twenty-four

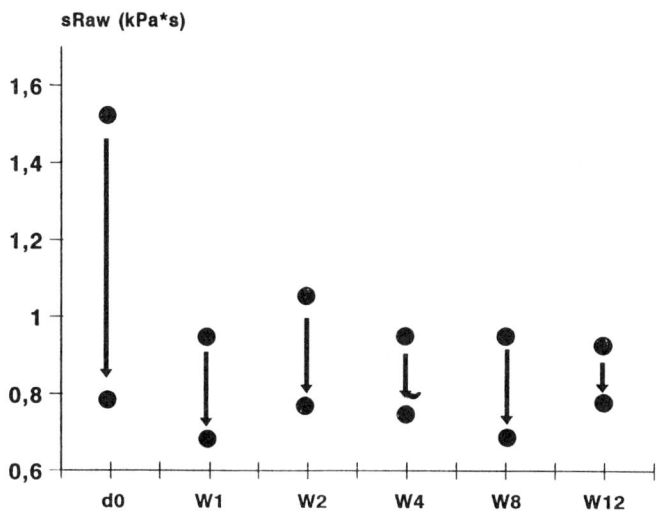

Figure D–1 Specific airway resistance (sRaw) before and 30 min after 12 μg formoterol before (d0) and during treatment with 2 × 12 μg formoterol for 12 weeks (w1–w12) (1).

hours after the last dose (day 91), there was a slight increase in specific airway resistance (sRaw) above pretreatment values with both formoterol and salbutamol (Fig. D–2b). The bronchodilation effect of formoterol lost significance after 2 months of treatment (Fig. D–2c). Again this might indicate the development of tolerance and a possible rebound effect. Protection of formoterol against histamine challenge was significant on the first and last days of the 3 month's treatment 2 hr postdose but missed significance after 8 hr. Salbutamol provided protection on the first but not on the 90th day. Bronchial responsiveness after treatment with formoterol and salbutamol was not significantly different from baseline (Fig. D–2d).

C. Long-Term Studies with Salmeterol

Two similar multicenter double-blind studies, one parallel-group study in 394 young asthmatics (3), and the other a crossover study in 91 children (4), compared efficacy, bronchial responsiveness, and safety of 50 μg bd salmeterol with placebo. A 2-week run-in was followed by two 6-month treatment periods with a 2-week off-treatment and a 2-week follow-up. Salbutamol as "rescue" medication and anti-inflammatory concomitant medication was permitted.

Patients kept twice daily peak-flow (PEF) records and symptom scores throughout. Morning and night PEF increased significantly compared with

Schedule

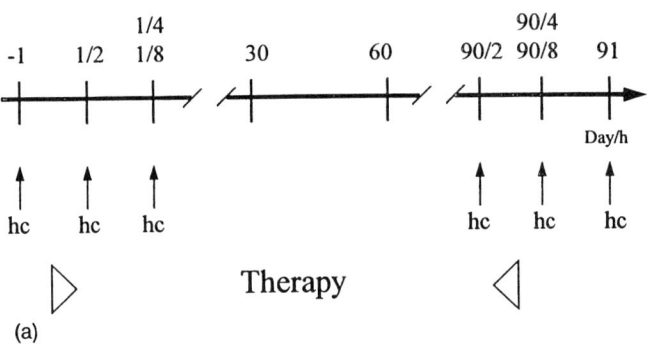

(a)

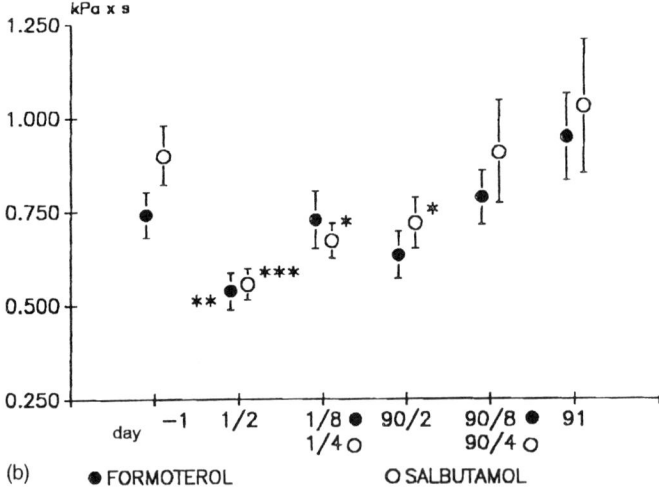

(b)   ● FORMOTEROL   O SALBUTAMOL

Figure D–2   (a) Schedule of the double-blind, parallel-group study in which 2 × 12 μg formoterol was compared versus 3 × 200 μg salbutamol over 90 days in 24 asthmatic children. Histamine challenges (hc) were performed before treatment (-1) and 24 hr after the last inhalation (91) and during treatment on the 1st and 90th day 2 and 8 hr after inhalation of formoterol (1/2, 1/8, 90/2, 90/8), respectively, 2 and 4 hr after inhalation of salbutamol (1/2, 1/4, 90/2, 90/4). A bronchodilation test with the respective drugs was performed on days 30 and 60. (b) Prechallenge lung function (sRaw) before histamine provocation. (c) Bronchodilating effect of additiional 12 μg formoterol and 200 μg salbutamol after 30 and 60 days of long-term treatment. (d) Bronchial responsiveness to histamine challenge before, during, and after long-term treatment with formoterol and salbutamol. Results: 2a, b, c (2).

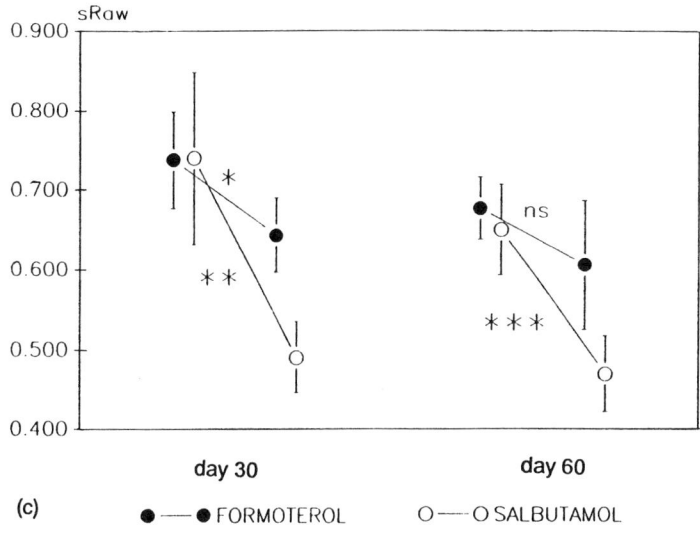

(c)

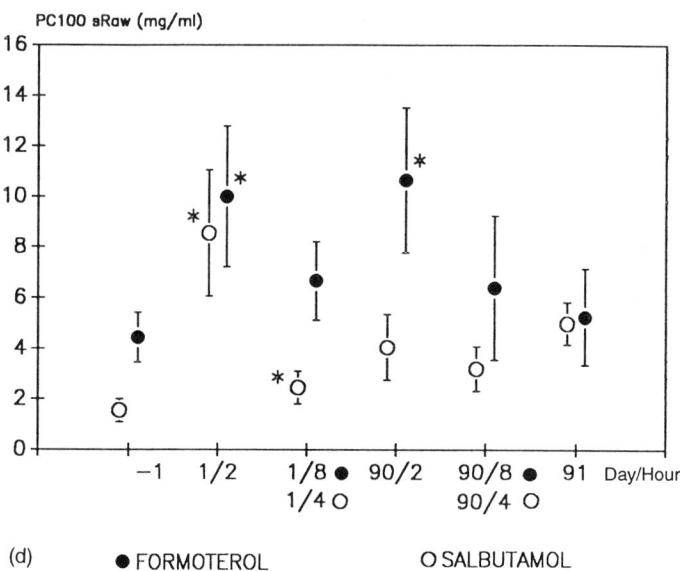

(d)

placebo. Neither treatment group caused a change of ≥ 1 doubling dose PC_{20}/PD_{20} FEV_1 during or after stopping treatment. Furthermore, the exacerbation rate did not differ between groups in both studies. However, the percentage of symptom-free days and nights and the use of rescue medication were significantly better in favor of salmeterol in the crossover study but not in the parallel-group study.

Two large multicenter studies, one using metered-dose inhalers (MDIs) and the other dry-powder inhalers (DPIs), showed that 50 μg bd salmeterol is the appropriate dose for asthmatic children with respect to efficacy and safety. These studies compared salmeterol, 25 μg bd, salmeterol, 50 μg bd, and salbutamol, 200 μg bd, in altogether 847 children with mild to moderate asthma. Because of the similarities in design and methodology, all statistical tests were conducted on the total population of both studies (5).

After 3 months salmeterol, 50 μg bd, was significantly better than salbutamol, 200 μg bd, at improving daily morning and evening PEF and also was better than salmeterol, 25 μg bd, in the change from baseline in morning PEF. The data from both studies showed that the improvement in lung function was maintained over 12 months. Patients on 50 μg salmeterol also had more symptom-free nights and a higher percentage of days without rescue medication. Asthma exacerbation rate and adverse event rate were not different between groups.

No direct comparisons between the effect of formoterol and salmeterol in childhood asthma exists. From receptor binding studies, we are, however, aware of differences between the two drugs regarding the binding to the receptor. These differences explain the faster onset of action of formoterol already after 2 min as shown in an earlier study (1). The duration of protection against metacholine challenge seems to be longer with salmeterol (6), although there is no study following consequently the time curve of protection of formoterol up to 24 hr postdose.

It would be of great interest for the position of the long-acting β_2-agonists in the treatment guidelines to know whether there are differences between formoterol and salmeterol in long-term treatment regarding development of tolerance, rebound lung function, rebound hyperresponsiveness, and the loss of protection against various unspecific stimuli, especially exericse-induced asthma. The studies discussed here are not comparable, because inhaled steroids were permitted in the salmeterol and not in the formoterol studies.

From the two monotherapy studies with formoterol, we have indications for the development of tolerance and a possible rebound effect in lung function but not in bronchial responsiveness. When anti-inflammatory medication was permitted, no such effects were observed (salmeterol study).

Since the goal of drug treatment is that patients should be free of asthmatic symptoms and not suffer from any disturbing side effects, and since no such deleterious effects known from long-term treatment with short-acting β_2-agonists occurred when combined with inhaled steroids, it is likely that long-acting β_2-agonists will play a role in the long-term treatment of children with asthma symptoms, especially symptoms from exercise-induced asthma not controlled by inhaled steroids in recommended doses. Further studies comparing the long-term effect of formoterol and salmeterol on exercise-induced asthma are needed.

References

1. von Berg A, Berdel D. Efficacy of formoterol metered aerosol in children. Lung 1990; 168(suppl):90–98, 180.
2. von Berg A, Peters S, Berdel D. Comparison of the effect of three months' treatment with formoterol and salbutamol on bronchodilatation and bronchial hyperresponsiveness (BHR) in children with asthma. Eur Respir J 1992; 5:283s.
3. Berdel D, von Berg A, Scheinmann P, Moorat A. Asthmatic children benefit from regular salmeterol xinofoate (50 mcg bd) compared with salbutamol as required. Eur Respir J 1995; 8(suppl):518s.
4. Götz MH, Zarkovic J, Taak NK. The efficacy and safety of inhaled salmeterol xinofoate (50 mcg bd) compared with salbutamol (200 mcg prn) in children with asthma. Eur Respir J 1995; 8(suppl):517s.
5. Lenney W, Pedessen S, Boner AL, Ebbutt A, Jenkins MM. Efficacy and safety of salmeterol in childhood asthma. Eur J Pediatr 1995; 154:983–990.
6. Verberne A, Hop WCJ, Bos AB, Kerrebijn KF. Effect of a single dose of inhaled salmeterol on baseline airway calibre and metacholin-induced airway obstruction in asthmatic children. J Allergy Clin Immunol 1993; 91:127–134.

14

Tolerance with Beta₂-Agonists

A Clinical Problem?

BRIAN JONATHON LIPWORTH

Ninewells Hospital and Medical School
University of Dundee
Dundee, Scotland

I. Introduction

Beta₂-agonists have played a pivotal role as bronchodilator therapy for asthma over the past three decades. They have an established place in therapeutic guidelines as an effective and safe form of reliever therapy for bronchospasm both in terms of chronic maintenance therapy as well as during acute attacks (1). There have, however, been some concerns raised as to a possible link between the regular use of β_2-agonists and asthma mortality, as well as a putative association between regular use and disease control. More recently, longer-acting β_2-agonists have become available, and their use has become increasingly widespread in many countries. The issue of safety, particularly with these newer long-acting β_2-agonists, has been linked to the possible development of tolerance and associated β_2-receptor down-regulation which may occur owing to prolonged receptor occupancy. This issue may become an increasing problem, as long-acting β_2-agonists are often used in an attempt to obviate the requirement for high doses of inhaled corticosteroid in view of concerns regarding systemic adverse effects with the latter.

The agenda for this chapter is to discuss clinical studies which have investigated tolerance with β_2-agonists and in particular to focus on the long-acting drugs. In order to do this, however, it is first of all important briefly to overview some of the key studies with short-acting β_2-agonists, as this will then facilitate interpretation of more recent data with the long-acting drugs.

II. Requisites for Clinical Studies

There are some simple, yet fundamental, principles of clinical study design which are required in order to detect tolerance. First, it is important to distinguish as to whether the aim is to detect tolerance to bronchodilator activity or tolerance to antibronchoconstrictor activity (functional antagonism) of the β_2-agonist. These are two completely different situations in that bronchodilator activity occurs in the setting of resting bronchomotor tone, whereas antibronchoconstrictor activity occurs in the presence of increased airway tone, usually induced by a spasmogen. With respect to the latter, it is possible that susceptibility to tolerance occurring may differ between different stimuli such as histamine, methacholine, allergen, or exercise challenge. In terms of bronchodilator activity, it is necessary to distinguish between the peak and duration of the response, particularly with long-acting drugs. Also, it is more likely that tolerance due to β_2-receptor downregulation will most likely be uncovered in the presence of a high degree of receptor occupancy, as would be achieved during a dose-response curve. A run-in period prior to the study without β_2-agonists is preferable to ensure that downregulation has not already occurred as a result of previous exposure to β_2-agonists (2,3). Likewise, if a crossover-type design is employed, then a washout period between treatments without β_2-agonists may also be required, along with the inclusion of a placebo control period. The type of patients selected for inclusion into the study may also have a bearing on the results and their interpretation. For example, preventative drugs such as corticosteroids may up-regulate β_2-receptors (4). However, the early use of inhaled corticosteroid in asthma management guidelines may mean that their concomitant use is mandatory in order to impart any clinical relevance on a given study with long-acting β_2-agonists. Finally, it should be borne in mind that it may not be possible to extrapolate results showing tolerance, for example, from a group of mild asthmatics to what might occur in more severe patients, not only because of differences in therapy, but also because of other effects such as altered airways geometry.

III. Studies with Short-Acting β_2-Agonists

A. Bronchodilator Effects

There are few proper dose-response studies with placebo control which have evaluated tolerance with short-acting β_2-agonists. However, in general, it has not been possible to demonstrate tolerance in asthmatic airways. Harvey et al. (5) showed with inhaled salbutamol tolerance to develop in a normal but not in an asthmatic group of subjects. Even with a higher dose of inhaled salbutamol, it appears that bronchodilator tolerance does not occur in asthmatic subjects. Lipworth et al. reported a crossover study whereby placebo, low-dose inhaled salbutamol (800 μg daily) or high-dose inhaled salbutamol (4000 μg daily) was given each for 2 weeks along with 2-week run-in and washout periods without β_2-agonists (6). A dose-response curve to inhaled salbutamol performed after each of the treatment periods showed a right shift in extrapulmonary but not airway β_2-receptor dose-response curves even with the higher dose. This apparent tissue dissociation in β_2-receptor subsensitivity may reflect differences in numbers of spare receptors or possibly receptor turnover between airway and other extrapulmonary tissues. It should also be pointed out that there is no difference in β_2-receptor density on circulating lymphocytes when comparing normal subjects with asthmatic subjects who have not been exposed to exogenous β_2-agonists (3).

B. Antibronchoconstrictor Effects

With respect to antibronchoconstrictor properties it is important to distinguish between tolerance to this protection which occurs with regular use and the rebound increase in airway activity which occurs after stopping regular therapy. Vathenen et al. showed a significant reduction in the protective effect of inhaled terbutaline against histamine-induced bronchoconstriction following 2 weeks of treatment (7). In addition, an increase in airway reactivity amounting to 1.5 doubling doses was found at 23 hr after cessation of therapy. This rebound effect is similar to that described by Larsson and coworkers (8), where a trend toward enhanced reactivity was found with allergen challenge at 48 hr after stopping therapy with oral terbutaline.

In terms of comparing different spasmogens, it has been shown that the loss of protection occurs more readily with adenosine monophosphate (AMP) than with methacholine (9). After 7 days' treatment of inhaled terbutaline, this reduction in protection amounted to 2.1 doubling doses of AMP. Finally, Cockcroft et al. (10) showed that after 2 weeks of treatment with inhaled salbutamol, there was an attenuation of the acute protective effect of salbutamol against both allergen and methacholine challenge, with the effect being more pronounced with the former (1.9 doubling doses). In addition, having withheld salbutamol, a small rebound increase occurred with allergen only, equivalent to 0.9 doubling doses. It is of course important to consider these results in the light of known intrinsic biological variability of bronchial hyperreactivity which amounts to approximately one doubling dose. In other words, changes which are shown to be statistically significant may not necessarily translate into clinically relevant differences. However, the conclusion from the above studies is clearly that with short-acting β-agonists after a period of 1–2 weeks, it is easy to demonstrate loss of protection against a number of bronchoconstrictor stimuli along with a rebound effect after stopping treatment.

C. Tolerance and Related Effects on Disease Control

There have been studies suggesting that regular treatment with short-acting β-agonists may result in a deterioration in parameters of disease control (11–12). Sears et al. reported that regular compared with on-demand β2-agonist produced a deterioration in disease control, although this was only associated with increased airway reactivity to methacholine in 34% of cases (11). Furthermore, changes in reactivity were of relatively small magnitude, suggesting that the loss of airway protection was not the main factor in causing worsening disease control. Interestingly a subgroup analysis showed that the deterioration occurred equally for those receiving β2-agonist monotherapy as compared with those receiving concomitant inhaled steroid, suggesting that the latter did not exhibit any facilitatory effect on airway β2-receptors. In the study of Van Shayck et al. comparing regular ipratropium bromide and salbutamol, a decline in FEV_1 occurred in regular as compared with on-demand treatment, although this was small (52 ml/year) and not associated with any changes in airway reactivity (12). More recently, Chapman et al. demonstrated improved symptom control with regular salbutamol compared with as-required therapy, although disease activity parameters other than peak flow were not measured as part of this study (13). On the basis of the available evidence, it would therefore appear that tolerance as such is probably not the explanation for observations of impaired disease control associated with the regular use of β2-agonists. Indeed it is questionable whether impaired disease control would be observed where patients were optimally treated with inhaled corticosteroid, which is in keeping with published asthma management guidelines.

IV. Studies with Long-Acting β2-Agonists

A. Bronchodilator Effects

Early attempts at evaluating bronchodilator subsensitivity with salmeterol and formoterol have been flawed because of inherent problems with methodological design. Ullman et al. compared 2 weeks of treatment with salmeterol, 50 μg, twice daily or salbutamol, 200 mg, four times daily without a placebo control period. No run-in or washout period without β2-agonist was employed in this study. A salbutamol dose-response curve was constructed before and after each treatment period. The baseline FEV_1 was significantly higher after treatment with salmeterol compared with before treatment, reflecting the use of a 12-hr washout period after the last dose. This confounding effect on the baseline FEV_1 after salmeterol, along with a ceiling being reached in the salbutamol dose-response curve, makes it difficult to draw any valid conclusions as to whether tolerance actually occurred or not. Since it was also not possible to demonstrate tolerance to extrapulmonary β_2 effects, this further suggests that the methodology employed was at best suspect. In a similar study, formoterol, 12 μg, twice daily was compared in a crossover study with salbutamol, 200 μg, twice daily, each given for 2 weeks, again without placebo control or a run-in period (15). As in the study of Ullman et al., the baseline FEV_1 was significantly increased 12 hr after the last dose of formoterol prior to the salbutamol dose-response curve, and the ceiling in the salbutamol in the dose-response was reached, thus making interpretation difficult to evaluate properly.

We have in our own laboratory attempted to resolve some of these problems by performing studies with both formoterol and salmeterol using appropriate methodology employing a placebo control period, adequate run-in without β_2-agonists and a longer washout prior to the dose-response curve. Two separate studies were performed with aerosol and dry-powder formulations of formoterol, 24 μg, twice daily given for 4 weeks compared with placebo in a double-blind randomized crossover design. A dose-response curve to repeated doses of inhaled formoterol was constructed after each 4-week treatment period (16,17). Since formoterol is fast acting, it is inconceivable that patients might use it repeatedly in this way for "rescue" relief of bronchoconstriction as might occur during an acute attack. In the first of these studies, baseline FEV_1 showed a nonsignificant trend toward a higher value 12 hr after the last dose of formoterol compared with placebo, suggesting there may have been a small carryover effect (16). This criticism was dealt with in the second study by employing a 24-hr washout period after the last dose of formoterol where baseline values were almost identical (17).

In both studies, there was a clear rightward shift in the dose-response curve after prior treatment with formoterol compared with placebo, and a plateau in the response curve was not achieved after the final cumulative dose. Bronchodilator subsensitivity was found to be greatest when measured at 6 hr after the final dose of the cumulative formoterol dose-response curve. This was observed both in terms of FEV_1 and FEF_{25-75}, perhaps inferring that subsensitivity had occurred in both large and small airway β_2-receptors (Fig. 1). Also as expected, formoterol produced subsensitivity of extrapulmonary β_2 responses compared with placebo. It is relevant that in both of these studies, most of the patients were receiving concomitant inhaled corticosteroid therapy, suggesting that this does not fully protect against the development of β_2-receptor subsensitivity in asthmatic airways. The finding of airway β_2-receptor subsensitivity was associated with significant downregulation of lymphocyte β_2-receptor density. In this respect, there is now data using positron emission tomography to show that downregulation of lung β_2-receptors closely

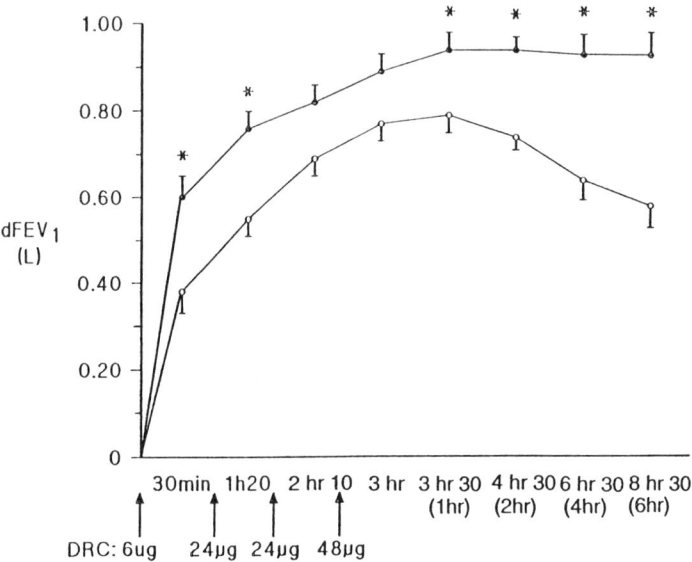

Figure 1 Cumulative dose-response curve and response time profile after last-dose for change in FEV₁ (dFEV₁) after treatment for 4 weeks with either placebo (solid circles) or formoterol, 24 μg, twice daily (open circles). Asterisks denote a significant difference between formoterol and placebo. (From Ref. 17.)

follows that of lymphocyte β_2-receptors following exposure to β_2-agonists, suggesting that lymphocyte β_2-receptors may be used as a surrogate for following airway β_2-receptors (18).

The effects of regular salmeterol therapy have also been studied using a similar design. Seventeen patients with moderately severe asthma all receiving inhaled corticosteroids were randomized to receive salmeterol dry-powder, 50 μg, twice daily or placebo in a double-blind crossover design (19). Salbutamol was given in repeated cumulative doses to construct the dose-response curve to mimic what might happen in an acute attack, since salmeterol would not be used for this purpose because of its slow onset of action. A 36-hr washout period was used after the last dose of salmeterol prior to the salbutamol dose-response curve, and this resulted in baseline FEV1 values showing no significant difference. There was a rightward shift in the salbutamol dose-response curve after prior treatment with salmeterol compared with placebo. This reduction in bronchodilator response equated to a 2.5-fold and a 4.0-fold greater dose of salbutamol being required to produce a given FEV₁ and a peak flow response, respectively (Fig. 2). This was associated with a significant reduction

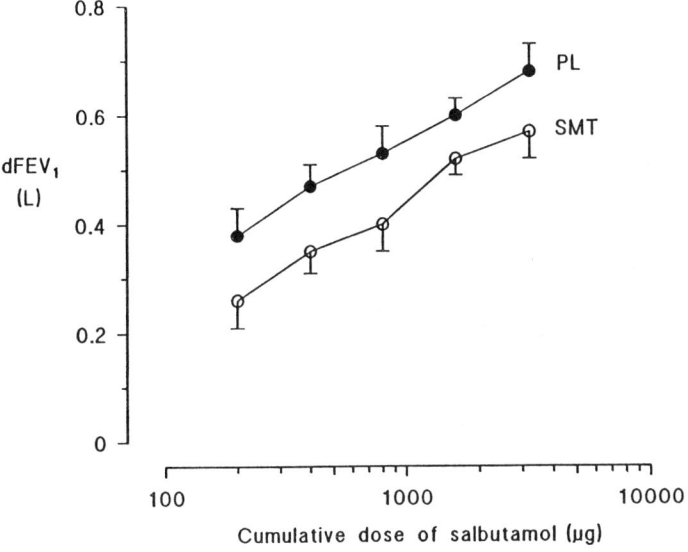

Figure 2 Dose-response curve for change in FEV₁ (dFEV₁) in response to cumulative doubling doses of inhaled salbutamol after 4 weeks' treatment with either placebo (PL) or salmeterol, 50 μg, twice daily (SMT). (From Ref. 19.)

in lymphocyte β₂-receptor density after salmeterol as compared with placebo or run-in (Fig. 3).

Taken together, these three studies (16,17,19) clearly indicate that prolonged receptor occupancy with long-acting β₂-agonists results in down-regulation and associated airway β₂-receptor subsensitivity in terms of bronchodilator response. These findings were all in stable patients with moderately severe asthma, and the relevance of these effects in patients with more severe asthma or during episodes of acute airflow obstruction is as yet unknown. It is, however, evident, perhaps concerning, that the concomitant use of inhaled corticosteroids does not appear to fully protect patients from developing tolerance.

B. Antibronchoconstrictor Effects

Since it is possible to demonstrate tolerance to the protective effects of short-acting β₂-agonists against bronchoconstrictor stimuli, it is perhaps not surprising that the same phenomenon has also been reported with long-acting β₂-agonists. In discussing studies which have looked at antibronchoconstrictor effects with long-acting β₂-agonists, it is important to consider whether

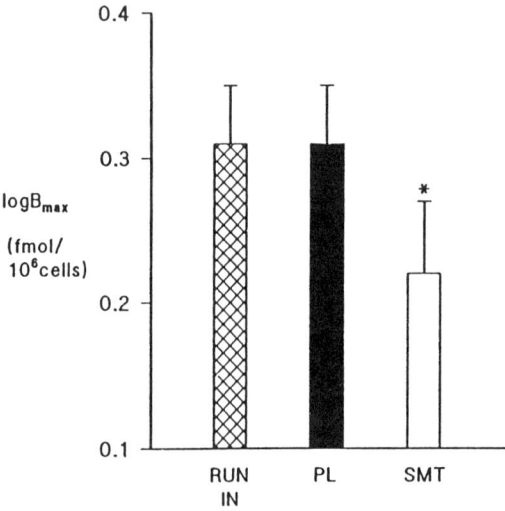

Figure 3 Lymphocyte β_2-receptor density at the end of the run-in period without β_2-agonists and after 4 weeks' treatment with either placebo or salmeterol, 50 μg, twice daily. Asterisk denotes a significant difference comparing salmeterol with run-in or placebo. (From Ref. 19.)

tolerance occurs not only at peak effects but also toward the end of its action at 12 hr, given that these drugs are usually used with a twice daily dosing regimen.

Cheung and colleagues evaluated a group of patients with mild asthma who were not receiving inhaled corticosteroid and who used salbutamol as required (20). In a parallel-group study, patients received treatment for 8 weeks with either salmeterol, 50 μg, twice daily or placebo. Methacholine challenges were performed after the first dose and repeated at 4 and 8 weeks of treatment. The challenges were performed at 1 hr after receiving a dose of salmeterol, having withheld treatment for 36 hr previously. The results showed that after the first dose of salmeterol, there was a 10-fold protection with salmeterol which had diminished after 4 weeks to only a 2-fold protection. There was no rebound increase in methacholine reactivity for up to 4 days after stopping the treatment. It could be argued that this study has little clinical relevance in that these patients were not on inhaled steroids and hence would not normally have been given salmeterol therapy. Furthermore, patients do not usually stop their salmeterol for 36 hr prior to inhaling a further dose as was the case in this particular study.

In this respect, it is perhaps more relevant to discuss those studies in which the protective effect of salmeterol has been assessed within the normal dosing interval at 12 hr after inhalation. Booth et al. studied a group of patients with mild to moderate asthma in whom 19 out of 26 were taking inhaled corticosteroid therapy (21). In a parallel-group study, patients were given treatment for 8 weeks with either salmeterol, 50 μg, twice daily or placebo, with a methacholine challenge performed at 12 hr after the first dose and again at 4 and 8 weeks of treatment, as well as after a 2-week washout without salmeterol. The protection afforded by salmeterol was not significantly altered when comparing the first dose (0.9 doubling dose difference from baseline) with subsequent repeated dosing at 4 weeks (1.2 doubling doses) or 8 weeks (0.6 doubling doses). Also, there was no rebound increase in reactivity after stopping methacholine. A failure to demonstrate tolerance may reflect the small degree of protection afforded by salmeterol at 12 hr, and indeed there was no significant bronchodilator effect at this time point either. The same investigators have since reported (in abstract form) a comparison of salmeterol, 50 μg, twice daily or placebo on methacholine reactivity using the same design as Cheung et al. by performing the methacholine challenge 1 hr after inhalation of the test drug following a 36-hr test drug washout period (22). In this case, unlike the Cheung study, all of the patients were inhaling regular corticosteroids. It was also found that the protection afforded by salmeterol had reduced (1–3 doubling doses) after 4 weeks of treatment compared with the first dose effect. Yates et al. have also reported data with formoterol, 24 μg, twice daily in steroid-naive asthmatic patients showing a significant loss of protection against methacholine at 12 hr after the first dose compared with the last dose after 2 weeks of therapy (23).

There is also evidence to show that tolerance develops to the protective effect of salmeterol against exercise-induced bronchoconstriction in a study comparing 50 μg of salmeterol twice daily with placebo given for 4 weeks, with an exercise challenge being performed at 6 and 12 hr after the first dose and again at 12 weeks (24). Although salmeterol afforded protection against exercise compared with placebo at 6 and 12 hr after the first dose, no significant difference between salmeterol and placebo was apparent after 4 weeks of continuous therapy (Fig. 4). In the study of Grove et al. reported above (19), as well as evaluating bronchodilator dose response, a histamine challenge performed at 12 hr after the last dose of each treatment period showed only minimal protection amounting to 0.7 doubling dose difference comparing salmeterol with placebo; again inferring the development of tolerance. Finally, Gustafsson et al. (abstracted data) showed a loss to the protective effect of salmeterol, 50 μg, twice daily at 12 hr after dosing in terms of protection against bronchial cold air challenge in a group of asthmatics receiving inhaled corticosteroid therapy (25).

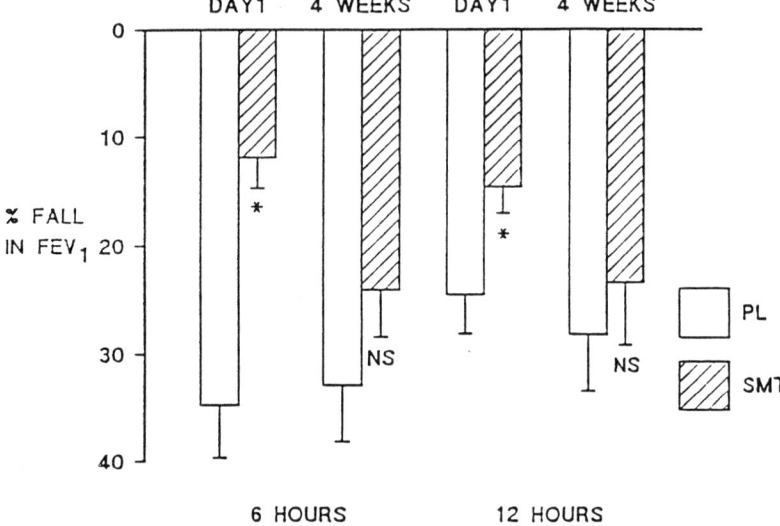

Figure 4 Percentage fall in FEV₁ after exercise challenge performed at 6 and 12 hr after the first dose (day 1) and after 4 weeks of continuous inhaled salmeterol, 50 μg, twice daily (hatched bars) or placebo (open bars). Asterisks denote a significant difference between salmeterol or placebo. (From Ref. 24.)

Tying together all of the above challenge studies, it would appear that long-acting β_2-agonists, and in particular salmeterol, exhibit a loss of protection to a variety of bronchoconstrictor stimuli, including methacholine, histamine, cold air, and exercise. Furthermore, as with bronchodilator tolerance, this effect does not appear to be fully prevented by concomitant treatment with inhaled corticosteroids.

V. Conclusions

There is good evidence to show that tolerance develops to the protective effects of both short- and long-acting β_2-agonists against a number of bronchoconstrictor stimuli. It appears that this effect occurs even in patients who are receiving inhaled corticosteroid therapy. Whether or not this phenomenon is related to adverse effects of β_2-agonists on disease control remains unclear at present. Despite the fact that there are differences in intrinsic agonist activity between formoterol and salmeterol, it appears that both drugs have a similar propensity for inducing tolerance to antibronchoconstrictor effects of these long-acting β_2-agonists.

Regular twice-daily treatment with either salmeterol or formoterol produces a downregulation of β_2-receptors as a consequence of prolonged receptor exposure. This results in subsensitivity of airway β_2-receptors in terms of an acute bronchodilator response to repeated doses of β_2-agonist as might occur during an acute asthma situation. At least when using repeated doses of formoterol after prior exposure to regular formoterol, it appears that the diminution in its response is greatest for duration rather than peak response. Such studies have been performed in stable patients with moderate disease severity and it is unknown as to the possible clinical relevance of these findings in patients with more severe asthma in the setting of an acute exacerbation. As with tolerance to antibronchoconstrictor effects, it appears that concomitant treatment with inhaled corticosteroids does not appear to fully protect against the development of bronchodilator tolerance. That it is more difficult to demonstrate bronchodilator tolerance following regular exposure to short-acting β_2-agonists (e.g., salbutamol) may reflect periods of unoccupied airway β_2-receptors which obviates the development of downregulation and hence bronchodilator subsensitivity. This of course would not explain why tolerance develops readily to antibronchoconstrictor activity with short-acting β_2-agonists.

Although there are clearly unresolved questions regarding tolerance with long-acting β_2-agonists, several studies have shown that the use of these drugs is often associated with an overall improvement in symptom control, reduced requirement for short-acting reliever therapy, and improvement in lung function parameters. It is possible that these effects, along with masking of underlying inflammation in patients suboptimally treated with inhaled corticosteroids, might result in patients being lulled into a perceived false sense of security in that their airway β_2-receptors may be subsensitized during the downhill spiral of an acute asthma attack. However, since systemic corticosteroids are known to upregulate β_2-receptors, it is possible that during an acute attack of asthma, there may be a left shift in the airway β_2-receptor dose-response curve which might obviate the phenomenon of downregulation and subsensitivity. Clearly, studies are warranted to further investigate these important issues. It also is unknown whether the use of long-acting β_2-agonists on a once-daily basis at night with a drug-free interval might obviate the development of downregulation and subsensitivity due to a period of receptor-free occupancy.

Current asthma management guidelines stress the importance of optimally suppressing the underlying inflammatory process. In this respect, from first principles it would appear rational to consider the use of long-acting β_2-agonists only in the context of such combined therapy once patients have been optimally titrated with a dose of inhaled corticosteroid. Providing that such guidelines are adhered to, there is no cause for concern regarding the use of long-acting β_2-agonists and particularly with reference to the developments of tolerance.

References

1. British Thoracic Society guidelines for the management of asthma. Thorax 1993; 48:S1–S24.
2. Lipworth BJ, Clark RA, Dhillon DP, McDevitt DG. Subsensitivity of β-adrenoceptor responses in asthmatic patients taking regular low-dose inhaled salbutamol. Eur J Clin Pharmacol 1990; 38:203–205.
3. Newnham DM, Coutie WJR, McFarlane LC, Lipworth BJ. Comparison of parameters of in vitro lymphocyte beta-2 adrenoceptor function in normal and asthmatic subjects. Eur J Clin Pharmacol 1993; 43:535–538.
4. Brodde OE, Brinkmann M, Schemuth R, O'Hara N, Daul A. Terbutaline-induced desensitisation of human lymphocyte beta-2 adrenoceptors. Accelerated restoration of beta-adrenoceptor responsiveness by prednisone and ketotifen. J Clin Invest 1985; 76:1096–1101.
5. Harvey JE, Tattersfield AE. Airway response to salbutamol: effective regular salbutamol inhalation inormal atopic and asthmatic subjects. Thorax 1982; 37:280–287.
6. Lipworth BJ, Struthers AD, McDevitt DG. Tachyphylaxis to systemic but not airways responses during prolonged therapy with high dose salbutamol in asthmatics. Am Rev Respir Dis 1989; 140:586–592.
7. Vathenen AS, Knox AJ, Higgins BG, Britton JRS, Tattersfield AE. Rebound increase in bronchial responsiveness after treatment with inhaled terbutaline. Lancet 1988; 1:554–558.
8. Larsson S, Svedmyr N, Thiringer GJ. Lack of bronchial beta-adrenoceptor resistance in asthmatics during long term treatment with terbutaline. J Clin Allergy Clin Immunol 1977; 59:93–100.
9. O'Connor BJ, Aikman S, Barnes PJ. Tolerance to the non-bronchodilator effects of inhaled beta-2 agonists in asthma. N Engl J Med 1992; 327:1204–1208.
10. Cockcroft DW, McFarland CP, Britto SA, Swystun VA. Regular inhaled salbutamol and airway responsiveness to allergen. Lancet 1993; 342:833–836.
11. Sears MR, Taylor DR, Print CG, Lake DC, Li Q, Flanery EM, Yates DM, Lucas MK, Herbison GP. Regular inhaled beta-agonist treatment in bronchial asthma. Lancet 1990; 336:1391–1396.
12. Van Schayck DP, Dompeling E, van Herwaarden CLA, Folgering H, Verbeek ALM, van der Haagen HJM, van Weel C. Bronchodilator treatment in moderate asthma or chronic bronchitis: continuous or on demand? A randomised controlled study. Br Med J 1991; 303:1426–1431.
13. Chapman KR, Kesten S, Szalai JP. Regular vs as-needed inhaled salbutamol in asthma control. Lancet 1994; 343:1379–1382.
14. Ullman A, Hedner J, Svedmyr N. Inhaled salmeterol and salbutamol in asthmatic patients. An evaluation of tachyphylaxis. Am Rev Respir Dis 1990; 142:571–575.
15. Arvidsson P, Larsson S, Lofdahl CG, Melander B, Wahlender L, Svedmyr N. Formoterol, a new long acting bronchodilator for inhalation. Eur Respir J 1989; 2:325–330.
16. Newnham DM, McDevitt DG, Lipworth BJ. Bronchodialtor subsensitivity after chronic dosing with eformoterol in patients with asthma. Am J Med 1994; 97:29–37.

17. Newnham DM, Grove A, McDevitt DG, Lipworth BJ. Subsensitivity of bronchodilator and systemic β_2-adrenoreceptor responses after regular twice-daily treatment with eformoterol dry powder in asthmatic patients. Thorax 1995; 50:497–504.
18. Quing F, Hayes M, Rhodes CG, Ind PW, Jones T, Hughes JMB. The effects of chronic salbutamol therapy on β-adrenergic receptors: peripheral mononuclear leucocytes compared to lung tissue. Thorax 1994; 49:1046–1047P.
19. Grove A, Lipworth BJ. Bronchodilator subsensitivity to salbutamol after twice-daily salmeterol in asthmatic patients. Lancet 1995; 346:201–206.
20. Cheung D, Timmers MC, Zwindermann AH, Bel E, Dijkman J, Sterk P. Long term effects of a long acting beta-2 adrenoceptor agonist, salmeterol on airway hyperresponsiveness in patients with mild asthma. N Engl J Med 1992; 327:1198–1203.
21. Booth H, Fishwick K, Harkawat R, Devereux G, Hendrick DJ, Walters EH. Changes in methacholine induced bronchoconstriction with the long acting beta-2 agonist salmeterol in mild to moderate asthmatic patients. Thorax 1993; 48:1121–1124.
22. Booth H, Bish R, Walters J, Whitehead F, Walters EH. Salmeterol tachyphylaxis in steroid neared asthmatic subjects. Thorax 1996; 51:1100–1109.
23. Yates DH, Sussman H, Shaw M, Barnes PJ, Cheung KF. Regular formoterol treatment in mild asthma: effect on bronchial responsiveness during and after treatment. Am J Respir Crit Care Med 1995; 152:1170–1174.
24. Ramage L, Lipworth BJ, Ingram CG, Cree IA, Dhillon DP. Reduced protection against exercise induced bronchoconstriction after chronic dosing with salmeterol. Respir Med 1994; 88:363–368.
25. Gustafsson P, Ekstrom T, Forsstrom E, Ramas M. Bronchial hyper-responsiveness (BHR) and protection by salmeterol against bronchial cold air challenge (CACH) during regular salmeterol treatment in steroid treated asthmatics. Eur Respir J 1995; 8(suppl 9):455S.

Discussion

PETER J. STERK

Leiden University Medical Centre, Leiden, The Netherlands

A. Introduction

As a discussant of B. Lipworth's overview of the studies showing the development of tolerance to inhaled β_2-agonists in patients with asthma in vivo, I will concentrate on the second part of the title that we had been appointed to; namely, whether or not this should be considered as being a clinical problem. To that end, we first have to delineate the conditions at which tolerance will be of clinical relevance. And second, we have to add the latest information on experimental or clinical studies in this area. Such a short inventory will allow us to assess whether the current findings on tolerance are indeed indicative of a real clinical problem.

B. Clinical Problem

Tolerance to inhaled β_2-agonists in asthma occurs at various conditions. Table D–1 summarizes conditions which should be met in order to consider tolerance to be of clinical relevance. These relate to the response measures, the patient characteristics, and the concomitant treatment in the experimental and clinical studies addressing this issue.

Response Measures

As Dr. Lipworth has shown, there is little doubt that short- as well as long-acting β_2-agonists produce tolerance for their protective effects against physiological (exercise) or pharmacological (histamine, methacholine, AMP) bronchoconstrictor challenges in asthma. In addition, he has shown data from his own laboratory suggesting tolerance regarding the bronchodilatory properties. Even though the method of analysis of the latter studies is an issue of current debate, this has been confirmed by other investigators when analyzing the change in FEV_1 expressed as percentage of prediced value (1).

However, to my knowledge, there is not a single study showing a relationship or even an association between such development of tolerance to β_2-agonists and worsening of the clinical control (morbidity, mortality) or the long-term prognosis of the disease. So far, this question has not been specifically addressed in long-term prospective studies. Therefore, it remains to be

Table D–1 Criteria to Be Fulfilled in Order to Consider Tolerance to β_2-Agonists as a Clinical Problem in Asthma

1. Response measures
   - ✓ bronchodilation
   - ✓ bronchoprotection
   - ? clinical control and prognosis
2. Patient characteristics
   - ✓ intermittent to mild persistent asthma
   - ? moderate to severe persistent asthma
3. Concomitant regular therapy
   - ✓ inhaled steroids
   - ? oral steroids
   - ✓ oral theophylline

established as to whether the loss of bronchoprotection and/or bronchodilation by short- or long-acting β_2-agonists after regular usage in asthma is related to deterioration of clinical indices such as daytime and nighttime symptoms, peak-flow variability, steroid usage, quality of life, exacerbation rate, hospital admission, and mortality.

Subject Characteristics

The second point of importance when considering the clinical relevance of tolerance to β_2-agonists in asthma is the selection of patients in the currently available studies (see Table D–1). Are all the classes of asthma severity (as presently recommended by GINA/WHO) represented in these studies? For instance, including our own study on salmeterol (2), the loss of bronchoprotective activity has exclusively been shown in patients with intermittent or mild persistent asthma, well controlled by short-acting β_2-agonists on demand, normal baseline FEV1 values, and mild airway hyperresponsiveness. In addition, the studies reporting the loss of bronchodilatory properties have all been done on in mild to moderate persistent asthma.

Even though such patients had been purposely selected for the benefit of clinical stability and uncomplicated analysis, it is questionable as to whether this selection of patients will adequately allow inference on the clinical relevance of tolerance to β_2-agonists in asthma. Hence, there is no doubt that we need data on the development of such tolerance in patients with severe persistent asthma, who are likely to be most vulnerable to the loss of β_2-agonist activity during acute life-threatening exacerbations.

Concomitant Regular Therapy

The initial studies on the development of tolerance to the bronchoprotective or bronchodilatory activity of β_2-agonists in asthma have been criticized for their design; namely, the investigation of monotherapy with regular β_2-agonists. First, this is clinically unrealistic, since this type of therapy is presently considered to be obsolete. Second, it has been shown that other drugs can prevent or reverse β-adrenoceptor downregulation in vitro. Even though some of the reports in the literature on tolerance to β_2-agonists have been done with patients on regular inhaled steroids, until recently, there were no randomized, placebo-controlled studies addressing the issue of concomitant treatment. However, at least three of such studies have become available in 1996, which are discussed below (see Table D–1).

It is well-known that steroids can upregulate β_2-receptor density in various tissues in vitro, including human lung (3). Therefore, it had been postulated that concomitant treatment with inhaled steroids would prevent the development of tolerance to β_2-agonists in asthma in vivo. Surprisingly, the available studies show that it does not! Using 1-week treatment with short- or long-acting β_2-agonists, either combined or not with inhaled steroids, Cockcroft and coworkers (4,5) demonstrated that the reduction in protective activity by the β_2-agonists against methacholine challenge could not be prevented by an inhaled steroid. In addition, Yates et al. (6) showed recently that 3 weeks of budesonide treatment does not influence the development of tolerance for the bronchoprotective activity by salbutamol against methacholine, as obtained by regular treatment with the long-acting β_2-agonist salmeterol during the third week of treatment. Hence, inhaled steroids do not seem to be able to protect against β_2-agonist tolerance in asthma. This underlines the clinical relevance of this phenomenon even though it remains to be investigated as to whether systemic steroids are more successful in this respect.

The other common regular treatment in asthma is theophylline. If tolerance to β_2-agonists results from a cAMP-mediated mechanism, one might postulate that concomitant regular theophylline treatment can even aggravate the loss in bronchoprotection or bronchodilation by β_2-agonists. Alternatively, however, cAMP might enhance the transcription of the β_2-receptor gene by CREB. Indeed there is some evidence from a study in asthmatic children by Otto et al. (7) that theophylline might prevent the β_2-agonist–induced reduction in β_2-receptor density, as measured on peripheral blood polymorphonuclear leukocytes in vitro. Therefore, Cheung et al. (8) recently finished a study on the interaction between regular theophylline and salmeterol on bronchoprotection against methacholine in a parallel study in 25 patients with asthma. They found that oral theophylline (mean plasma level: 9.9 mg/L) as compared with placebo did not affect the development of tolerance for the bronchoprotective effect of salmeterol during 4 weeks of concomitant treatment. Hence, the good news is that theophylline does not worsen tolerance to β_2-agonists in asthma. However, the bad news is that it does not prevent it either.

C. Conclusions

When ticking off the criteria that need to be fulfilled in order to consider tolerance to β_2-agonists to be a clinical problem, the number of question marks is rapidly decreasing (see Table D–1). Particularly, this holds for the development of tolerance even in the presence of widely used concomitant treatment. Does this mean that this phenomenon should be considered as a clinical problem? No, I don't think so, because there are no confirmative data yet regarding the three most important clinical conditions: (1) an association between β_2-agonist tolerance and worsening of clinical control or prognosis; (2) the development of such tolerance in patients with severe persistent asthma; and (3) the potential modulation of it by concomitant treatment with oral steroids. Further studies in these areas are needed definitively to exclude the possibility that tolerance to β_2-agonist is a clinical problem in asthma.

References

1. Yates DH, Sussman HS, Shaw MJ, Barnes PJ, Chung KF. Regular formoterol treatment in mild asthma. Effects on bronchial responsiveness during and after treatment. Am J Respir Crit Care Med 1995; 152:1170–1174.
2. Cheung D, Timmers MC, Zwinderman AE, Bel EH, Dijkman JH, Sterk PJ. Long-term effects of a long-acting β₂-adrenoceptor agonist, salmeterol, on airway hyper-responsiveness in patients with mild asthma. N Engl J Med 1992; 327:1198–1203.
3. Mak JCW, Nishikawa M, Barnes PJ. Glucocorticosteroids increase beta-2-adrenergic receptor transcription in human lung. Am J Physiol 1995; 268:L41–L46.
4. Cockcroft DW, Swystun VA, Bhagat R. Interaction of inhaled β₂ agonists and inhaled corticosteroid on airway responsiveness to allergen and methacholine. Am J Respir Crit Care Med 1995; 152:1485–1489.
5. Kalra S, Swystun VA, Bhagat R, Cockcroft DW. Inhaled corticosteroids do not prevent the development of tolerance to the bronchoprotective effect of salmeterol. Chest 1996; 109:953–956.
6. Yates DH, Kharitonov SA, Barnes PJ. An inhaled glucocorticosteroid does not prevent salmeterol-induced loss of bronchoprotection in mild asthma. Am J Respir Crit Care Med 1996. In press.
7. Otto J, Gunther S, Urbanek R. The effects of theophylline on beta2-adrenoceptors on polymorphonuclear leukocytes of asthmatic children and juveniles. Eur J Pediatr 1990; 149:661–664.
8. Cheung D, Wever AMJ, de Goeij JA, de Graaff CS, Engelstätter R, Steen R, Sterk PJ. The effect of theophylline on tolerance to the bronchoprotective action of salmeterol in asthmatics in vivo (abstr). Am J Respir Crit Care Med 1996; 153:A805.

15

Role of Beta$_2$-Agonists in the Treatment of Asthma in Adults

ROMAIN PAUWELS

University Hospital
Ghent, Belgium

I. Introduction

Guidelines for the management of asthma have been developed and published over the last 10 years (1–6). The therapeutic recommendations that they contain are based on the results of controlled clinical trials, clinical experience, and scientific concepts. The place of short-acting and long-acting inhaled beta$_2$-agonists in the treatment of bronchial asthma has undergone considerable changes over the last years. Despite the fact that these guidelines suggest a restriction in the use of short-acting inhaled β_2-agonists, they remain the most widely prescribed antiasthma class of medications in the world. The aim of this chapter is to summarize our current knowledge about the most appropriate use of β_2-agonists in the management of asthma in adults.

II. Inhaled Sympathomimetics in the Chronic Treatment of Asthma

The recommendation that chronic treatment with anti-inflammatory therapy and especially inhaled steroids should be started in all patients with persistent asthma is based on the results from clinical studies showing that such a treatment is more effective than regular treatment with short-acting bronchodilators (7,8). This therapeutic attitude is also supported by the demonstration of the presence of chronic inflammatory changes in the airways of asthmatics and by several studies that observed a significant parallel effect of inhaled steroids on the asthmatic airway inflammation and on the clinical symptoms and functional abnormalities of asthma (9–12).

The role of short-acting inhaled β_2-agonists in the chronic treatment of asthma has therefore been restricted to the treatment of acute symptoms that occur despite chronic anti-inflammatory therapy and to the prevention of exercise-induced asthma. This change to the use of short-acting inhaled β_2-agonists when needed has the supplementary advantage that the use of these drugs can be monitored as a parameter of the efficacy of the anti-inflammatory therapy and of the changing severity of the underlying asthmatic disease. The recommendation that short-acting inhaled β_2-agonists should only be used when needed also reflects the concern that regular treatment with these drugs might result in a worsening control of chronic asthma (13).

Long-acting inhaled β_2-agonists have been shown to be clearly superior to the short-acting inhaled β_2-agonists with regard to their clinical efficacy when used on a regular basis in the treatment of chronic asthma (see Chapter 12). The fact that treatment with long-acting inhaled β_2-agonists does not modify the chronic asthmatic airway inflammation (14) has resulted in the recommendation that these drugs should only be used in association with regular anti-inflammatory therapy. The current knowledge does not, however, allow a final judgment about the optimal combination between inhaled steroids and long-acting inhaled β_2-agonists in the treatment of moderate persistent asthma.

Mild persistent asthma can usually be well controlled with a low dose of inhaled steroids and a short-acting inhaled β_2-agonist when needed. Severe persistent asthma requires the regular administration of the combination of high doses of inhaled steroids and a long-acting bronchodilator such as a long-acting inhaled β_2-agonist eventually combined with other bronchodilators and oral steroids. Two 6-month studies in moderate asthma have shown that asthma in most individuals is better controlled by a combination of inhaled steroids and long-acting inhaled sympathomimetics than by a double dose of inhaled steroids (15).

The most acceptable explanation for these findings is that the symptoms of asthma are not only due to the airway inflammation that is present but also to inflammation-induced changes in the airway that are poorly or not at all reversible by inhaled steroids over a 6-month treatment period. It has indeed been demonstrated that even prolonged treatment with inhaled steroids in mild to moderate asthma in children does not result in a complete disappearance of the symptoms and the airway hyperresponsiveness (8). Along the same line, it has been suggested that delayed avoidance of the responsible sensitizer (16) or delayed introduction of inhaled steroids (17,18) results in irreversible changes in the airways. The incomplete control of the symptoms and functional abnormalities of moderate to persistent asthma by increasing doses of inhaled steroids is probably due to a limitation to the anti-inflammatory activity of these drugs, the presence of inflammatory changes that are not or are poorly reversible, and to some irreversible remodeling of the airways (19). The persistent airway inflammation and the airway remodeling are responsible for the brief symptoms that are observed in asthma despite the regular intake of inhaled steroids (Fig. 1). The symptoms can be explained by an abnormal acute airway response to various triggers. The fact that nonspecific airway responsiveness is still present despite prolonged treatment with inhaled steroids is an argument for this hypothesis. The brief symptoms are generally better controlled with a regular treatment with a long-acting inhaled β_2-agonist.

The difficulty arises how to balance the anti-inflammatory and the bronchodilator therapy in an individual patient. A rational choice is almost impossible owing to the lack of a reliable parameter of airway inflammation, the individual variability in the response to various antiasthma drugs, and the not yet fully evaluated risk of side effects for high-dose inhaled steroids and/or long-acting inhaled β_2-agonists.

Although clearly further large-scale long-term studies are needed, one could currently recommend that in moderate persistent asthma not well controlled with inhaled steroids up to 1 mg of beclomethasone or budesonide or equivalent, a combination with long-acting inhaled β_2-agonists should be started especially directed at the control of brief symptoms and the remaining variable airflow obstruction. Further improvement over months due to the delayed effects of inhaled steroids on airway inflammation might allow one to decrease or stop the additional long-acting inhaled β_2-agonists.

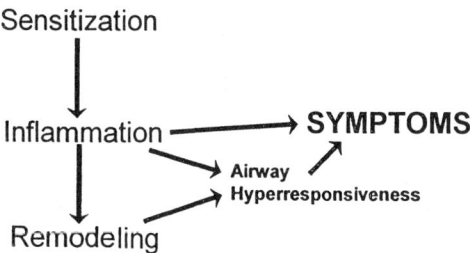

Figure 1   Pathogenesis of asthma.

However, if recurrent more severe exacerbations still persist, then the dose of inhaled steroids should be increased. Indeed, although it has been rather difficult to demonstrate a dose-response effect at higher doses of inhaled steroids (20), exacerbations of asthma, defined as a progressive worsening of asthma over hours to days and poorly responsive to short-acting inhaled sympathomimetics, seem to be responsive to an increase in the dose of inhaled steroids (21). The risks that are linked to these exacerbations justify the increase in dose of the inhaled steroids and on the potential risk of side effects from the higher doses of inhaled steroids.

III. Inhaled Sympathomimetics in the Treatment of Acute Severe Asthma

Inhaled β_2-agonists are the preferred initial treatment for acute asthma attacks (22,23). Of all existing antiasthma medications, they are the most effective and rapidly acting relievers of asthmatic symptoms. In acute severe asthma, they are generally administered in high dose via nebulizer either intermittently or continuously for 1–2 hr. Two recent studies have shown that continuous nebulization of high doses of β_2-agonists in subjects with a severe acute asthma exacerbation results in a significantly higher increase of the lung function parameters within 2 hr after starting the treatment in comparison with an intermittent administration of the same dose (24,25).

The dose of nebulized β_2-agonists for the treatment of acute severe asthma is not firmly established. No proper dose-response studies have been performed. The rather high doses that are currently used have been determined empirically based on the concept that the lack of response to standard doses of β_2-agonists is due to the poor pulmonary deposition of these drugs during a severe asthma attack. However, studies comparing administration via nebulization with the administration of β_2-agonists from a pressurized metered-dose device using a spacer have shown that the latter method is as effective as the former but with a much lower total dose of the β_2-agonists (26). This observation suggests that either the dose of β_2-agonists required might be lower than the one recommended for nebulization or that nebulization is a very ineffective way of administration of the drug.

Several studies have shown that the intravenous administration of β_2-agonists in acute asthma does not result in a higher or quicker therapeutic effect but causes significantly more side effects (27–30). The routine use of intravenous β_2-agonists in the management of acute severe asthma can therefore not be recommended but, as is the case for some other treatment modalities, there is a tendency to use them when the patient does not respond to the standard treatment with high doses of inhaled β_2-agonists and systemic glucocorticosteroids.

IV. Place of Oral β₂-Agonists in the Treatment of Asthma

Long-acting β₂-agonists have been shown to cause a significant and prolonged bronchodilation. Their therapeutic index (ratio between effects and side effects) is, however, unfavorable compared with the long-acting inhaled β₂-agonists. They might be used in patients who cannot use an inhaler or prefer oral treatment. Oral short-acting β₂-agonists are sometimes used for the treatment of acute bronchoconstriction. They are, however, less active and slower in onset than the short-acting inhaled β₂-agonists and can therefore not be recommended except for patients who cannot use an inhaler or prefer oral treatment.

References

1. British Thoracic Society, Research Unit of Royal College of Physicians of London, King's Fund Centre, National Asthma Campaign. Guidelines for management of asthma in adults. I. Chronic persistent asthma. Br Med J 1990; 301:651–653.
2. Sheffer ALE. International Consensus Report on Diagnosis and Management of Asthma. Eur Respir J 1992; 5:601–641.
3. Sheffer AL. National Heart Lung and Blood Institute National Asthma Education Programme Expert Panel Report: guidelines for the diagnosis and management of asthma. J Allergy Clin Immunol 1991; 88:425–534.
4. Warner JO, Gotz M, Landau LI, Milner AD, Pedersen S, Silverman M. Management of asthma: a consensus statement. Arch Dis Child 1989; 64:1065–1079.
5. Warner J, et al. Asthma: a follow up statement from an international pediatric asthma consensus group. Arch Dis Child 1992; 67:240–248.
6. Hargreave FE, Dolovich J, Newhouse MT. The assessment and treatment of asthma: a conference report. J Allergy Clin Immunol 1990; 85:1098–1111.
7. Haahtela T, Jarvinen M, Kava T, et al. Comparison of beta2-agonist, terbutaline, with an inhaled corticosteroid, budesonide, in newly detected asthma. N Engl J Med 1991; 325:388–392.
8. Van Essen-Zandvliet EE, Hughes MD, Waalkens HJ, Duiverman EJ, Pocock SJ, Kerrebijn KF. Effects of 22 months of treatment with inhaled corticosteroids and/or beta-2-agonists on lung function, airway responsiveness, and symptoms in children with asthma. Am Rev Respir Dis 1992; 146:547–554.
9. Djukanovic R, Roche WR, Wilson JW, et al. Mucosal inflammation in asthma. Am Rev Respir Dis 1990; 142:434–457.
10. Djukanovic R, Wilson JW, Britten KM, et al. Effect of an inhaled corticosteroid on airway inflammation and symptoms in asthma. Am Rev Respir Dis 1992; 145:669–674.
11. Laitinen LA, Laitinen A, Haahtela T. A comparative study of the effects of an inhaled corticosteroid, budesonide, and a beta2-agonist, terbutaline, on airway inflammation in newly diagnosed asthma: a randomized, double-blind, parallel-group controlled trial. J Allergy Clin Immunol 1992; 90:32–42.

12. Jeffery PK, Godrey RW, Adelroth E, et al. Effects of treatment on airway inflammation and thickening of basement membrane reticular collagen in asthma. Am Rev Respir Dis 1992; 145:890–899.

13. Sears MR, Taylor DR, Pruit CG, et al. Regular inhaled beta-agonist treatment in bronchial asthma. Lancet 1990; 336:1391–1396.

14. Gardiner PV, Ward C, Booth H, Allison A, Hendrick DJ, Walters EH. Effect of eight weeks of treatment with salmeterol on bronchoalveolar lavage inflammatory indices in asthmatics. Amer J Respir Crit Care Med 1994; 150:1006–1011.

15. Greening AP, Ind PW, Northfield M, Shaw G. Added salmeterol versus higher-dose corticosteroid in asthma patients with symptoms on existing inhaled corticosteroid. Lancet 1994; 344:219–224.

16. Chan-Yeung M, Leriche J, Maclean L, Lam S. Comparison of cellular and protein changes in bronchial lavage fluid of symptomatic and asymptomatic patients with red cedar asthma on follow-up examination. Clin Allergy 1988; 18:359–365.

17. Agertoft L, Pedersen S. Effects of long-term treatment with an inhaled corticosteroid on growth and pulmonary function in asthmatic children. Respir Med 1994; 88:373–381.

18. Haahtela T, Jarvinen M, Kava T, et al. Effects of reducing or discontinuing inhaled budesonide in patients with mild asthma. N Engl J Med 1994; 331:700–705.

19. Kuwano K, Bosken CH, Pare PD, Bai TR, Wiggs BR, Hogg JC. Small airways dimensions in asthma and in chronic obstructive pulmonary disease. Am Rev Respir Dis 1993; 148:1220–1225.

20. Boe J, Bakke P, Rodolen T, Skovlund E, Gulsvik A. High-dose inhaled steroids in asthmatics: moderate efficacy gain and suppression of the hypothalamic-pituitary-adrenal (HPA) axis. Eur Respir J 1994; 7:2179–2184.

21. Chervinsky P, Vanas A, Bronsky EA, et al. Fluticasone propionate aerosol for the treatment of adults with mild to moderate asthma. J Allergy Clin Immunol 1994; 94:676–683.

22. McFadden ER, Hejal R. Asthma. Lancet 1995; 345:1215–1220.

23. Manthous CA. Management of severe exacerbations of asthma. Am J Med 1995; 99:298–308.

24. Lin TY, Sauter D, Newman T, Sirleaf J, Walters J, Tavakol M. Continuous versus intermittent albuterol nebulization in the treatment of acute asthma. Ann Emerg Med 1993; 22:1847–1853.

25. Rudnitsky GS, Eberlein RS, Schoffstall JM, Mazur JE, Spivey WH. Comparison of intermittent and continuously nebulized albuterol for treatment of asthma in an urban emergency department. Ann Emerg Med 1993; 22:1842–1846.

26. Idris AH, Mcdermott MF, Raucci JC, Morrabel A, Mcgorray S, Hendeles L. Emergency department treatment of severe asthma. Metered dose inhaler plus holding chamber is equivalent in effectiveness to nebulizer. Chest 1993; 103:665–672.

27. Lawford P, Jones BMJ, Milledge JS. Comparison of intravenous and nebulised salbutamol in initial treatment of severe asthma. Br Med J 1978; 1:84.

28. Williams SJ, Winner SJ, Clark TJH. Comparison of inhaled and intravenous terbutaline in acute severe asthma. Thorax 1981; 36:629–631.

29. Bloomfield PJ, Carmichael J, Petrie GR, Jewel NP, Crompton GK. Comparison of salbutamol given intravenously and by intermittent positive-pressure breathing in life-threatening asthma. Br Med J 1979; 1:848–850.
30. Salmeron S, Brochard L, Mal H, et al. Nebulized versus intravenous albuterol in hypercapnic acute asthma: a multicenter, double-blind, randomized study. Am J Respir Crit Care Med 1994; 149:1466–1470.

Discussion

ALBERT L. SHEFFER

Harvard Medical School and Brigham and Women's Hospital, Boston, Massachusetts

Asthma is underdiagnosed and undertreated worldwide. As a consequence, asthma morbidity and mortality remains unacceptably high. No cure for asthma is available, but with appropriate care, mortality can be avoided and morbidity significantly reduced. Such control of asthma includes ideally:

1. Minimal; ideally no chronic symptoms, including nocturnal asthma
2. Infrequent exacerbations
3. No emergency visits
4. Minimal requirement for as-needed β_2-agonist therapy
5. No limitations on activities, including exercise
6. Diurnal variation of pulmonary function (PEFR or FEV_1) less than 20%
7. Near-normal pulmonary function
8. Minimal adverse effects from medications
9. Prevent asthma mortality
10. Prevent development of irreversible airway obstruction

In the stepwise approach (Fig. D–1) to asthma therapy enunciated by the National Heart, Lung, and Blood Institute–World Health Organization (NHLBI-WHO) Panel, Global Strategy for Asthma, progression to the next step is indicated when control is not achieved or lost at the current step. The occurrence of symptoms more than three times a week, that is, cough, wheezing, and/or dyspnea requiring short-acting β_2-agonists, is further evidence of inadequate control of asthma symptoms. If short-acting β_2-agonists are required more than three times weekly, or if theophylline agents are required daily, anti-inflammatory treatment is required. The rationale for this decision is based on the following observations. Figure D–2 demonstrates a carinal biopsy (courtesy of Professor Stephen Holgate, University of Southampton School of Medicine, Southampton, England) from a nonasthmatic subject. Note the tall columnar epithelium positioned on a thin basement membrane

**Classify Severity
of Asthma**

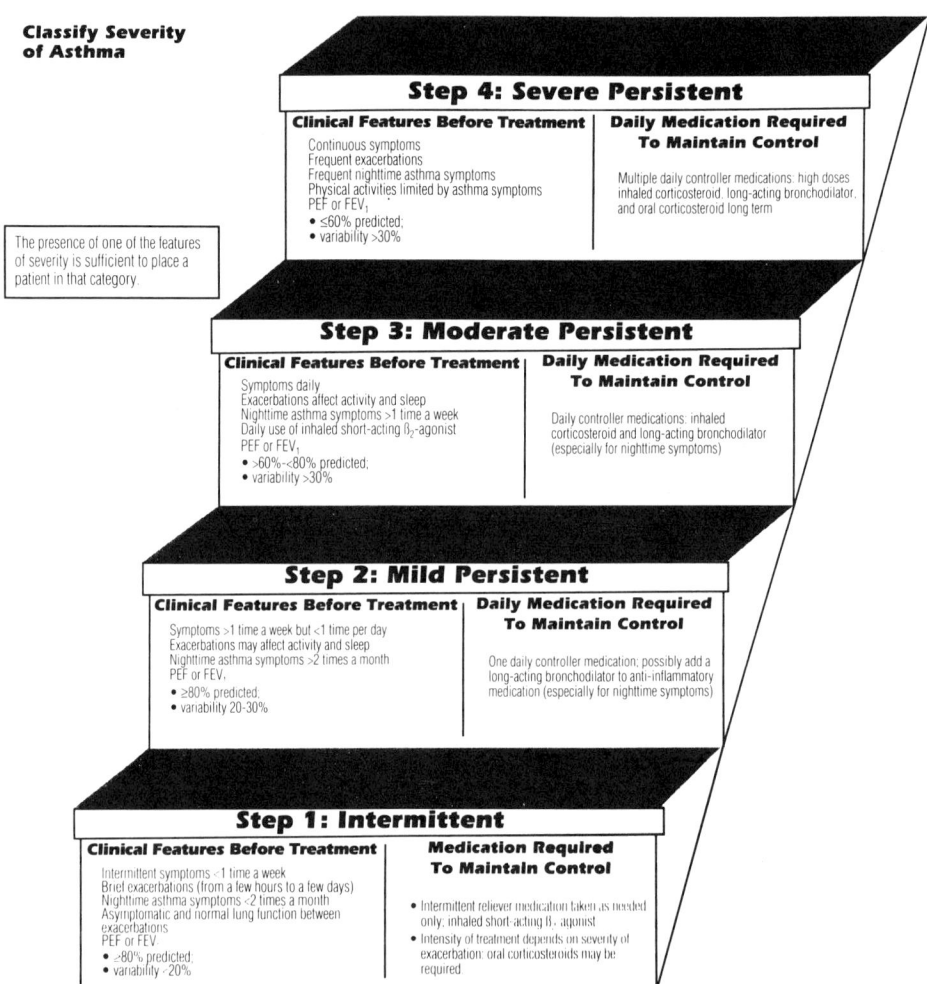

The presence of one of the features
of severity is sufficient to place a
patient in that category.

Step 4: Severe Persistent

Clinical Features Before Treatment	**Daily Medication Required To Maintain Control**
Continuous symptoms Frequent exacerbations Frequent nighttime asthma symptoms Physical activities limited by asthma symptoms PEF or FEV$_1$ • ≤60% predicted; • variability >30%	Multiple daily controller medications: high doses inhaled corticosteroid, long-acting bronchodilator, and oral corticosteroid long term

Step 3: Moderate Persistent

Clinical Features Before Treatment	**Daily Medication Required To Maintain Control**
Symptoms daily Exacerbations affect activity and sleep Nighttime asthma symptoms >1 time a week Daily use of inhaled short-acting ß$_2$-agonist PEF or FEV$_1$ • >60%-<80% predicted; • variability >30%	Daily controller medications: inhaled corticosteroid and long-acting bronchodilator (especially for nighttime symptoms)

Step 2: Mild Persistent

Clinical Features Before Treatment	**Daily Medication Required To Maintain Control**
Symptoms >1 time a week but <1 time per day Exacerbations may affect activity and sleep Nighttime asthma symptoms >2 times a month PEF or FEV$_1$ • ≥80% predicted; • variability 20-30%	One daily controller medication; possibly add a long-acting bronchodilator to anti-inflammatory medication (especially for nighttime symptoms)

Step 1: Intermittent

Clinical Features Before Treatment	**Medication Required To Maintain Control**
Intermittent symptoms <1 time a week Brief exacerbations (from a few hours to a few days) Nighttime asthma symptoms <2 times a month Asymptomatic and normal lung function between exacerbations PEF or FEV$_1$ • >80% predicted; • variability <20%	• Intermittent reliever medication taken as needed only; inhaled short-acting ß$_2$-agonist • Intensity of treatment depends on severity of exacerbation: oral corticosteroids may be required

Figure D–1 Stepwise asthma therapy (1).

with an intact ciliated epithelium. The biopsy obtained from the same location
(carinal) from a mild asthmatic (Fig. D–3) with pulmonary function greater
than 80% (FEV$_1$ and PEFR) and mild symptoms reveals the loss of columnar
epithelium, including the ciliated epithelium. The basement membrane is thick-
ened and there is a significant infiltration of inflammatory cells into the sub-

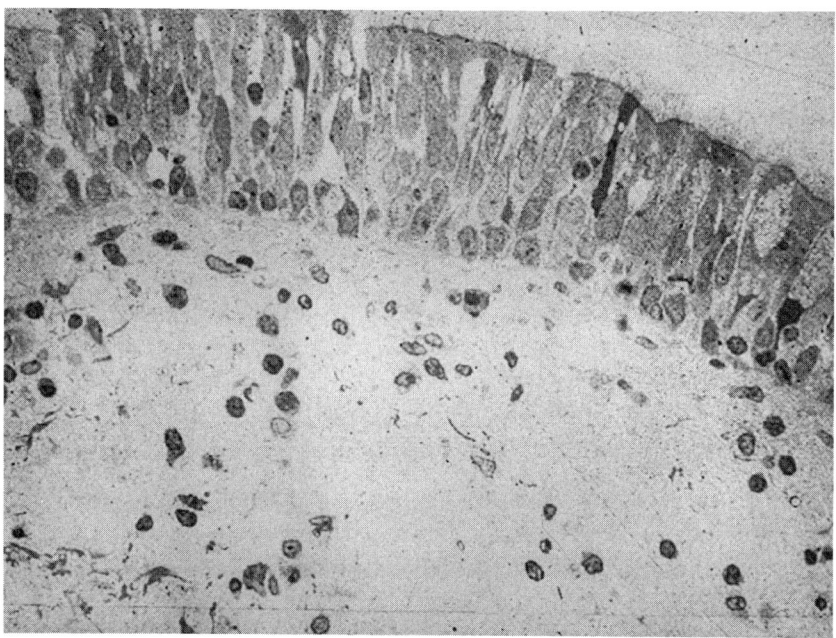

Figure D–2   Carinal biopsy–nonasthma sufferer.

mucosa (mainly eosinophils and mast cells), which is consistent with early re-modelling of the airways. The conclusion is that even in mild persistent and possibly intermittent asthma, significant inflammation is present, thus confirming the need for early anti-inflamamtory therapy in treating even mild asthma, particularly when short-acting β_2-agonists are required more than three times a week.

Another decision to be considered is the placement of the long-acting β_2-agonists in the zonal-stepwise therapy scheme. Patients with moderate persistent asthma are characterized by daily symptoms over a prolonged period of time or nocturnal asthma more than once a week. Such affected patients have had a pretreatment baseline PEF of more than 60%, but less than 80% of predicted or personal best and PEF variability of 20–30%. Patients with moderate persistent asthma require daily medication to maintain asthma control. In addition to daily inhaled corticosteroids, long-acting β_2-agonists should be considered, particularly to control nocturnal symptoms. Such drugs may have a complementary effect with

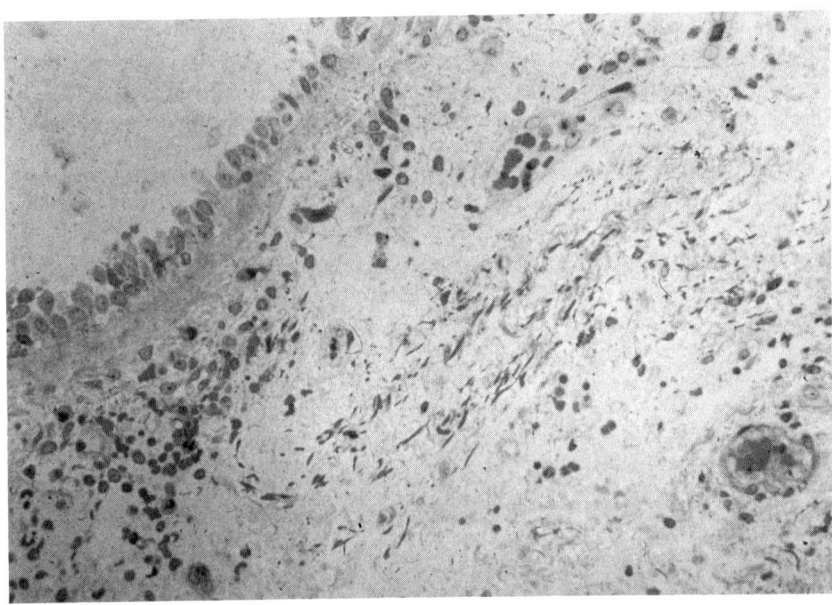

Figure D–3   Carinal biopsy–mild asthma sufferer.

inhaled corticosteroids. However, the place of long-acting β_2-agonists in asthma therapy is being further defined.

The last point in reviewing the zonal-stepwise program of therapy is the reduction of maintenance therapy or stepdown treatment when control of asthma is achieved and maintained for a suitable period of time (i.e., 3 months). A gradual stepwise reduction of the maintenance therapy should be attempted. The minimum therapy required to maintain control should be established. Bronchodialtors, including β_2-agonists, should be the first drugs deleted, but they should be reserved for "rescue." Anti-inflammatory therapy should be maintained indefinitely or interrupted when newer data reflect valid indicators for interruption of such asthma treatment.

Thus, an asthma management zone system provides patients with a program of therapy based on clinical and pulmonary function assessment. They can identify early deterioration and implement appropriate therapy.

In summary, asthma is a chronic persistent inflammatory reaction of the airways. Therefore, anti-inflammatory therapy should be considered for most asthma patients with moderate to severe symptoms and even for some with mild asthma. β_2-Agonists are the most dependable agents available for the prompt reversal of bronchospasm. However, β_2-agonists should not be administered on a scheduled regular therapy but rather on an as-needed basis.

Reference

1. Global Strategy for Asthma Management and Prevention. NHLBI/WHO Workshop Report, NIH, NNLBI, January 1995, Publication #95-3659:89.

16

The Role of Beta$_2$-Agonists in the Treatment of Asthma in Children

SØREN PEDERSEN

University of Odense
Odense, Denmark

I. Introduction

Beta-adrenergic agents are by far the most effective bronchodilators available and therefore the drug of choice in acute asthma in children in all age groups. In addition, β-adrenoceptor agonists have also been the mainstay of chronic asthma treatment in children for many years and given on a regular basis four to six times per day and/or as required. However, when the importance of airway inflammation was appreciated and studies suggesting that regular β-agonist use may not be beneficial or even make asthma worse, the pendulum swung to the other extreme; that is, β-agonists were only recommended used as needed medication, and if more than three such treatments were required per week, inhaled corticosteroids should be added or increased in dose. Today, however, the exact role of β-agonists in the maintenance treatment of asthma in children is undergoing reappraisal after the introduction of long-acting inhaled β-agonists and the publication of dose-response studies with inhaled corticosteroids which show that only small increases are seen in symptom control in the day-to-day treatment with increasing doses of inhaled corticosteroids.

In this chapter, the present role of β_2-agonist therapy in children is briefly discussed with the main emphasis on four main indications where such therapy has been shown to be particularly beneficial:

Treatment of acute severe asthma
Reversal of acute bronchoconstriction
Inhibition of acute bronchoconstriction
Chronic treatment of symptoms

In addition, the route of administration is discussed.

II. Acute Severe Asthma

The value of inhaled β_2-agonists in the treatment of acute, severe asthma in schoolchildren and preschoolchildren has been demonstrated in several controlled trials (1–16). Such treatment is superior to treatment with all other bronchodilators, since the β-agonist works effectively within minutes after administration. Similarly, subcutaneous, intramuscular, or intravenous administration of β-agonists is associated with a significant effect (17,18).

A. Modes of Administration in Acute Asthma

No direct comparisons between inhaled and systemic administration of β_2-agonists have been performed in children. However, in general, the inhaled route provides a better clinical effect to side effect ratio than the systemic route in adults with severe acute symptoms (19). Furthermore, the inhaled route appears to be less affected by the pretreatment given prior to admission (20). For these reasons *inhalations are the best way to administer β_2-agonists to children with acute asthma attacks.*

B. Inhalation Systems

Nebulizers are simple to use and in the acute situation it is advantageous that oxygen can be administered through the nebulizer at the same time as the β_2-agonist. Therefore, *nebulizers are still the delivery system of choice in the treatment of acute severe asthma in all age groups of hospitalized children* even though most studies show that the same results can be obtained with other inhalation systems in schoolchildren (1,2,10,11,13,21). Normally, lower doses are required from spacers to produce the same response as from a nebulizer (13,21–23).

Simply varying the choice of compressor, jet nebulizer, and volume fill has been shown to vary the mass of drug in respirable particles over a 10-fold range (24). Therefore, conclusions from one nebulizer may not be transferred to other nebulizers or comparisons with other inhalers. It is also important to realize that the inhalations should take place through a tightly fitting face mask or a mouthpiece. Inhalation through a face mask 2–3 cm from the face, which is often seen, will reduce drug delivery to the patient by approximately 50% in schoolchildren, with a corresponding increase in the release of aerosol to the environment.

Fast inhalations are required to produce a maximum effect from dry powder inhalers (DPIs) (25–28), and therefore it is sometimes suggested that they are ineffective during acute attacks of wheezing. However, the majority of schoolchildren can also generate a sufficient inspiratory flow rate during episodes of acute wheezing (27,29) and therefore dry powder inhalers (DPIs) can also be used in such situations in schoolchildren (29). In contrast, many preschoolchildren may not be able to generate sufficiently high inspiratory flow rates during acute episodes of bronchoconstriction (26,27). Therefore *DPIs should be reserved for children older than 5 years*. The same is true for conventional metered-dose inhalers, which can normally only be used effectively in schoolchildren after careful instructions for their use are given (26,30). However, even if a child can use a MDI in the day to day treatment, this may not be the case during episodes of acute wheeze (31).

C. Dose Recommendations

It is always dangerous to recommend doses of β-agonists for acute severe asthma. This is because the dose required depends on the response. The correct strategy is to administer enough drug for each individual patient under guidance of careful monitoring for adverse effects and measurement of the clinical response. Therefore, dose recommendations should be considered suggestions for an average patient. Furthermore, not all selective $β_2$-agonists have been extensively studied in children. When conclusions from studies with one drug are transferred to the others, it must be remembered that some differences exist between the various agents.

D. Nebulized Therapy

The optimal dose of nebulized $β_2$-agonists for acute asthma not only depends on the nebulizer brand but also on volume fill: More drug will be delivered if the same amount of drug is given in 4 ml than in 2 ml in the chamber. However, high doses of salbutamol (0.30 mg/kg) were better than low doses (0.15 mg/kg) when given at 3-hr intervals (8). No significant difference was observed in the effect on heart rate or potassium levels between the two treatments. Furthermore, continuous nebulizations of 0.3 mg salbutamol/kg/hr produced better results than the same dose nebulized intermittently over 20 min every hour (32). The value of continuous or frequent administration has also been emphasized by other investigators (33–35).

A dose-response study found that 5–10 mg of nebulized metaproterenol seems to be the optimal bronchodilating dose for acute asthma in schoolchildren (36).

Inhalation of high doses of β_2-agonists causes significant systemic absorption, so that after some inhalations, plasma drug levels are in the same range as after continuous systemic administration. As a consequence, the same side effects may be seen (21,37,38). So this treatment combines the effects of local and systemic administration.

E. Spacers

The optimal dose from a spacer is not known. Doses from 2 to 6 mg and doses around 0.1 mg/kg have been used without unacceptable side effects (1,2,10,11, 13,21,22). In agreement with the nebulizer studies, frequent administration seems to be better than single high-dose administration: A single dose of six puffs of terbutaline (1500 μg) from a spacer was less effective than three puffs given twice at 15-min intervals (4). In addition, one dose of 500 μg of terbutaline was less effective than two doses of 250 μg given 5 min apart (39).

F. Systemic Administration

A significant correlation is seen between plasma drug levels and bronchodilating effect after systemic administration of a β-agonist (17,40). However, considerable interindividual variations exist—also in plasma levels obtained after a given dose (17,40). Therefore, standard doses are not feasible for effective therapy. Dosing should be individualized under the monitoring of the therapeutic response and the occurrence of side effects (41).

In a dose-response trial, an intravenous loading dose of 2 μg terbutaline/kg followed by a continuous infusion of 5 μg/kg/hr was optimal for the majority of children not receiving other therapy (17). Furthermore, inhalation of 1 mg terbutaline from a Nebuhaler did not further improve bronchodilation, indicating that maximum effect in these children could be achieved by systemic administration of drug. The same intravenous doses seem to apply when salbutamol is used (42–44). When systemic administration is combined with high-dose inhaled therapy, the systemic doses should probably be reduced.

Finally, doses around 10 μg/kg of terbutaline or salbutamol given subcutaneously or intramuscularly have produced significant clinical effect without unacceptable side effects (18,45). In one of these studies, 12 μg/kg was better than 3 and 6 μg/kg (45).

G. Special Considerations in Infants

Several early studies failed to find any bronchodilator response to nebulized β_2-agonists in infants (46–49), and for many years, it was believed that β-agonists are ineffective in this age group although functioning β-adrenoceptors are present. In agreement with these observations, two recent studies assessing transcutaneous oxygen pressure and/or oxygen saturation found a fall in these parameters after treatment of acute wheezing in infants with nebulized salbutamol (50,51). One of these studies suggested that some of the fall in PO_2 might be caused by the acidity of the aerosol (50). In contrast, another study found an increase in $tcPO_2$ after nebulized salbutamol in children aged 11–30 months (52). In accordance with this, recent placebo-controlled double-blind studies have demonstrated significant bronchodilator effects (53–58), protective effects against bronchoconstrictor agents (51,59–61) and clinical improvement in infants treated with β2-agonists either alone or in combination with steroids (49,62). The reason for this discrepancy is not clear. The various studies have differed with respect to dose, inhaler (spacer, nebulizer), baseline lung function, duration of symptoms, and method of lung function measurement. The discrepancy is only seen in studies assessing bronchodilator effects. All studies find a significant protection against bronchoconstriction induced by various challenges. *Thus, it seems that infants have functionating β2-receptors from birth and that stimulation of these receptors can produce the same effects as in older children.* However, often the response is rather small and marked interindividual differences are seen. As a consequence, further studies are needed to assess the optimal use during episodes of acute wheeze.

III. Reversal of Acute Bronchoconstriction

The main action of β-agonists is to reverse bronchoconstriction, and inhaled β2-agonists have repeatedly proved their superiority to other drugs in the treatment of episodes of wheezing (31,63). A measurable bronchodilator effect is seen within 1 min and >90% of the maximal is normally measured within 10 min (26). Generally, quite low doses (25% of the normal dose in the inhaler) produce marked bronchodilation, whereas somewhat higher doses are required to protect effectively against various challenges (64).

The normal duration of bronchodilatation of a standard dose of a conventional inhaled β2-agonist is 1–6 hr (65). New selective β2-agonists with a much longer duration of action after inhalation have now been developed (salmeterol and formoterol). Both drugs have been shown to have a significant bronchodilatory effect and a protective effect against various challenges for 10 hr or more (66–71). This prolonged action is only seen after inhalation and not after oral or systemic dosing, so these drugs are only given by the inhaled route. Although the duration of bronchodilatation is longer than for conventional β2-agonists, these drugs have not been evaluated in the treatment of acute episodes of bronchoconstriction in children, and until further studies are available, their use should be reserved mainly for chronic treatment or for the prevention of acute bronchoconstriction.

A. Preschoolchildren

The number of double-blind placebo-controlled studies in these age groups is lower than in schoolchildren, and the well-known problems with accurate lung function measurements and challenge tests makes it more difficult objectively to demonstrate the beneficial effects of the treatment. However, the studies that have been performed indicate that inhaled and oral treatment produces the same bronchodilatory, protective, and clinical effects as in schoolchildren (43,72–76). The long-acting β_2-agonists have not yet been studied in pre-schoolchildren.

IV. Inhibition of Acute Bronchoconstriction

Pretreatment with an inhaled β_2-agonist protects against virtually all broncho-constrictor stimuli, including histamine, methacloline, hyperventilation, cold air, exercise, adenosine monophosphate (AMP), and allergen (77,78). This is clinically very useful. Normally, a parallel shift to the right in the dose-response curve is seen so that higher doses of the constrictor are required to produce a certain fall in lung function. However, sometimes the treatment may not only cause a parallel shift in the curve but may also change its shape so that the slope becomes steeper and the magnitude of the response is unaffected or increased (79).

Continuous treatment with oral β_2-agonists does not protect effectively against exercise-induced asthma (80), although it improves symptoms and peak expiratory flow rates and protects against nocturnal asthma, particularly when slow-release products are used (80,81). Continuous oral therapy seems to be as effective as treatment with cromoglycate and theophylline (81).

Generally, somewhat higher doses are required to protect effectively against various challenges (64), and the duration of the protective effect is markedly shorter than the duration of the bronchodilatory effect (78). Typically, a clinically significant protection against exercise-induced asthma is achieved for only 0.5–2.0 hr after inhalation of a standard dose of a conventional β_2-agonist. As a result, some children are not sufficiently protected to be able to participate in sports. This problem can be overcome by using one of the long-acting β_2-agonists, which provide significant protection for several hours (77,78), and one of the main indications for these drugs in children is prophylactic use before exercise to inhibit exercise-induced bronchoconstriction. Many children are sufficiently protected against exercise-induced asthma during most of the day if they inhale a long-acting β_2-agonist in the morning.

If this is not sufficient, many children will achieve a sufficient effect if the drug is taken 10 min prior to exercise. Furthermore, when this treatment is given regularly on a daily basis, the protective effect is reduced as compared with the effect seen during the first hour after a single dose. This should be remembered when athletes require treatment. They may be better protected when they really need it (competition) if they do not use the long-acting β_2-agonists on a regular basis.

V. Chronic Treatment of Symptoms

Asthma symptoms such as episodic wheezing, cough, breathlessness, restriction of activity during the day, and disturbed sleep and awakenings during the night indicate an abnormality in the bronchial wall and may present a risk factor for exacerbations. Symptoms are normally associated with a degree of lung function abnormality, airway hyperreactivity, and inflammation, but the interrelationship is complex and not direct. Airway inflammation of bronchial asthma may exist without giving rise to symptoms or airway hyperreactivity. Airway hyperreactivity may also exist without giving rise to symptoms in some patients.

Asthma symptoms diminish and/or disappear completely when regular inhaled corticosteroids are given—especially in mild and moderate cases treated early after the debut of symptoms. However, in some moderate and severe cases, corticosteroid only reduces symptoms to a certain extent even if the dose of corticosteroid is increased to high-dose therapy. The addition of a long-acting β_2-agonist to such adult patients normally produces better and a more rapid symptom control during day and night than increasing the daily dose of inhaled corticosteroid two to three times. This speaks for adding a long-acting inhaled β_2-agonist to patients with unacceptable residual symptoms on a certain dose of inhaled steroid rather than increasing the steroid dose. No such studies have been conducted in children, so it is not known if the same would apply for these age groups.

It must be remembered, however, that there is more to asthma control than symptoms and lung functions, including reduction in frequency and severity of acute exacerbations, reduction in mortality, cost effectiveness, control of airway hyperresponsiveness, normalization of the chronic inflammatory changes in the airways, prevention of irreversible airway obstruction, and normal growth (children) or decline (adults) in lung function. Furthermore, the question of whether treatment can change the natural course or even cure the asthma disease is important to consider when the response to treatment is studied. It is probably not correct or optimal only to select a single outcome parameter when assessing the response to a treatment. Further studies are still needed to define the best and most important parameter(s) to assess. Only inhaled corticosteroids have been shown to have marked beneficial effects on the majority of the outcome parameters mentioned. This should also be considered when making therapeutic decisions. However, if unacceptable residual symptoms are the only or the main problem in a patient receiving the highest dose of inhaled corticosteroid which is considered safe, treatment with an inhaled long-acting β_2-agonist is normally indicated. Regular treatment has been shown to reduce symptoms and increase peak expiratory flow rates (82,83). This is also achieved by twice-daily treatment with the long-acting β_2-agonists, which also reduces nocturnal symptoms. The latter therapy is normally more effective than treatment with a short-acting β_2-agonist given four times a day (66,82).

In the day-to-day clinical setting, the vast majority of children treated with inhaled corticosteroids have no nocturnal symptoms. Therefore, once-daily treatment in the morning is often sufficient. Once-daily dosing may also reduce the risk of tachyphylaxis to bronchodilation, which has recently been suggested to occur in children (84) (but not adults [85,86]) treated twice daily with salmeterol.

If there are indications that airway inflammation is not controlled by the dose of inhaled steroid taken, it would probably be better to increase the steroid dose or to increase the steroid dose and add a long-acting β_2-agonist rather than just adding a long-acting β_2-agonist. Further studies are needed to assess the appropriateness of these considerations.

VI. Modes of Administration

A. Inhalation

β_2-Agonists should preferably be given by inhalation, since this allows bronchodilatation to be achieved more rapidly and at a lower dose and with fewer side effects than either oral or intravenous administration (87,88). After inhalation, a measurable bronchodilator effect is seen within 1 min and >90% of the maximal is measured within 10 min (26). Normally, the various inhalers deliver rather large doses, so one dose results in near maximum bronchodilation when the patient is not suffering from acute wheezing. Furthermore, inhalation offers significant protection against exercise-induced asthma and other challenges (78), which is not seen after systemic administration (80). Generally, quite low doses (25% of the normal dose in the inhaler) produce marked bronchodilatation, whereas higher doses are required to protect effectively against various challenges (64).

B. Systemic Administration

A significant correlation is seen between plasma drug levels and the bronchodilating effect after the systemic administration of a β-agonist (17,40). However, considerable interindividual variations exist—also in plasma levels obtained after a given dose (17,40). Therefore, standard doses are not feasible for effective therapy. Dosing should be individualized under the monitoring of the therapeutic response and the occurrence of side effects (41). A rational approach would be to start at a dose around 0.15 mg/kg/day and then gradually increase the dose until a sufficient clinical effect or systemic side effects are seen. Studies doing so indicate that oral doses of terbutaline of around 0.5 mg/kg/day are probably required to produce significant clinical effects (40,80). This is higher than the normally recommended doses and emphasizes the importance of individual dose titration.

VII. Conclusions

β₂-Agonists should preferably be given by the inhaled route. Conventional β₂-agonists are the drugs of choice for the treatment of acute severe asthma and occasional episodes of bronchoconstriction in children. Both conventional and long-acting inhaled β₂-agonists are effective in preventing bronchoconstriction when given prophylactically prior to a challenge such as exercise. However, many children prefer the long-acting agents which protect for a longer period of time. The continuous use of long-acting β₂-agonists is associated with a small reduction in protection, so many physicians and patients prefer intermittent prophylactic use prior to exercise only on days when high protection is needed. Chronic treatment either given once or twice daily is mainly reserved for children in whom unacceptable residual symptoms are the only or the main problem even if they receive the highest dose of inhaled corticosteroid which is considered safe.

References

1. Pendergast J, Hopkins J, Timms B, Van Asperen PP. Comparative efficacy of terbutaline administered by Nebuhaler and by nebulizer in young children with acute asthma. Med J Aust 1989; 151:406–408.
2. Fuglsang G, Pedersen S. Comparison of a new multidose powder inhaler with a pressurized aerosol in children with asthma. Pediatr Pulmonol 1989; 7:112–115.
3. Watson WT, Becker AB, Simons FE. Comparison of ipratropium solution, fenoterol solution, and their combination administered by nebulizer and face mask to children with acute asthma. J Allergy Clin Immunol 1988; 82:1012–1018.
4. Phanichyakarn P, Kraisarin C, Sasisakulporn C, Kittikool J. A comparison of different intervals of administration of inhaled terbutaline in children with acute asthma. Asia Pac J Allergy Immunol 1992; 10:89–94.
5. Kelly HW, McWilliams BC, Katz R, Murphy S. Safety of frequent high dose nebulized terbutaline in children with acute severe asthma. Ann Allergy 1990; 64:229–233.

6. Victoria MS, Battista CJ, Nangia BS. Comparison between epinephrine and terbutaline injections in the acute management of asthma. J Asthma 1989; 26:287–290.
7. Portnoy J, Aggarwal J. Continuous terbutaline nebulization for the treatment of severe exacerbations of asthma in children. Ann Allergy 1988; 60:368–371.
8. Schuh S, Reider MJ, Canny G, et al. Nebulized albuterol in acute childhood asthma: comparison of two doses. Pediatrics 1990; 86:509–513.
9. Pool JB, Greenough A, Price JF. Abnormalities of functional residual capacity in symptomatic and asymptomatic young asthmatics. Acta Paediatr Scand 1988; 77:419–423.
10. Scalabrin DM, Naspitz CK. Efficacy and side effects of salbutamol in acute asthma in children: comparison of oral route and two different nebulizer systems. J Asthma 1993; 30:51–59.
11. Lowenthal D, Kattan M. Facemasks versus mouthpieces for aerosol treatment of asthmatic children. Pediatr Pulmonol 1992; 14:192–196.
12. Ben-Zvi Z, Lam C, Hoffman J, Teets-Grimm KC, Kattan M. An evaluation of the initial treatment of acute asthma. Pediatrics 1982; 70(suppl 3):348–553.
13. Kerem E, Levison H, Schuh S, et al. Efficacy of albuterol administered by nebulizer versus spacer device in children with acute asthma. J Pediatr 1993; 123:313–317.
14. Turpeinen M, Kuokkanen J, Backman A. Adrenaline and nebulized salbutamol in acute asthma. Arch Dis Child 1984; 59:666–668.
15. Becker AB, Nelson NA, Simons FER. Inhaled salbutamol (albuterol) vs injected epinephrine in treatment of acute asthma in children. J Pediatr 1983; 102:465–469.
16. Kelly HW, McWilliams BC, Katz R, Murphy S. Safety of frequent dose nebulized terbutaline in children with acute severe asthma. Ann Allergy 1990; 64:229–233.
17. Fuglsang G, Pedersen S, Borgstrom L. Dose-response relationships of intravenously administered terbutaline in children with asthma. J Pediatr 1989; 114:315–320.
18. Davis WJ, Pang LM, Chernack WJ, Mellins RB. Terbutaline in the treatment of acute asthma in childhood. Chest 1977; 72:614–617.
19. Janson C. The role of adrenergics in the management of severe, acute asthma. Res Clin Forums 1993; 15(no 4 part 2):9–14.
20. Swedish Society of Chest Medicine. High dose inhaled versus intravenous salbutamol combined with theophylline in acute severe asthma. Eur Respir J 1990; 3:163–170.
21. Fuglsang G, Pedersen S. Comparison of Nebuhaler and Nebulizer treatment of acute severe asthma in children. Eur J Respir Dis 1986; 69:109–113.
22. Blackhall MI, O'Donnell SR. A dose-response study of inhaled terbutaline administered via nebuhaler or nebuliser to asthmatic children. Eur J Respir Dis 1987; 71:96–101.
23. Freelander M, Van Asperen PP. Nebuhaler versus nebuliser in children with acute asthma. Br Med J 1984; 288:1873–1874.
24. Newman SP, Pellow PGD, Clay MM, Clarke SW. Evaluation of jet nebulizers for use with gentamycin solution. Thorax 1985; 40:671–676.
25. Pedersen S, Steffensen G. Fenoterol powder inhalator technique in children: Influence of inspiratory flow rate and breath-holding. Eur J Respir Dis 1986; 68:207–214.

26. Pedersen S. Inhalere use in children with asthma. Dan Med Bull 1987; 34:234–249.
27. Pedersen S, Hansen OR, Fuglsang G. Influence of inspiratory flow rate upon the effect of a Turbuhaler. Arch Dis Child 1990; 65:308–310.
28. Richards R, Dickson CR, Renwick AG, Lewis RA, Holgate ST. Absorption and disposition kinetics of cromolyn sodium and the influence of inhalation technique. J Pharmacol Exp Ther 1987; 241:1028–1032.
29. Rufin P, Benoist MR, de Blic J, Braunstein G, Scheinmann P. Terbutaline powder in asthma exacerbations. Arch Dis Child 1991; 66:1465–1466.
30. Pedersen S, Frost L, Arnfred T. Errors in inhalation technique and efficacy of inhaler use in asthmatic children. Allergy 1986; 41:118–124.
31. Pedersen S. Aerosol treatment of bronchoconstriction in children, with or without a tube spacer. N Engl J Med 1983; 308:1328–1330.
32. Papo MC, Frank J, Thompson AE. A prospective, randomized study of continuous versus intermittent nebulized albuterol for severe status asthmaticus in children. Crit Care Med 1993; 21:1479–1486.
33. Robertson CF, Smith F, Beck R, Levison H. Response to frequent low doses of nebulized salbutamol in acute asthma. J Pediatr 1985; 106:672–674.
34. Portnoy J, Nadel G, Amado M, Willsie-Ediger S. Continuous nebulization for status asthmaticus. Ann Allergy 1992; 69:71–79.
35. Singh M, Kumar L. Continuous nebulized salbutamol and oral once a day prednisolone in status asthmaticus. Arch Dis Child 1993; 69:416–419.
36. Shapiro GG, Furukawa CT, Pierson WE, Chapko MK, Sharpe M, Bierman CW. Double-blind, dose-response study of metaproterenol inhalant solution in children with acute asthma. J Allergy Clin Immunol 1987; 79:378–386.
37. Janson C, Herala M. Plasma terbutaline levels in nebulisation treatment of acute asthma. Pulmon Pharmacol 1991; 4:135–139.
38. Pedersen S. Treatment strategies for acute asthma in infants and children. Res Clin Forums 1993; 15(no 4 part 2):55–61.
39. Pedersen S. The importance of a pause between the inhalation of two puffs of terbutaline from a pressurized aerosol with a tube spacer. J All Clin Immunol 1986; 77:505–509.
40. Lonnerholm G, Foucard T, Lindstrom B. Oral terbutaline in chronic childhood asthma; effects related to plasma concentrations. Eur J Respir Dis 1984; 65(suppl 134):205–210.
41. Morgan DJ. Clinical pharmacokinetics of beta-agonists. Clin Pharmacokinet 1990; 18:270–294.
42. Bohn D, Kalloghlian A, Jenkins J, Edmunds J, Barker G. Intravenous salbutamol in the treatment of status asthmaticus in children. Crit Care Med 1984; 12:892–896.
43. Ahlström H, Svenonius E, Svensson M. Treatment of asthma in children with inhalation of terbutaline Turbuhaler compared with Nebuhaler. Allergy 1989; 44: 515–518.
44. Edmunds AT, Godfrey S. Cardiovascular response during severe acute asthma and its treatment in children. Thorax 1981; 36:534–540.
45. Estelle F, Simons R, Gillies JD. Dose response of subcutaneous terbutaline and epinephrine in children with acute asthma. Am J Dis Child 1981; 135:214–217.

46. Lenney W, Evans NAP. Nebulised salbutamol and ipratropium bromide in asthmatic children. Br J Dis Chest 1986; 80:59–65.
47. Lenney W, Milner AD. At what age do bronchodilator drugs work? Arch Dis Child 1978; 53:532–535.
48. O'Callaghan C, Milner AD, Swardbrick A. Paradoxical deterioration in lung function after nebulised salbutamol in wheezy infants. Lancet 1986; 1:1424–1425.
49. Tal A, Bavilski C, Yohai D, Bearman JE, Gorodischer R, Moses SW. Dexamethasone and salbutamol in the treatment of acute wheezing in infants. Pediatrics 1983; 71:13–18.
50. Seidenberg J, Mir Y, Von der Hardt H. Hypoxaemia after nebulized salbutamol in wheezy infants: the importance of aerosol acidity. Arch Dis Child 1991; 66:672–675.
51. Ho L, Collis G, Landau LI, Le Souef PN. Effect of salbutamol on oxygen saturation in bronchiolitis. Arch Dis Child 1981; 66:1061–1064.
52. Holmgren D, Bjure J, Engstrom I, Sixt R, Sten G, Wennergren G. Transcutaneous blood gas monitoring during salbutamol inhalations in young children with acute asthmatic symptoms. Pediatr Pulmonol 1992; 14:75–79.
53. Yuksel B, Greenough A. Effect of nebulized salbutamol in preterm infants during the first year of life. Eur Respir J 1991; 4:1088–1092.
54. Wilkie RA, Bryan MH. Effect of bronchodilator on airway resistance in ventilator-dependent neonates with chronic lung disease. J Pediatr 1987; 111:278–282.
55. Sosulski R, Abbasi S, Bhutani V, Fox W. Physiological effects of terbutaline on pulmonary function in infants with bronchopulmonary dysplasia. Pediatr Pulmonol 1986; 2:269–273.
56. Kao LC, Durand DJ, Nickerson GB. Effects of inhaled metaproterenol and atropine on the pulmonary mechanics of infants with bronchopulmonary dysplasia. Pediatr Pulmonol 1989; 7:74–80.
57. Cabal LA, Lanazabal C, Ramanathan R, et al. Effects of metraproterenol on pulmonary mechanics, oxygenation and ventilation in infants with chronic lung disease. J Pediatr 1987; 110:116–119.
58. Kraemer R, Frey U, Sommer CW, Russi E. Short term effect of albuterol, delivered via a new auxiliary device, in wheezy infants. Am Rev Respir Dis 1991; 144:347–351.
59. Prendiville A, Green S, Silverman M. Airway responsiveness in wheezy infants. Thorax 1987; 42:100–104.
60. O'Callaghan C, Milner AD, Swarbrick A. Nebulised salbutamol does have a protective effect on airways in children under one year old. Arch Dis Child 1988; 63:479–483.
61. Prendiville A, Green S, Silverman M. Airway responsiveness in wheezy infants: evidence for functional beta adrenergic receptors. Thorax 1987; 42:100–108.
62. Daugbjerg P, Brenoe E, Forchammer H, et al. A comparison between nebulized terbutaline, nebulized corticosteroid and systemic corticosteroid for acute wheezing in children up to 18 months of age. Acta Paediatr 1993; 82:547–551.
63. Pedersen S. Treatment of acute bronchoconstriction in children with use of a tube spacer aerosol and a dry powder inhaler. Allergy 1985; 40:300–304.
64. Henriksen JM, Dahl R. Effects of inhaled budesonide alone and in combination with low-dose terbutaline in children with exercise-induced asthma. Am Rev Respir Dis 1983; 128:993–997.

65. Formgren H. Clinical comparison of inhaled terbutaline and orciprenaline in asthmatic patients. Scand J Respir Dis 1970; 51:203–211.
66. Brogden RN, Faulds D. Salmeterol xinofoate. A review of its pharmacological properties and therapeutic potential in reversible obstructive airways disease. Drugs 1991; 42:895–912.
67. Faulds D, Hollingshead LM, Goa KL. Formoterol. A review of its pharmacological properties and therapeutic potential in reversible obstructive airways disease. Drugs 1991; 42:115–137.
68. Jack D. A way of looking at agonism and antagonism: lessons from salbutamol, salmeterol and other beta-adrenoceptor agonists. Br J Clin Pharmacol 1991; 31:501–514.
69. Green CP, Price JF. Prevention of exercise induced asthma by inhaled salmeterol xinofoate. Arch Dis Child 1992; 67:1014–1017.
70. Lötvall J, Svedmyr N. Salmeterol: an inhaled β_2-agonist with prolonged duration of action. Lung 1993; 171:249–264.
71. Verberne AAPH, Hop WCJ, Bos AB, Kerrebijn KF. Effect of a single dose of inhaled salmeterol on baseline airway caliber and methacholine-induced airway obstruction in asthmatic children. J Allergy Clin Immunol 1993; 91:127–134.
72. Nussbaum E, Eyzaguirre M, Galant SP. Dose-response relationship of inhaled metaproterenol sulfate in preschool children with mild asthma. Pediatrics 1990; 85:1072–1075.
73. Ahlstrom H, Svenonius E, Svensson M. Treatment of asthma in pre-school children with inhalation of terbutaline in Turbuhaler compared with Nebuhaler. Allergy 1989; 44:515–518.
74. Pool JB, Greenough A, Gleeson JG, Price JF. Inhaled bronchodilator treatment via the nebuhaler in young asthmatic patients. Arch Dis Child 1988; 63:288–291.
75. Yuksel B, Greenough A, Maconochie I. Effective bronchodilator therapy by a simple spacer device for wheezy premature infants in the first two years of life. Arch Dis Child 1990; 65:782–785.
76. Conner WT, Dolovich MB, Frame RA, Newhouse MT. Reliable salbutamol administration in 6 to 36 month old children by means of a metered dose inhaler and aerochamber with mask. Pediatr Pulmonol 1989; 6:263–267.
77. Dinh Xuan AT, Lebeau C, Roche R, Ferriere A, Chaussain M. Inhaled terbutaline administered via a spacer fully prevents exercise-induced asthma in young asthmatic subjects: a double-blind, randomized, placebo-controlled study. J Int Med Res 1989; 17:506–513.
78. Henriksen JM, Agertoft L, Pedersen S. Protective effect and duration of action of inhaled formoterol and salbutamol on exercise-induced asthma in children. J Allergy Clin Immunol 1992; 89:1176–1182.
79. Bel EH, Zwinderman AH, Timmers MC, Dijkman JH, Sterk PJ. The effect of beta-adrenergic bronchodilator on maximal airway narrowing to bronchoconstrictor stimuli in asthma and chronic obstructive pulmonary disease. Thorax 1991; 46:9–14.
80. Fuglsang G, Hertz B, Holm B. No protection by oral terbutaline against exercise-induced asthma in children: a dose response study. Eur Respir J 1993; 6:527–530.

81. Chow OK, Fung KP. Slow-release terbutaline and theophylline for the long-term therapy of children with asthma: a Latin square and factorial study of drug effects and interactions. Pediatrics 1989; 84:119–125.
82. Simmons FE, Soni NR, Watson WT, Becker AB. Bronchodilator and bronchoprotective effects of salmeterol in young patients with asthma [see comments]. J Allergy Clin Immunol 1992; 90:840–846.
83. Shapiro GG, Furukawa CT, Pierson WE, Sharpe MJ, Menendez R, Bierman CW. Double-blind evaluation of nebulized cromolyn, terbutaline, and the combination for childhood asthma. J Allergy Clin Immunol 1988; 81:449–454.
84. Fuglsang G, Agertoft L, Vikre-Jørgensen J, Pedersen S. Influence of budesonide on the response to inhaled terbutaline in children with mild asthma. Pediatr Allergy Immunol 1995; 6:103–108.
85. O'Connor BJ, Aikman SL, Barnes RJ. Tolerance to the non-bronchodilator effects of inhaled beta-2-agonists in asthma. N Engl J Med 1992; 237:1204–1208.
86. McGivern DV, Ward M, Revill S, Sechiari A, Macfarlane J, Davies D. Home nebulizers in severe chronic asthma. Br J Dis Chest 1984; 78:376–378.
87. Thiringer G, Svedmyr N. Comparison of infused and inhaled terbutaline in patients with asthma. Scand J Respir Dis 1976; 57:17–24.
88. Williams SJ, Winner SJ, Clark TJH. Comparison of inhaled and intravenous terbutaline in acute severe asthma. Thorax 1981; 36:629–631.

Discussion

JAMES P. KEMP

University of California School of Medicine, San Diego, California

In the chapter presentation by S. Pedersen, we have been given an excellent review of the use of β_2-agonists in the treatment of children with asthma. As has been pointed out, there are many good and some excellent studies reported in the literature evaluating the use of β_2-agonists in older children. However, many children, especially preschoolchildren and infants, are treated with β_2-agonists and other asthma therapies without adequate documentation of the beneficial effects or the adverse effects of the doses that are prescribed. This unacceptable state is not limited to the treatment of asthma. In a 1990 survey by the American Academy of Pediatrics, only 20% of the newly approved drugs by the U.S. Food and Drug Administration in the United States had information on how to use these new drugs in children.

Clinical research trials in children with asthma will never be easy and commonly have the following underlying issues with which the investigator and pharmaceutical industry must contend:

> Approval of regulatory and/or ethics committees who take an overly protective attitude toward children
> Protocol Design
>> Blinding of drugs, especially inhalers or liquids (taste).

Use of a placebo in children which is thought in some countries to be
unethical no matter what the disease

Obtaining adequate numbers of subjects with similar age, weight, or
disease characteristics

Determining the optimal length of treatment, the dose to be given, and
the frequency and route of administration

Dosing of an investigational medication at school

Difficulty in obtaining blood/urine specimens

Concern about x-rays

Data collection

Subjective

Who is the reporter—the parent/guardian? Teacher? and/or child?

What is being reported and how is it being quantified?

Objective

Ability to perform effort dependent maneuvers such as spirometry
and challenge tests

Appropriate compensation (if any)

Despite these obstacles, good clinical studies can be and must be performed in children, especially when the response to the drug can be determined within a short period of time. Certainly, this is the case in asthma where
the therapeutic response to a β_2-agonist is apparent within a few minutes to
hours after administration. This is true regardless of whether the drug is administered by injection, inhalation, or orally. Fortunately, many oral formulated β_2-agonist drugs are available as syrups and suspensions. These are pleas-
ant-tasting drugs which allows them to be administered to any age child or
infant. Although the onset of activity is longer than with inhaled β_2-agonist
therapy, there is a greater degree of assurance as to the dose that the child has
received. The response to treatment can be and should be objectively evaluated with peak expiratory flow measurements when possible.

Generally, it is agreed by asthma specialists that the inhaled route of
administration is preferred for the delivery of β_2-agonists to the airway. This
presents a problem for some pediatric patients with asthma, as well as their
parents and the physicians who treat them. Often, it is unclear as to how much
of the dose delivered to the young children is actually inhaled. Neither is it
clear where the inhaled dose is deposited in the airway. This problem is not
overcome when spacers or chamber devices are attached to metered-dose inhalers (MDIs). These devices vary greatly in size and shape, which greatly
affects the dose delivered to the patient (1,2).

Older children who can consistently inhale at a velocity of 30 L/min can
be taught to use dry-powder breath-activated inhalers such as the Rotahaler
(Glaxo Wellcome, Research Triangle Park, North Carolina) which has a very

low resistance to inspiratory flow. This simple device, which must be loaded with a capsule each time, allows 200 μg of albuterol dry powder to be administered with one or two breaths. The Turbuhaler (Astra Draco, Lund, Sweden), a somewhat higher-resistance device, is able to be used by some children as young as 2–3 years of age and has the added advantage of multiple dosing. However, these devices still do not solve all the problems of delivering β_2-agonists (and other drugs such as cromolyn, nedocromil, and corticosteroids) to the large number of very young children and infants who have asthma. Some of these patients can be given β_2-agonists inhaled via a jet nebulizer. Here too, information on the proper dose of β_2-agonists to be given by nebulization and the effects in children are minimal. Even though there are older studies failing to demonstrate improvement in airway obstruction when β_2-agonists have been administered to infants and young children (3–6) and studies indicating a worsening or paradoxical response (7,8), there are two studies in children under 2 years of age that showed a response to nebulized albuterol (salbutamol) (9,10). These studies were both performed in an emergency department, and although one was not a controlled study (9), the second (10) was blinded and placebo controlled and only enrolled patients who had a history of recurrent wheezing. These acute care studies of course do not establish either the efficacy or safety of β_2-agonists as maintenance treatment in this patient population. Also, neither study evaluated with electrocardiography possible effects on the QTc intervals with the doses used nor effects on serum potassium. Therefore, these studies do not help us to understand the optimal dose that should be administered to young children.

Because of the reports in the medical literature concerning the possible adverse effects of regularly administered β_2-agonists in adults and what has become to be called "the β-agonist controversy" (11,12), it would seem even more important that adequate dose-determination studies with these drugs be done in children with asthma. Fortunately, the mortality rate from asthma in children is very low and no "epidemics" of asthma deaths in children have been reported. Also, the administration of these drugs by the oral route has not been associated with increased mortality or increased airway responsiveness (13), even in adults. Nevertheless, there has been a true increase in the prevalence of severe childhood asthma over the past 15 years (14). More information on the effects of current therapy in children is clearly needed.

In recent years, there has been a trend to use jet nebulizers for the delivery of inhaled therapy to children with asthma who are unable adequately to use MDIs with or without spacers. The drugs that are most used are β_2-agonists and cromolyn, although the availability of a budesonide nebulizer suspension in some countries has allowed inhaled corticosteroids to be delivered by inhalation even to infants. This method of delivery of β_2-agonists at home has in my experience decreased the frequency of acute care asthma visits to the physician's office and emergency departments. However, it seems paradoxical that what was primarily an inpatient treatment and later determined to be effective in the outpatient setting is being challenged by some recent acute treatment studies (15–17). In some centers, jet nebulizers are being replaced by the use of β_2-agonist MDIs attached to a spacer device. In general, most studies that have been published comparing these two techniques of inhalation therapy have shown equal therapeutic response or a response which favors the MDI-spacer. This information has resulted in many hospital administrators and respiratory therapists recommending this method of delivering β_2-agonist drugs, primarily because it offers a savings in both time and money (17). However, it should be remembered that many children present to a clinic or hospital in acute respiratory distress because their β_2-agonist MDI with a spacer has not been effective in relieving their airway obstruction. These children, particularly those who are young, apprehensive, and in rather marked respiratory distress, should be given nebulized β_2-agonists. This is especially important if excessive mucous secretions are present. In such settings, nebulizers should be driven by pressurized oxygen and not room air to decrease the potential for worsening hypoxemia.

It is now clear that even in infancy bronchial smooth muscle (18) and functioning β_2-receptors are present (19). Although a varying degree of inflammation and mucous secretions may in some young children diminish the response to β_2-agonists, bronchospasm does contribute to airway narrowing in this age group (20,21).

Despite concerns based on a plausity of scientific data on the dose of β_2-agonist drugs to be used in children with asthma, especially those under the age of 4 or 5 years, clinical experience has demonstrated that, as in adults, β_2-agonists are the best bronchodilator drugs for children of all ages whether given intermittently for acute increases in symptoms, regularly with short- or long-acting drugs for maintenance bronchodilation, or for the prevention of exercise-induced bronchospasm. However, until further information is available, β_2-agonists must be considered drugs which only treat the symptoms of asthma and not the underlying pathology of the disease—inflammation.

References

1. Ahrens R, Lux C, Bahl T, Han S. Choosing the metered dose inhaler spacer or holding chamber that matches the patient's need: Evidence that the specific drug being delivered is an important consideration. J Allergy Clin Immunol 1995; 96:288–235.
2. Newhouse MT. Pulmonary drug targeting with aerosols: principles and clinical application in adult and children. Am J Asthma Allergy Pediatr 1993; 1:23–35.
3. Rutner N, Milner AD, Hiller EJ. Effects of bronchodilators on respiratory resistance in infants and young children with bronchiolitis and wheezy bronchitis. Arch Dis Child 1975; 50:719–722.

4. Lenney W, Milner AD. At what age do bronchodilator drugs work? Arch Dis Child 1978; 53:532–535.
5. Lenney W, Milner AD. Alpha and beta adrenergic stimulants in bronchiolitis and wheezy bronchitis in children under 18 months of age. Arch Dis Child 1978; 53: 707–709.
6. Silverman M. Bronchodilators for wheezy infants? Arch Dis Child 1984; 59:84–87.
7. Prendiville A, Green S, Silverman M. Paradoxical response to nebulized salbutamol in wheezy infants, assessed by partial expiratory flow volume curves. Thorax 1987; 42:86–91.
8. O'Callaghan C, Milner AD, Swarbrick A. Paradoxical deterioration in lung function after nebulized salbutamol in wheezy infants. Lancet 1986; 2:1424–1425.
9. Bentur L, Kerem E, Canny G, et al. Response of acute asthma to a beta$_2$-agonist in children less than 2 years of age. Ann Allergy 1990; 65:122–126.
10. Bentur L, Canny G, Shilds M, et al. Controlled trial of nebulized albuterol in children younger than 2 years of age with asthma. Pediatrics 1992; 89:133–137.
11. Crane J, Burgess C, Pearce N, Beasley R. The B-agonist controversy: a perspective. Eur Respir Rev 1993; 3:15,475–482.
12. Warner J. The beta2 agonist controversy and its relevance to the treatment of children. Eur Respir Rev 1994; 4:17,21–26.
13. Herdman MJ, Ferguson H, Thomas K, et al. The effect of salbutamol controlled release on airways responsiveness to inhaled methacholine in mild asthmatic subjects. Respir Med 1993; 87:23–27.
14. Burney PGJ, Chinn S, Rona R. Has the prevalence of asthma increased in children? Evidence from the national study of health and growth. Br Med J 1990; 300:1306–1309.
15. Fuglsang G, Pedersen S. Comparison of nebuhaler and nebulizer treatment of acute severe asthma in children. J Respir Dis 1986; 69:109–113.
16. Benton G, Thomas RC, Nickerson BG, et al. Experience with a metered dose inhaler with a spacer in a pediatric emergency department. Am J Dis Child 1989; 143:678–681.
17. Bowton DL, Goldsmith WM, Haponik EF. Substitution of metered dose inhaler for hand held nebulizers. Chest 1992; 101:305–308.
18. Matsuba K, Thurlbeck WM. A morphometric study of bronchial and bronchiolar walls in children. Am Rev Respir D 1972; 105:908–913.
19. Prendiville A, Green S, Silverman M. Airway responsiveness in wheezy infants: evidence for functional beta adrenergic receptors. Thorax 1987; 42:100–104.
20. Prendiville A, Green S, Silverman M. Bronchial hyperresponsiveness to histamine in wheezy infants. Thorax 1987; 42:92–99.
21. O'Callaghan C, Milner AD, Swarbrick A. Nebulized salbutamol does have a protective effect on airways in children under 1 year old. Arch Dis Child 1988; 63:479–483.

AUTHOR INDEX

Italic numbers give the page on which the complete reference is listed.

397

SUBJECT INDEX

A

Acetylcholine, 39, 169, 181, 192
Activating protein, 52
Acute severe asthma, 164, 370, 380
Adenosine, 181, 209
Adenosine-monophosphate, 43, 44,
48, 187, 285, 306, 312, 351,
362, 384
Adenosine triphosphate, 20
Adenyl cyclase, 20, 49, 50, 51, 137
Adrenal extract, 4, 5, 8
Adrenaline, 1, 2, 4, 7, 8, 9, 12, 15, 16,
19, 30, 70, 143, 161, 164, 223,
259, 266, 271, 334
Adrenergic transmitters, 11
Aerosol holding chamber, 240
Affinity, 131, 136, 152
Agitation, 335
Agonist, 150

Airway hyperresponsiveness, 363, 369,
385
Airway remodeling, 314, 369
Airway responsiveness, 181, 185, 305,
306, 307, 308, 394
Albuterol (*see* Salbutamol)
Allergen, 2, 44, 70, 71, 72, 74, 183, 187,
188, 259, 306, 312, 350, 351, 384
Allergen challenge, 73, 84
Allergen exposure, 75
Alveolar walls, 36
Aminophylline, 169, 171, 330
Antibronchoconstrictor, 351, 355, 358,
359
Anticholinergic, 1, 47, 169
Antigen, 285
Apanin, 37
Arrhythmias, 259
Asthma deaths, 10
Atenolol, 277